BREVERTON'S
Complete
Herbal

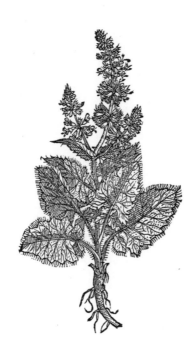

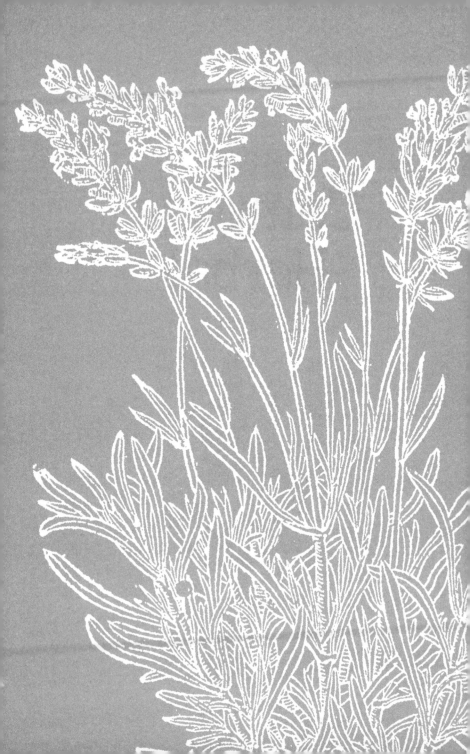

BREVERTON'S

Complete
Herbal

A book of
remarkable plants
and their uses

Based on Culpeper's *The English Physitian*
and *Compleat Herball* of 1653

TERRY BREVERTON

LYONS PRESS
Guilford, Connecticut
An imprint of Globe Pequot Press

CONTENTS

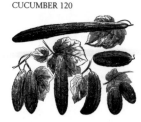

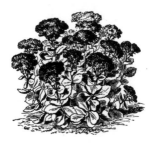

INTRODUCTION

This book is intended to be both entertaining and informative. It is written in part as a homage to the knowledge of our forebears and to the memory of a remarkable 'maverick', a man who wished to bring medical knowledge to those who could not afford the prices and fees of apothecaries and doctors. Apart from three pages devoted to this polymath, Nicholas Culpeper (see pages 122–124), whose *The English Physitian* (1652) and *Compleat Herball* (1653) have been continuously in print since the 17th century, it consists of either single-page or double-page entries about all the most interesting herbs, spices and associated herb gardens and gardeners. The book is arranged in alphabetical order by common name, with just a very few entries being slightly out of sequence to ensure that each double-page entry appears on a natural spread of the book. Most spellings have been modernized.

Please note: do not try any of these remedies without first consulting a qualified doctor.

Nicholas Culpeper (1616–54) not only gave very full descriptions of the *Government and Virtues* of each herb or spice that he described, but also its other common names, astrological notes, a full description of all its parts so one could recognize it when gathering herbs, the places where it grew and when to pick it. In his books, he listed all the known

herbal remedies of the time, wishing to create a book that would help ordinary people make their own herbal remedies. An astrologer, herbalist, physician and botanist, Culpeper gathered and catalogued hundreds of medicinal herbs, and severely criticized his medical contemporaries for their restrictive practices, writing in his foreword: *'This not being pleasing, and less profitable to me, I consulted with my two brothers, DR. REASON and DR. EXPERIENCE, and took a voyage to visit my mother NATURE, by whose advice, together with the help of DR. DILIGENCE, I at last obtained my desire; and, being warned by MR. HONESTY, a stranger in our days, to publish it to the world, I have done it.'* Of course, he was hated by the medical men – the surgeons, doctors and apothecaries of his time – and his name was blackened in his lifetime and his reputation besmirched after his early death.

Herbalism is the oldest known method of systematic healing. Many of today's herbs are known to have been used therapeutically for thousands of years. The word 'herb' refers to a plant of which the leaves, flowers, stems or roots are used for food, flavouring, scent or medicine. Many have multiple uses, e.g. marjoram can be used for flavouring, scent, healing and dyeing. So-called *'pot herbs'* could be used in 'pottage' the staple stew of the people, and in cooking pots; 'salets' or salad herbs went into salads with olive oil and vinegar. Apart from their use as remedies and preventative medicines and in cooking, herbs have long been employed as disinfectants, as perfumes and air fresheners, dyes, cosmetics, as companion plants, as insect and animal repellents and attractors, and even as currency. The distinction between a herb and a spice is this: herbs are the fresh and dried leaves generally of temperate plants, often green in colour. Spices are the flowers, fruit, seeds, bark and roots typically of tropical plants, which range from brown to black to red in colour. Usually, spices have a more pungent flavour than herbs, but it is possible for one plant to provide both a herb and a spice, e.g. *Coriandrum sativum*'s leaves are used as the herb *cilantro* and the seed is the spice *coriander*.

The first botanic gardens for educating schools of herbalists were founded in Padua, Italy in 1545 and in Oxford, England in 1621. These schools effectively took medicine out of the hands of the monks tending the monastic gardens, and placed it under the control of physicians. Newly trained doctors began to lecture on the healing properties of herbs, and their reliance on leeching, or bleeding, and chemical alchemy was largely replaced by the study of herbal alchemy. Alongside them, apothecaries, the chemists of the Middle Ages, had a near monopoly upon the supply of herbs and spices, and worked closely with the physicians. In the 17th century there was a great influx of herbs from the New World as a result of the Spanish and Portuguese conquests, and a number of herbals were published, written by doctors for doctors and apothecaries. It signalled a breakthrough in healing, with the authors focusing upon the botanical properties and characteristics of plants themselves rather than on '*humours*', planetary influences and the Doctrine of Signatures (the belief that some plants had been 'signed' by God to indicate their uses by virtue of the way they appeared).

The common people had traditionally been forced to rely upon local 'wise women' for cheap treatment of illnesses, and many of these women, who relied upon the oral herbal tradition, were burned as witches across Europe. With the publication of Culpeper's works, people could begin to treat themselves, often for free, rather than go to an apothecary's shop. Many plants have the Latin suffix '*officinalis*' in their botanic name signifying that they were '*of the shop*', i.e. approved for sale by apothecaries. Culpeper's publications combined traditional plant lore with descriptions of the medicinal properties of the herbs and their astrological indicators. Many of his herbs and spices have been found to have extremely valuable properties in treating illnesses, and multiple other uses, and they remain as valuable to us today as they were in Culpeper's own time.

ADDER'S TONGUE

OPHIOGLOSSUM VULGATUM
Family Ophioglossaceae

OTHER NAMES: Adder's tongue fern, common adder's tongue, English adder's tongue, snake's tongue, viper's tongue, serpent's tongue, adder's-tongue fern, southern adder's tongue, adder's spear, Christ's spear. (This is not the American adder's-tongue, which is an *Erythronium*, but O. *vulgatum* is native across much of the USA).

DESCRIPTION: A genus of about 25–30 species, the perennial adder's tongues are so named because the spore-bearing stalk resembles a snake's tongue. It has no resemblance to any other fern, and has much the appearance of a small arum flower. The plant grows from a central, budding, fleshy structure to 3–6 inches (8–15 cm) tall and has a two-part frond, forming a rounded diamond-shaped sheath and a narrow spore-bearing spike which can grow taller than its leaf. Culpeper's description indicates that his variety was the O. *vulgatum* which '*grows in moist meadows, and such like places*'.

PROPERTIES AND USES: The leaves and rhizomes have been used across Europe as a poultice for wounds. The fresh leaves make an effective and comforting poultice for ulcers and tumours. This remedy was sometimes called the '*Green Oil of Charity*'. The juice of the leaves, drunk alone, or with distilled water of horsetail, used to be

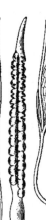

popular for internal wounds and bruises, vomiting or bleeding at the mouth or nose. The distilled water was also considered good for sore eyes. Culpeper calls it a '*herb under the dominion of the Moon and Cancer…The juice of the leaves drank with the distilled water of horse tail, is a singular remedy for all manner of wounds in the breasts, bowels, or other parts of the body, and is given with good success unto those that are troubled with casting, vomiting, or bleeding at the mouth or nose, or otherwise downwards…For ruptures or burst bellies, take as much of the powder of the dried leaves as will lie on a sixpence, or less, according to the age of the patient, in two ounces of horse-tail or oak-bud water, sweetened with syrup of quinces. Use it every morning for the space of fifteen days. But, before you enter upon the use of this or any other medicine, the gut, if it fall into the scrotum, must be reduced by a surgeon, and a truss must be worn to keep it up, and the patient must avoid all violent motions, and lie as much as may be, in bed or on a couch. Fabricius Hildanus* [the 'Father of German Surgery' 1560–1634] *says that some have been cured of great ruptures by lying in bed, when they could be cured no other way.*'
A salve was made to massage into the blocked or inflamed udders of cows.

HISTORY: The name *Ophioglossum* comes from the Greek *ophios* (serpent), and *glossa* (tongue). Medieval herbalists called it '*a fine cooling herb*', but if anyone picking the hard-to-find herb risked being followed by snakes. In witchcraft, the herb's use is said to stop slander and gossip. Adder's-spear ointment was sold by apothecaries from the 18th century. Adder's tongue was a popular treatment for scrofula, a form of tuberculosis that affects the lymph nodes in the neck, and it is still used by herbalists for skin ailments. The name 'Christ's spear' comes from its appearance, and the fact that Jesus' side was pierced by a spear. Thus, according to Paracelsus's 16th-century Doctrine of Signatures the plant was used to cure wounds. In flower language it is a symbol of jealousy.

NOTE: Chromosomes are complex structures containing a single molecule of DNA and many DNA packaging proteins. This packaging of DNA ensures that the whole genome can fit in the nucleus of a cell, and also that the genome can be faithfully divided during cell divisions. Chromosomes are present in all cells which have a complex structure between the membranes (such cells are called eukaryotes). Their number varies enormously and is characteristic for each species. The parasitic worm *Ascaris lumbricoides* has only four chromosomes whereas some ferns, such as the adder's tongue fern *(Ophioglossum vulgatum)*, have more than 1000 chromosomes. *Ophioglossum vulgatum* has the highest chromosome count of any known British plant, and other ophioglossums have even higher chromosome counts. For example *Ophioglossum reticulatum* has the highest chromosome number of any organism on Earth. This appears to represent an evolutionary dead end through repeated cycles of polyploidy (having extra sets of chromosomes), so it seems highly likely that this ancient group of ferns is on the verge of extinction.

Wounds and Witch's Brew

This ancient recipe using adder's tongue is recommended as an ointment for wounds: '*Put two pounds of leaves chopped very fine into a half-pint of oil and one and a half pounds of suet melted together. Boil the whole till the herb is crisp, then strain off from the leaves.*' A witchcraft alternative for treating wounds and bruising is: '*Soak some adder's tongue in cold water, wrap it in a cloth, and apply it to the wound or bruise it until the herb grows warm. Bury the wet herb in a muddy place. The wound will be cured.*'

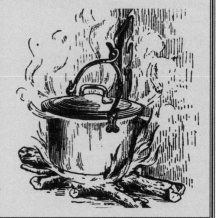

AGRIMONY

AGRIMONIA EUPATORIA
Family Rosaceae, Rose

OTHER NAMES: Harvest lice, rat's tail(s), liverwort, sticklewort, stickwort, stickweed, sweethearts, tea plant, liverwort, cockeburr, cockleburr, clot bur, fairy's wand, lemonwort, church steeples, salt and pepper, Aaron's rod, beggar's lice, beggar's ticks, money-in-both-pockets, philanthropos, garclive (Saxon).

DESCRIPTION: A hardy 24-inch (61-cm) perennial with downy leaves which smell faintly of apricot and small yellow flowers which grow up the erect spike at the end of the stem.

PROPERTIES AND USES: An infusion of the leaves and flowers can be taken as a tonic or diuretic, and used for bathing wounds or skin conditions. It is useful for alleviating the symptoms of coughs, bronchitis and asthma.

HISTORY: Agrimony is best known as a wound herb used on medieval battlefields to staunch bleeding, and Anglo-Saxons taught that it would heal wounds, snake bites, warts, etc. The Ancient Roman author Pliny described it as a *'herb of princely authority'* and Dioscorides recommended it as a general purgative, stating that it was *'a remedy for those that have bad livers'*, and also *'for such as are bitten with serpents.'* Galen recommended it for jaundice and as an astringent of the bowels. In the 13th century, the 'Physicians of Myddfai' in Wales used it for mastitis, which they called *'Inflammation of the Mammae'*, in the following way: *'Take agrimony, betony and vervain, and pound well, then mix with strong old ale, strain well, and set some milk on the fire; when this boils add the liquor thereto and make a posset thereof, giving it to the woman to drink warm. Let her do this frequently and she will be cured.'* In witchcraft it is still used to help create a deep, undisturbed sleep, by slipping dried leaves inside the sleeper's pillow. One recipe suggests agrimony in a mixture of pounded frogs and human blood as a remedy for all internal haemorrhages.

Good for Naughty Livers

The herbalist John Gerard wrote: *'A decoction of the leaves is good for them that have naughty livers'*, hence its name of *'liverwort'*. The long flower-spikes of agrimony have caused it to be called *'church steeples'*, and it was also known as *'cockeburr'*, *'sticklewort'* or *'Stickwort'*, because its seed-vessels cling by the hooked ends of their stiff hairs to any person or animal coming into contact with it. Gerard also informs us that it was once called *'philanthropos'*, on account of its beneficial properties.

ALDER

ALNUS GLUTINOSA
Family Betulaceae, Birch

OTHER NAMES: Common alder, black alder, owler, fever bush (n.b. the black alder in America is a different family, *Ilex verticillata*).

DESCRIPTION: Alder is the most common tree in riparian (stream-edge) forests, and *Love's Martyr* (1601) tells us: *'The alder, alnus, is so called because it is nourished by water; for it grows near water and survives with difficulty away from water. For this reason it is a delicate and soft because it is nourished in a wet environment.'* It can reach 75 feet (23 m) in height.

PROPERTIES AND USES: Alder greatly improves soil fertility through its ability to fix nitrogen from the air. A bacterium *(Frankia alni)* forms nodules on the tree's roots, absorbing nitrogen from the air and makes it available to the tree. Alder, in turn, provides the bacterium with carbon, which it produces through photosynthesis. Alder bark contains the anti-inflammatory salicin which is metabolized into salicylic acid in the body. It seems that Culpeper recognized this effect. He recommended bathing burns and inflammation with distilled water of the leaves to reduce swelling and for ague: *'...the leaves, put under the bare feet galled with travelling, are a great refreshing to them; the said leaves gathered while the morning dew is on them, and brought into a chamber troubled with fleas, will gather them thereinto, which, being suddenly cast out, will rid the chamber of those troublesome bed-fellows.'* The wood used to be made into clogs in mill-towns, for cart and spinning wheels, bowls, spoons, wooden heels, herring-barrel staves, etc. The bark was used by dyers, tanners, leather dressers, and for fishermen's nets.

HISTORY: The Physicians of Myddfai recommended the use of alder twigs for cleaning the teeth. In Celtic mythology, the alder is said to be the tree of Bran the Blessed, god of the Underworld. He was also known as the god of Prophecy, Arts, War and Writing. Possessing the size of a giant, it was impossible for King Bran to fit in a house or in a boat.

Durable Under Water

Under water the alder is very durable, and it was therefore valuable for pumps, troughs, sluices, and particularly for piles. It is the wood used in Venice as piles for the Rialto Bridge and other buildings, and was used widely for similar purposes in Amsterdam and France. Alder is commonly found supporting ancient crannogs, defensive artificial islands on lakes.

ALDER BUCKTHORN

FRANGULA ALNUS
Family Rhamnaceae, Buckthorn

OTHER NAMES: Black alder tree, dogwood (both Culpeper), frangula bark, black dogwood, alder dogwood, European black alder, European buckthorn, columnar buckthorn, black alder, Persian berries, stinking Roger, arrow wood.

DESCRIPTION: A small bushy tree with oval glossy leaves, which grows to 20 feet (6 m), with attractive berries which change from red to purple. The tree prefers damp acidic areas, including woodlands, wet heathlands and river banks. This is one of the two main food plants for the caterpillars of the brimstone butterfly, the other being the common buckthorn, *Rhamnus cathartica*.

PROPERTIES AND USES: The berries are toxic and the sap is an irritant. Alder buckthorn can be used as a tonic, is said to be antiparasitic, and is used as a local antiseptic. Fresh bark, powdered and mixed with vinegar, can treat fungal diseases of the skin and acne. An infusion of the bark can treat constipation and haemorrhoids, and as a treatment for chronic constipation is milder than its close relative, the significantly named purging buckthorn *(Rhamnus cathartica)*. Its green leaves make tumours less inflamed, and were put inside travellers' shoes to '*ease pain and remove weariness.*' Culpeper calls it '*a tree of Saturn*' and recommends the bark for those with the choler, phlegm and dropsy. Culpeper gives several other uses, including boiling the inner bark in vinegar '*to kill lice, to cure the itch, and to take away scabs by drying them up for a short time; it is singularly good to wash the teeth, to take away the pains, to fasten those that are loose, to cleanse them and keep them sound.*' One supposes that in the 17th century, anything was preferable to a trip to a tooth-puller.

HISTORY: The name *rhamnus* is derived from the Greek *rhamnos*, meaning a branch. In the 13th century it was a herbal laxative (hence purging buckthorn), and its wood was used to make arrows (hence the name arrow wood), shoe lasts, wooden nails, and veneers. The bark and leaves make a yellow dye, which turns black when mixed with iron salts, and unripe berries make a green dye.

NOTE: It is thought that the name 'alder' buckthorn comes about because the leaves look similar to that of alder, and the two trees/shrubs often grow in similar places, but they are not related. It has no thorns, so its name of alder buckthorn is doubly misleading. Its light, inflammable charcoal was highly prized for making the best gunpowder in medieval times, and it is known as *Pulverholz* – powder wood – in Germany.

ALECOST

TANACETUM BALSAMITA
Family Asteraceae/Compositae, Daisy/Sunflower

OTHER NAMES: Alecost, costmarie, sweet Mary, mintys mair (Mary's mint), alespice, lady's balsam, lady's herb, bitter buttons, goose tongue, allspice (not to be confused with the spice), sweet tongue, tongue plant, balsam herb, mint geranium, mace (not to be confused with nutmeg mace), Bible plant, Bible leaf.

DESCRIPTION: Attractive large-leaved perennial herb, reaching 4 feet (1.2 m) or more in height and producing pretty, yellow, button-like flowers. The leaves have a minty, balsam-like fragrance reminiscent of the taste of spearmint chewing gum.

PROPERTIES AND USES: Costmary was once a popular herb for scenting bath water and rinsing hair. Culpeper noted: '*It is under the dominion of Jupiter. It is astringent to the stomach, and strengthens the liver…it is very profitable for pains of the head that are continual…it cleanses that* which is foul, and hinders putrefaction and corruption'. Alecost was grown extensively for the treatment of burns and insect stings, when a fresh leaf was rubbed on the bite.

HISTORY: It was taken to the New World by early English colonists who combined it with lavender to scent linens and blankets. It was also used in wardrobes and clothes' stores to deter clothes moths. The dried leaves of alecost retain their minty-balsam perfume for a long time and make a sweet addition to pot pourris. A small amount of the leaf can be added to soups and salads, or added to melted butter and new potatoes. Alecost is recommended in modern herbals to relieve a stuffed-up nose. Place a handful of the leaves in a bowl of boiling water, cover the head with a towel and inhale for five to ten minutes. In flower language it is the symbol of impatience.

Spicy Herb for Ale

This aromatic herb has two common names, costmary and alecost. '*Cost*' refers to costus, a spicy Asian plant related to ginger, which has a slightly similar flavour. '*Mary*' refers to an association with the Virgin Mary, perhaps because it was used in medieval times as an infusion to relieve the pain of childbirth. '*Alecost*' translates into ale-cost or 'spicy herb for ale' as it was once an important flavouring of ales. The large, oblong leaves of costmary make neat, fragrant bookmarks, a use that gives us the old names Bible leaf or Bible plant. The minty odour might help to repel silverfish or insects from the family Bible, and the leaf could be smelt or chewed secretly during long sermons to stay awake.

ALE-HOOF

NEPETA GLECHOMA (syn. *GLECHOMA HEDERACEA*)
Family Lamiaceae/Labiatae, Mint

OTHER NAMES: Culpeper calls it ground ivy, cat's-foot, gill-go-by-the-ground, gill-creep-by-ground, tun-hoof and hay-maids. Also known as hedge-maids, hedgehove, hen and chickens, rat's foot, rabbit's mouth, ale gill, gill-run, gill-run-over, gill-go-over-the-ground, coin grass, creeping charlie, run-away-robin, field balm, wandering Jew, wild snakeroot (US), run-away-robin (US), hedgehove (Anglo-Saxon) etc.

DESCRIPTION: This creeping and trailing evergreen perennial has rounded leaves and small purplish flowers, sometimes being grown in hanging baskets. It grows 6 inches (15 cm) tall, and leaves form in pairs, looking like a string of coins, so the plant was sometimes called 'coin grass'. 'Cat's-foot' relates to its scalloped leaves resembling the size and shape of a kitten's paw. The leaves release a slightly balsamic aroma when crushed. It can be used as ground cover, but can be a nuisance as a lawn weed.

PROPERTIES AND USES: Ale-hoof is a stimulant and tonic, and was used for chest infections. Ale-hoof was made into 'gill tea' prescribed for: jaundice, arthritis, coughs and respiratory ailments, indigestion, fevers, headaches, stomach pains, gout, sciatica, vertigo, weak backs, nervous disorders and depression, hypochondria, normalizing heart beat, stones in the urinary tract, stimulating the circulation, detoxifying the body and strengthening the stomach, spleen, gall, glands, kidneys, liver, and even to prevent premature ageing. '*Traditionally, leaf tea* [was] *used for lung ailments, asthma, jaundice, kidney ailments, "blood purifier". Externally, a folk remedy for cancer, backaches, bruises, piles.*' Cooling and stimulating, this remarkable tea was also used as a wash for eye complaints and failing eyesight.

HISTORY: The herb has for recorded history been considered a panacea or 'cure-all'. Dioscorides said that its tea was a remedy for sciatica, and Gerard wrote that, boiled in a mutton broth, it was good for weak backs. For eye ailments, Gerard wrote that when mixed with daisies, celandines, rose water and sugar, alehoof removed '*any grief whatsoever in the eyes…it is proved to be the best medicine in the world.*' Ground ivy was also given to children to clear lingering congestion and to treat conditions such as 'glue ear' and sinusitis. Culpeper recommended the tea for tinnitus, poor hearing, stomach aches, indigestion, yellow jaundice, sciatica, mouth ulcers,

Adding the Bitter to Beer

'*Hofe*' was Old English for herb. '*Ale-hoof*' was one of the main plants used by the early Saxons to clarify their beers, the leaves being steeped in the hot liquor, hence the 'ale' nomenclature. The plant was used to improve the flavour, clarify and preserve the brew, until it was superseded by hops in medieval times. It was the main bitter before the use of hops in beer, a process known as 'tunning'. A tun was also the large cask in which ale was brewed, thus '*Tun-hoof*'. In Tudor times we read that ale-hoof '*is good to tun up with new drink, for it will clarify it in a night that it will be the fitter to be drank the next morning; or if any drink be thick with removing or any other accident, it will do the like in a few hours.*' The plant also acquired the name of '*gill*' from the French '*guiller*' – to ferment beer. The stronger ale of yesteryear was often served in gill measures of ¼ pint (142 ml), but in some areas a gill was ½ pint (284 ml) of ale. As a gill also meant a girl, ale-hoof also came to be called 'hedgemaids' and various combinations featuring the word gill. '*Alehoof Grut*' is a traditional ale presently brewed in Pennsylvania. In the Middle Ages, brewing was mainly carried out by women known as brewsters or ale-wives, who made beer from whatever grain was available, whether barley, oats, rye or wheat, and '*gruit*', a mixture of herbs such as ale-hoof, bog myrtle, rosemary, yarrow or ivy, or even fine, selected tree bark.

wounds, itching etc. Decocted in wine, with honey added, he advised its use '*to wash the sores and ulcers in the privy parts of man or woman*'. The ancient herbalists praised it greatly, saying it would cure insanity and melancholia by opening the stopping of the spleen. It also regulated the heart beat by making the blood more fluid. In the 13th century, the Physicians of Myddfai used it for fevers and snake bites, and the juice for inflamed eyes. In Wales it was used as a hair rinse, and it has been employed to prevent scurvy because of its high vitamin C content. It was a popular spring tonic, being considered beneficial in kidney disorders. The herb found its way to America and became a part of the pharmacopoeia of the settlers. 'Ground ivy!' was at one time one of the 'cries of London' and recommended for making a tea to purify the blood. Doctors also prescribed the tea to treat painter's colic, or lead poisoning. An infusion of the leaves was used for sufferers so '*painters who make use of it are seldom, if ever, troubled with that affection. The fresh juice snuffed up the nose often cures the most inveterate headache.*'

ALEXANDERS

SMYRNIUM OLUSATRUM
Family Apiaceae/Umbelliferae, Carrot/Parsley

OTHER NAMES: Alexander, Alexander's herb, alisander, horse-parsley, wild parsley and black pot-herb are all in Culpeper. Black lovage, black pot-herb, hell root, alick, megweed, Roman celery, Macedonian parsley, Alexandrian parsley.

DESCRIPTION: A pungent biennial, with yellow-green flowers and black fruits, similar to celery in appearance and taste, and up to 5 feet (1.5 m) in height. Alexanders grows in greatest profusion on sea cliffs and within a few miles of the sea. When found inland it is often near old monastery garden sites.

PROPERTIES AND USES: One of Europe's forgotten vegetables, it was grown as a salad and pot herb before being replaced in many dishes by celery. One can steam the stems, shoots and buds, ideally just before the flowers have opened, for an absolutely distinctive vegetable, a little like celery, parsley or chervil to use in fish dishes and soups. For some reason it has, over the last ten years, exploded in its range of sites, becoming invasive in many places.

HISTORY: Known to Theophrastus and Pliny the Elder, its roots are diuretics, its leaves make a healing juice for cuts and its crushed seeds were a popular condiment. Pliny recommended chewing 'Alexander's herb' with aniseed and a little honey in the morning to sweeten the breath. Alexanders was introduced into Britain by the Romans (hence the name 'Roman celery') but fell out of fashion with the introduction of new varieties of celery in the 19th century. John Evelyn, in his 1699 *Acetaria: A Discourse of Sallets* [Salads] describes Alexanders as a *'moderately hot, and of a cleansing faculty'*, comparing it favourably to parsley. *'Ellicksander Pottage'* was described by Robert May in *The Accomplish't Cook* (1660): *'Chop ellicksanders and oatmeal together, being picked and washed, then set on a pipkin with fair water, and when it boils, put in your herbs, oatmeal, and salt, and boil it on a soft fire, and make it not too thick, being almost boil'd put in some butter.'* According to Culpeper it was a herb of Jupiter, and he recommended the aforementioned Alexander pottage. Alexanders was carried on ships as a remedy against scurvy.

Wind Breaker

Culpeper noted *'It warms a cold Stomach, and opens stoppages of the Liver and Spleen, it is good to move Women's Courses to expel the After-birth, to break Wind, to provoke Urine, and help the Strangury* [painful urination caused by bladder diseases or kidney-stones]...*it is also effectual against the biting of Serpents.'*

ALKANET

ANCHUSA OFFICINALIS
Family Boraginaceae, Borage

OTHER NAMES: Bugloss, true bugloss, common bugloss, common alkanet, summer forget-me-not, ox tongue, langue de boeuf.

DESCRIPTION: Bugloss is a showy plant covered with prickly hairs. It grows to about 1–4 feet (30 cm–1.2 m), and has dainty purplish-blue flowers in late summer which attract bees.

PROPERTIES AND USES: Culpeper called this a Venus herb and *'one of her darlings.'…'It helps old ulcers, hot inflammations, burnings by common fire, and St. Anthony's Fire* [erysipelas], *by antipathy to Mars; for these uses, your best way is to make it into an ointment; also, if you make a vinegar of it, as you make vinegar of roses, it helps the morphew* [blisters caused by scurvy] *and leprosy; if you apply the herb to the privities, it draws forth the dead child. It helps the yellow jaundice, spleen, and gravel in the kidneys…It stays the flux of the belly, kills worms, helps the fits of the mother. Its decoction made in wine, and drank, strengthens the back, and eases the pains thereof: It helps bruises and falls, and is as gallant a remedy to drive out the small pox and measles as any is; an ointment made of it, is excellent for green wounds, pricks or thrusts.'* Extracted into vinegar, it was even used against leprosy. The dry leaves emit a rich musky fragrance, rather like wild strawberry leaves drying. Leaves and young shoots can be cooked like spinach.

HISTORY: An effective wound ointment was made by pounding alkanet roots with olive oil and earthworms. Egyptians created a face paint using the red dye obtained from alkanet roots. The name alkanet comes from Arabic, *al khenna* (henna), from the red colour of the roots. The bark of the roots provides a weak brownish-red or lilac dye, which is not as strong as the dye of its cousin, *Alkanna tinctoria*, dyer's bugloss. It was grown in medieval gardens, but is considered a weed if found in cereal fields. The name bugloss, which is of Greek origin, signifies an ox's tongue, and was applied to the plant because of the roughness and shape of the leaves.

Deadly to Snakes

The flowers appear in curling spikes that resemble scorpions, so in Culpeper we read: *'Dioscorides says it helps such as are bitten by a venomous beast, whether it be taken inwardly, or applied to the wound; nay, he says further, if any one that hath newly eaten it, do but spit into the mouth of a serpent, the serpent instantly dies.'*

ALL-HEAL

OPOPANAX CHIRONIUM, FERULA OPOPANAX
Family Umbelliferae/Apiaceae, Carrot/Parsley

OTHER NAMES: Culpeper calls this *'Alheal, Hercules' Alheal, and Hercules' Woundwort...Some call it panay, and others opapanawort'*. Rough parsnip.

DESCRIPTION: This has a thick, yellow, fleshy, perennial root and grows to 9 feet (2.75 m) high. Its flowers are small, yellow, and form large flat umbels at the termination of the branches. The plant grows wild in the south of France, Italy and Greece. When the base of the stem or root is cut, a yellowish juice exudes. When dried in the sun, this constitutes the gum-resin opopanax. Its odour is strong, peculiar and unpleasant, and its taste bitter and acrid.

PROPERTIES AND USES: Culpeper tells us: *'It is under the dominion of Mars, hot, biting, and choleric, and remedies evils...It kills worms; helps the gout, cramp,* and seizures; provokes urine, and helps all joint aches; helps all cold griefs of the head, vertigo, fits and lethargy; obstructions of the liver and spleen, stone in the kidneys and bladder. It provokes menses, and expels the dead birth; it is excellent good for the grief of the sinews, itch, sores and toothache; also the biting of mad dogs and venomous beasts; and purges choler very gently.'* In later times it was used in plasters, and internally for bronchitis with abundant expectoration, asthma, hysteria, amenorrhoea, etc.

HISTORY: Culpeper believed that *'Hercules learned of the virtues of the herb from Chiron* [the centaur who was master of the healing arts], *when he learned physic of him...'*, hence *'Hercules' Alheal.'* It was one of the gum-resins thought to be applicable to almost all ills, hence the name opopanax, meaning 'all-healing juice'.

A Difficult Herb to Identify

This has been the most difficult of Culpeper's herbs to identify. The height of up to about ten feet, with leaves like those of an ash tree and its presence in British gardens at Culpeper's time, indicate to some researchers that the plant in question is *Valerian officinalis*, but Culpeper describes valerian elsewhere in his *Herbal*. Some writers identify *Prunella vulgaris* as the plant in question, and others have made various *Stachys* varieties identical with Culpeper's *Alheal*. The picture is even further confused because *Opopanax chironium/ herculeum /herculaneum* is a name also given to sweet myrrh *(Commiphora erythraea)* as well as to *Acacia farnesiana*. Linnaeus mentions the plant as *Pastinaca opopanax*. The French, according to Mrs C.F. Level *(Herbal Delights,* 1937) call it *opapanax* or *panais sauvage* (wild parsnip), whence we have Culpeper's *'panay'*.

ALLSPICE

PIMENTA DIOICA or *OFFICINALIS*
Family Myrtaceae, Myrtle

OTHER NAMES: Allspice tree, bayberry, Carolina allspice, clove pepper, Indian wood tree, Jamaican pepper, myrtle pepper, pimento, pineapple shrub, strawberry shrub, toute épice (French), whole spice, newspice.

DESCRIPTION: A tropical evergreen with an aromatic bark, leaves and berries, it has bunches of greenish white flowers with a far-reaching scent. The berries are picked when mature, then dried (usually in the sun), and ground to create the familiar spice.

PROPERTIES AND USES: The allspice which we buy is not a mixture of different spices, but the produce of this tree. Its hard pinkish wood was once employed for the manufacture of walking sticks and umbrella handles. The oil is used by the toiletry and perfumery industries. It provides a commercial source of eugenol and vanillin, and is valuable in the food industry, particularly in sausages, sauces, fish preserves, ketchups, pickles, ice cream and baked food. Medicinally, the powdered fruit has been used to treat flatulence, diarrhoea and rheumatism, and allspice has been used as a poultice to relieve the pain of arthritis. In Jamaican 'jerk spice' the seasoning relies principally upon allspice and the very hot Scotch Bonnet chilli peppers, along with cloves, cinnamon, nutmeg, scallions, thyme, garlic, salt and pepper.

HISTORY: Aztecs used to flavour chocolate with allspice seeds. It was first imported into Britain in the early 17th century, and was described as 'allspice' in 1621 because its flavour resembled a combination of cinnamon, cloves and nutmeg. Around 65 to 90 per cent of the oil extracted from the seeds of Jamaican trees is *eugenol*, the same oil found in the above three spices. This oil gives the distinctive flavouring to Chartreuse, Benedictine and other liqueurs which were made in European monasteries. During the American War of Independence, allspice was used as a substitute for previously imported spices that were no longer available, as it is one of the few spices that are native to the western hemisphere.

Confused With Pepper

When dry, the fruits are brown and resemble large peppercorns, so allspice is often confused with black pepper *(Piper nigrum)* and cubeb *(Piper cubeba)*. However, when fully dried the two-celled allspice is dark reddish-brown, while one-celled black pepper is black and one-celled cubeb is grey. The fruit's similarity in appearance to peppercorns (for which the Spanish is *pimienta* i.e. pepper nigrum), led to its Latin name pimenta.

ALMOND TREE

PRUNUS DULCIS
Family Rosaceae, Rose

OTHER NAMES: Culpeper describes the sweet almond and the bitter almond, calling the latter amigdalum. Common almond, Greek nuts, jordan (a corruption of the French *jardin*, or garden) almond, sweet almond, tonsil plum.

DESCRIPTION: The almond is a small deciduous tree, with pale pink flowers succeeded by pale green oval fruits. Each fruit contain one edible seed, the almond 'nut'. However, the edible part of the almond is not a true nut, but the seed of a *'drupe'* (a botanical name for a type of fruit). As Culpeper noted, there are two forms of the plant, one (often with white flowers) producing sweet almonds, and the other (often with pink flowers) producing bitter almonds.

PROPERTIES AND USES: It was considered a soothing and calming herb, used to treat constipation and to help in cases of gallstones and kidney stones. The nuts can be eaten raw or roasted, and marzipan is made from ground almond paste. Almond milk and almond butter help people with allergies, and almond oil is used to remedy dry skin conditions and as a soothing carrier oil. Culeper wrote: '*sweet almonds nourish the body, and increase the seed* [male fertility]; *they strengthen the breath, cleanse the kidneys and open the passages of urine…Bitter almonds also open obstructions of the liver and spleen, expel wind, cleanse the lungs from phlegm, and provoke urine and the menses; the oil of them kills worms, and helps pains of the womb…the oil of both cleans the skin.*' Magnesium-rich almonds help reduce symptoms of IBS through activating the muscle contractions required for correct digestive functions, and studies suggest they may reduce the risk of colon cancer. In witchcraft, to always have money, place seven almonds in your pocket each Thursday, and eat one at noon on each day of the week. For those readers who may win the lottery when taking this advice, please remember this author.

HISTORY: Domesticated almonds appeared first in the Near East, and were present in the Cretan palace of Knossos and in Tutankhamen's tomb (*c.*1325 BCE). The name almond refers to the early blossom, as it comes from the Greek *amygdale*, meaning 'to hasten or awake early'. This early spring flowering led to almond being an emblem of hope.

Busy Bees

The pollination of California's almonds is the largest annually managed pollination event in the world, with nearly a million hives (nearly half of all beehives in the USA) being transported in February to almond groves across the state.

THE APOTHECARIES' GARDEN

SWAN WALK, LONDON SW3 4HS

Chelsea Physic Garden was founded in 1673 as the Apothecaries' Garden to train apprentices to identify plants. Its situation near the River Thames created a warmer microclimate allowing the survival of many non-native plants, for example the largest outdoor fruiting olive tree in Britain. Many plants from milder climates could thus survive harsh British winters, especially during the 'Mini Ice Age' of the 17th century when the river froze so severely that fairs were held on its frozen surface.

The apothecaries instituted an international botanic garden seed exchange system, which still continues today. For instance in 1683, four cedar of Lebanon seedlings came from the professor of botany at Leiden University. Sir Hans Sloane (1660–1753) purchased the Manor of Chelsea and he leased the 4 acres (1.6 ha) of garden to the Society of Apothecaries. He charged a peppercorn rent of £5 a year in perpetuity, on the condition that '*it be forever kept up and maintained as a Physic Garden*'. Sloane had studied at the Physic Garden while a young man, and was sympathetic to the financial problems of the garden's upkeep. Dr Sloane, whose collections of antiquities formed the nucleus of the British Museum, was president both of the Royal Society and of the Royal Society of Physicians. Environments for

supporting different types of plants were built, including the pond rock garden that was constructed from a variety of rock types, namely stones from the Tower of London, Icelandic lava (brought to the garden by Sir Joseph Banks in 1772), fused bricks and flint. This has been listed Grade II* and is the oldest rock garden in England on view to the public. It was completed on 16 August 1773. By this time the Physic Garden had achieved fame across the world.

The layout of narrow rectilinear beds in the garden is the original pattern, allowing one to get close to each plant. There are systematic order beds which demonstrate the botanical relationship of plants which are labelled with their name, origin and uses. As well as the above-mentioned olive there are a number of important trees, including an ancient yew. At the end of the 19th century the trustees of the City Parochial Foundation agreed to take over the running of the garden from the Society of Apothecaries. The Chelsea Physic Garden has developed a major role in public education focusing on the renewed interest in natural medicine. The Garden of World Medicine is Britain's first *garden of ethnobotany* (study of the botany of different ethnic groups and indigenous peoples) and is laid out together with a new Pharmaceutical Garden.

ALOE VERA

ALOE VERA, ALOE BARBADENSIS
Family Asphodelaceae (formerly Liliaceae), Lily

OTHER NAMES: Aloes, medicine plant, medicine aloe, true aloe, burn plant, cape aloes, socotrine, house leek; sea houseleek, sea-ay-green (Culpeper).

DESCRIPTION: A rosette of fleshy evergreen leaves which needs warm temperatures to grow up to 2 feet (60 cm) high; when mature has yellow or orange bell-shaped flowers.

PROPERTIES AND USES: Aloes have been used in Europe for centuries, for the glutinous sap or gel present in the leaves, which has immediate healing properties for cuts, eczema and burns. Broken leaves can be rubbed on the affected parts. It is used in suntan lotions and skin lotions, and can be added to shampoo for an itching or dry scalp. The juice is even used to treat radiation burns. Culpeper advised its use for purging, calling it a martial plant, hot, dry and bitter, and *'the basis for almost all pills'*. Amongst many other uses, he advised that aloe *'boiled with wine and honey, heals rifts and outgoings of the fundament* [anus], *and stops the flux of the haemorrhoids'*. Research shows that drinking high potency aloe vera juice helps with inflammatory bowel conditions such as IBS, colitis and diverticulitis. It is one of the only known natural vegetarian sources of vitamin B12, and it contains many minerals vital to the growth process and healthy function of all the body's systems. Studies indicate that it is a general tonic for the immune system, and research is

ongoing to use it to fight HIV, and to treat diabetes and certain types of cancer. This author remembers having bitter aloes 'painted' on his fingernails as a child to stop biting them.

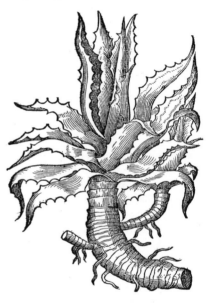

HISTORY: When a pharaoh died in Ancient Egypt, the funeral ceremony was by invitation only and each attendee had to bring aloes. A mixture of the powdered leaves of aloe and myrrh was used for embalming and also placed with the burial clothes. The Mesopotamians used aloe vera to keep the evil spirits from their residences. It was grown and used by King Solomon (reigned 971–931 BCE). Arabian records suggest that by the sixth century BCE aloe was being used as a laxative as well as for embalming. This is said to be referred to by John in the New Testament, when he describes how Nicodemus brings a pound of aloes to the garden tomb after Jesus' crucifixion. The Greeks believed aloe symbolized beauty, patience, fortune and good health. Hippocrates (c.460–370 BCE) declared that it was good for hair growth, healing of tumours, relief of dysentery and stomach aches. Cleopatra's beauty was attributed to the natural goodness of aloes, and she was supposed to have bathed in its juice before her first meeting with Mark Antony. By the time of the Greek physician Dioscorides, aloe was being recommended for many other medicinal purposes, including the treatment of digestive disorders, eye inflammation, kidney ailments and oral and skin diseases. Dioscorides wrote of it in his *De Materia Medica* in 41–68 CE describing how the Roman armies used it for boils, healing the foreskin, soothing dry itchy skin, ulcerated genitals, tonsils, gum and throat irritations, haemorrhoids, bruising, and to stop bleeding wounds. He also concurred with Hippocrates that the fresh pulp of aloe stopped the falling of hair.

Pliny the Elder said aloe cured leprosy sores and it reduced perspiration. Galen (c.130–201 CE) used aloes as a healing agent, drawing on the knowledge he had gained from being a doctor to gladiators. During the Crusades, the Knights Templar made a drink of palm wine, aloe pulp and hemp, which was named '*the Elixir of Jerusalem*'. They believed that it added years to their life. Hindus thought that aloe vera grew in the Garden of Eden and named it the '*silent healer*', and Russians called aloe '*the Elixir of Longevity*'. It would appear that the patriarch of Jerusalem recommended the plant for its medicinal qualities to Alfred the Great (849–99). In the tenth century CE, Moslem travellers noted that Socotra (islands lying to the east of the Horn of Africa) still seemed to be the only known source, and in the later centuries the British secured the monopoly from the sultan of Socotra.

Healing Alexander the Great's Wound

It is known as *Socotrine* as it originated in the Yemeni island of Socotra in the Indian Ocean. It is said that in 330 BCE, Alexander the Great had been wounded by an enemy arrow during the siege of Gaza. The wound became badly infected during his triumphal progress across Egypt and Libya. While at the oasis of Amon he was proclaimed son of Zeus. Here, a priest sent by Alexander's tutor Aristotle treated the injury with aloe vera which healed the wound. It is said that Aristotle convinced Alexander to conquer the island of Socotra in order to ensure the supply of aloes that grew there. Alexander then had his war wagons converted so that masses of fresh aloe could be loaded onto them and taken into battle to heal his wounded soldiers. Countries around the Mediterranean believed Socotra to be the only source of this precious drug at that time.

AMARANTHUS

AMARANTHUS CAUDATUS
Family Amaranthaceae, Amaranth

OTHER NAMES: Culpeper calls this flower-gentle, flower-velure, floramor and velvet-flower. Also known as flower of immortality, red cockscomb, quilete, foxtail amaranth, pendant amaranth, love-lies-bleeding, lady bleeding. There is some confusion, as the variety referred to in Culpeper may be *Amaranthus hypochondriacus*, prince's feather. The white amaranth mentioned by Culpeper is probably *Amaranthus albus*, white pigweed.

DESCRIPTION: A half-hardy annual originally from India, it can grow over 3 feet (90 cm) tall in full sun, and has remarkable tassels of red or purple inflorescences.

PROPERTIES AND USES: Because of its blood-red flowers, ancient medical practitioners used the herb to staunch bleeding, believing the Doctrine of Signatures whereby the colour or shape of a plant indicated its medical use. Even now, preparations are made with 'lady bleeding' to slow excessive bleeding during menstruation cycles. Culpeper calls it a herb of Mars and Venus, and applauds it for stopping the flow of blood in men or women. He also mentions an amaranthus with white flowers, *'which stops discharges in women, and gonorrhoea in men, and is a most singular remedy for the venereal disease.'* Recent research has shown that amaranth is an astringent, and it has been used over the centuries to heal diarrhoea and mouth ulcers.

HISTORY: The name *Amaranthus* stems from the Greek for 'unwithering', typifying immortality, as blooms of amaranth maintain their shape as well as their colour even after they are dried. In Greece, the amaranth was sacred to Artemis, and was supposed to have special healing properties, so it became a symbol of immortality used to decorate images of the gods and tombs. The amaranth was outlawed by Spanish colonial authorities in Mexico because it was used by Aztecs in their rituals, again as a symbol of immortality.

Bullet-proof Magic

Dried amaranth flowers have been used to call forth the dead, and are also carried to mend a broken heart. Other 'magical' uses include the cure of wearing a crown of amaranth flowers to speed healing. To make sure that you are never struck by a bullet, pull up a whole amaranth plant, preferably on a Friday at the full moon. Leave an offering to the plant and then fold it, including the roots, in a piece of white cloth. Wear this against your chest to be 'bullet-proof'.

(WOOD) ANEMONE

ANEMONE NEMOROSA
Family Ranunculaceae, Buttercup or Crowfoot

OTHER NAMES: Culpeper calls it the wind-flower on Pliny's advice, *'because they say that the flowers never open but when the wind blows'*. Thimbleweed, smell smock, smell fox (because of the musky smell of the leaves), American wood anemone, *blodyn y gwynt* (windflower, in Welsh), Bow bells, bread and cheese and cider, Candlemas caps, chimney smocks, crowfoot, drops of snow, Easter flower, evening twilight, fairies' windflower, flower of death, granny's nightcap, granny-thread-the-needle, jack o' lantern, lady's milk-cans, lady's nightcap, lady's petticoat, lady's purse, lady's shimmy, milkmaids, moggie nightgown, Moll o' the woods, moonflower, Nancy, nemony, nightcaps, old woman's nest, shame-faced maiden, shoes and slippers, silver bells, snake flower, snakes and adders, snake's eyes, soldiers, soldier's buttons, Star-of-Bethlehem, white soldiers, wild jessamine, wind plant, wood crowfoot.

DESCRIPTION: The foliage forms long spreading clumps in woodland, where drifts of the exquisite white flowers often carpet large areas in spring. The fragile white or pinkish flower is almost 1 inch (2.5 cm) in diameter, with six or seven petal-like segments. *Nemorosa* is derived from the Latin meaning 'covered with trees'.

PROPERTIES AND USES: The wood anemone is poisonous and can cause severe skin and gastrointestinal irritation. However, various parts of this herb used to be recommended for a variety of complaints such as headaches, gout and rheumatism. Culpeper calls it under the dominion of Mars, and recommends it to *'provoke menses mightily'* as well as for lethargy, headaches, leprosy, ulcers and eye inflammations.

HISTORY: For the Ancient Egyptians the wood anemone was an emblem of sickness, and it is still called the 'flower of death' by the Chinese. Greek legend says that Anemos, the wind, sent his namesakes, the anemones, in the earliest spring days as the heralds of his coming. The Romans viewed the first wood anemones they picked from the wild as charms against fever. In the first century CE Dioscorides recommended the plant to be used in external treatments for eye inflammation and ulcers.

Confirmation of Spring
'If primroses are the harbingers of spring, then wood anemones are its confirmation. The sight of shady banks and glades lit by their white stars on a sunny spring day leaves you in no doubt that spring is truly here...' (Carol Klein, the *Daily Telegraph* 16 March 2002).

ANGELICA

ANGELICA ARCHANGELICA
Family Apiaceae/Umbelliferae, Carrot/Parsley

OTHER NAMES: Angelic plant, angelic herb, archangel, Holy Ghost, the root of the Holy Ghost (Renaissance), garden angelica, herb of angels, angel's food, archangel, Aunt Jericho, Holy Ghost plant, holy plant, llys yr angel peraroglaidd (perfumed flower of the angel, Welsh), St Michael's flower.

DESCRIPTION: An aromatic large-leaved plant with large umbels of small yellow-green flowers, which can grow 3–8 feet (90 cm–2.4 m) tall. Angelica is unique amongst the Umbelliferae for its pervading aromatic odour, with a hint of aniseed. It is a biennial that will return year after year if you cut all but one flower. It can cause dermatitis and photosensitivity, and gloves should be used to handle the plant, particularly in quantity. For heaven's sake do not confuse it with hemlock, which has white flowers. The leaves of hemlock smell foul when it is crushed.

PROPERTIES AND USES: Its long, thick and fleshy roots are the part used in herbal medicine. Use the stems for flavouring stewed fruit. Hollow stems can be candied. The stem was a remedy for indigestion, for which at that time only

---

Angelica and Longevity

Lapps used the leaves to wrap and preserve fish transported on long journeys, and also believed that garden angelica could prolong life, so in Lapland it was smoked in the same manner as tobacco. Annibal Camoux was a former French soldier from Marseilles who was noted for his amazing longevity. A soldier in the service of the king of France, according to his biography Camoux reached 100 without losing his strength, which he attributed to his daily practice of chewing angelica root. He claimed to have gained his knowledge of herbs from the naturalist Joseph Pitton de Tournefort in 1681. Louis XV granted him a pension, and several artists painted his portrait. Camoux died in 1759 in Marseilles, at the claimed age of 121. Research in 1957, however, discovered that he was born in Nice in 1669, meaning that he was only 90 when he died.

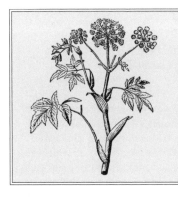

There is Angelica or Dwarf Gentian,
Whose root being dried in the hot shining Sun,
From death it doth preserve the poisoned man,
Whose extreme torment makes his life half gone,
That from death's mixed potion could not shun:
No Pestilence nor no infectious air,
Shall do him hurt, or cause him to despair.

Robert Chester

ginger was believed to be a better cure. Medicinally all the parts act as a digestive tonic and a circulatory stimulant, and is said to be 'a warming plant', suitable for people who feel the cold in winter. The fruit, leaf and root of angelica stimulate digestion, help dispel flatulence, circulate the blood and calm nerves. Culpeper states '*It is an herb of the Sun in Leo; let it be gathered when he is there, the Moon applying to his good aspect; let it be gathered either in his hour, or in the hour of Jupiter; let Sol be angular. In all epidemical diseases caused by Saturn, this is as good a preservative as grows; it resists poison by defending and comforting the heart, blood and spirits; it does the like against plague and all epidemical diseases…*'
He recommends it for curing virtually everything under the sun, including poisoning, pestilent airs, pestilence, ague, stomach ache, passing water, women in labour, expelling wind, eye problems, the biting of mad beasts, snake bites, ulcers, deafness, sores and rabies. And in flower language is said to be a symbol of ecstasy, inspiration and magic. The smell of garden angelica root is inviting for both fish and deer, so it was used as bait. It is said to create distaste for alcohol. However,

angelica is one of the flavourings used in vermouth, gin, Dubonnet, Benedictine and Chartreuse.

HISTORY: In legend, a monk was visited in a dream by the Archangel Raphael, who revealed the plant to be a cure for one of the many plagues that beset Europe in the Middle Ages. St Gabriel is also associated with the same legend. Thereafter the plant was called angelica and the belief grew that if chewed it could give protection against disease, as well as against evil and witchcraft. During the time of the Great Plague in London in 1665 angelica was chewed to protect against infection. Another source of its name of *St Michael's flower* is that angelica is said to flower on 8 May, when the Feast of the Apparition of St Michael was celebrated. This was believed by many to explain its protective qualities against evil and why it used also to be called *Root of the Holy Ghost*. Its virtues are praised by old writers, and the folklore of all North European countries demonstrate the ancient traditions of a belief in its use as a protection against contagion, for purifying the blood, and for curing every conceivable malady.

ANISE

PIMPINELLA ANISUM
Family Apiaceae/Umbelliferae, Carrot/Parsley

OTHER NAMES: Aniseed, anis, anneys, sweet fennel, sweet cumin, anise plant, common anise, green anise, Roman fennel, sweet Alice, sweet cumin. It is a spice, rather than a herb, and only its seeds are mentioned by Culpeper, in conjunction with a 'polypody of the oak' remedy.

DESCRIPTION: A feathery plant that grows about 2 feet (60 cm) high, with flat, white flower heads, small, aromatic brown seeds, and a distinctive liquorice taste.

PROPERTIES AND USES: The leaves of anise are a garnish for flavouring salads. The seeds are used as flavouring for various condiments, especially curry powders. Banckes's *Herbal* of 1525 suggests it to treat flatulence, induce sweating, and as diuretic and/or laxative, but tells us *'the seed must be parched or roasted in all manner'* to work better as a medicine. In William Turner's *New Herball* of 1551 it is said: *'Anise makes the breath sweeter and assuages pain.'* In India the end of a meal is often signalled when a dish of seeds is served as a digestive aid. William Langham, in the *Garden of Health* (1683), writes: *'For the dropsy, fill an old cock with Polypody and Aniseeds and seethe him well, and drink the broth.'* In Roman times, they were baked into a cake that was served at the end of the wedding feast, and the seeds became a herb of protection said to avert all evil. Inside a pillow anise is said to ward off nightmares. Many alcoholic drinks and cordials are flavoured with anise, particularly pastis, Pernod, Ricard, ouzo, raki and arrak. The seeds may be used to lay drag hunt trails and also by anti-blood sport movements to put hounds off the scent.

HISTORY: It is one of the oldest known spice plants used both for culinary and medicinal purposes by the Egyptians and it is mentioned by Dioscorides and Pliny. In the ninth century, Charlemagne (747–814 CE) commanded that it be grown upon the imperial farms. Edward IV of England in around 1480 had sachets of anise and orris root to perfume his linen. In England anise was in use from the 14th century, and was being cultivated in English gardens from the middle of the 16th century.

Poison Antidote

Aniseed was probably one of the 36 ingredients used by King Mithridates of Pontus (c.132–63 BCE) in a poison antidote (*Antidotum Mithradaticum*) which he took daily to acquire an overall immunity. It should be remembered that he gained his position of power by poisoning all rivals to the throne.

APPLE

MALUS species
Family Rosaceae, Rose

OTHER NAMES: Fruit of the gods, fruit of the underworld, silver branch, silver bough, tree of love.

DESCRIPTION: *Malus domestica* has almost 8000 known cultivars (cultivated variants), and is too well-known to describe in detail here.

PROPERTIES AND USES: Culpeper writes: '*They are very proper for hot and bilious stomachs, but not to the cold, moist, and flatulent. The more ripe ones eaten raw, move the belly a little; and unripe ones have the contrary effect. A poultice of roasted sweet apples, with powder of frankincense, removes pains of the side: and a poultice of the same apples boiled in plantain water to a pulp, then mixed with milk, and applied, take away fresh marks of gunpowder out of the skin…Roasted apples are good for the asthmatic; either raw, roasted or boiled, are good for the consumptive, in inflammations of the breasts or lungs…*' Apples are said to clean the liver, cure constipation, and tone the gums. A half and half mixture of apple cider vinegar and water make a rinse to restore hair, scalp and skin

HISTORY: To the druids the apple was sacred tree, a symbol of immortality. A branch of the apple which bore buds, flowers and fully ripened fruit (sometimes known as the *silver bough*) was a magical charm which enabled its possessor to enter into the the underworld of the gods. The tree originated in Kazakhstan, and the first analysis of the apple genome indicates that it underwent rapid genetic change around 60 million years ago, in the same period as dinosaurs vanished. This scientific research seems to resolve the mystery of why the apple is so different from its close botanical relatives, the strawberry and raspberry.

An Apple a Day Keeps the Doctor Away

The proverb is first recorded from Pembrokeshire, Wales in the 19th century. According to the *European Journal of Cancer Protection* eating apples regularly may reduce the risk of developing colorectal cancer. It seems to be the result of the high content of flavonoids, antioxidants found in the skin of apples, so the recommendation is to wash, but not to peel, them.

ARCHANGEL

LAMIUM ALBUM
Family Lamiaceae/Labiataea, Mint
Culpeper describes all three types of archangel

OTHER NAMES: Deadnettle, white deadnettle, white nettle, white archangel, stingless nettle, nettle flowers, blind nettle, bee nettle (bees are attracted to the flowers which contain nectar or pollen), Adam-and-Eve-in-the-bower, dog nettle, dumb nettle, honey-bee, snake's flower, suck-bottle, sucky Sue.

DESCRIPTION: It is an herbaceous perennial plant growing to 3 feet (90 cm), with green, four-angled stems. Like many other members of the Lamiaceae, the leaves appear similar to those of the unrelated stinging nettle *(Urtica dioica)* but do not sting, thus the common name 'deadnettle'. The flowers are white, with a lobed bottom lip and hooded top lip. They evolved like this to attract pollinating bees which use the lower lip as a landing pad while they take the nectar from the bottom of the flower tube. At the same time the bee brushes against the stamens that dangle from the hood, collecting pollen to transfer to the next flower.

PROPERTIES AND USES: Gerard described archangel thus: '*The flowers are baked with sugar as Roses are, which is called Sugar roset: as also the distilled water of them to make the heart merry, to make a good colour in the face, and to make the vital spirits more fresh and lively.*' Children used to make whistles from the stems, and the young leaves are edible and can be used in salads or cooked as a vegetable. The plant is also used in herbal medicine, for example as a dermatological remedy. Rich in tannin, the flowering plant has provided an astringent, anti-inflammatory dressing for cuts, wounds, and burns. When brewed as a tea, archangel has been used to halt internal bleeding. Archangel also is reported to cure diarrhoea.

HISTORY: Archangel formerly enjoyed prestige in England as a reputed cure for scrofula (a type of tuberculosis of the lymph nodes), the so-called king's evil, which was believed to respond to a monarch's touch. Archangel leaves mixed with grease were mentioned by the Roman naturalist Pliny the Elder (23–79 CE) as a remedy for the disease. Pliny also contended that the plant's smell was unpleasant enough to deter snakes from the surrounding area. John Gerard (1545–1612) wrote that the flowers were often baked in sugar. Children were known to have sucked the flowers for their nectar. Herbalists used a decoction of the plant primarily to stop internal haemorrhages but also prescribed it for some female ailments, and used it in the treatment of some forms of tuberculosis. It was also used externally for treating gout, sciatica and muscular pains, and for healing burns, bruises and wounds.

Chicken Feed

In Britain the white, yellow and red deadnettle are known as archangel, because it first blooms about 8 May, once a feast day of the Archangel Michael. Culpeper noted that physicians called it archangel *'to put a gloss on their practice'* rather than use the country people's more vulgar name of deadnettle. Another deadnettle, *Lamium amplexicaule*, is called henbit deadnettle as it is a favoured food of chickens.

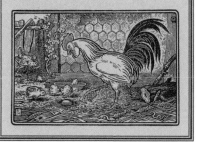

YELLOW ARCHANGEL
LAMIUM GALEOBDOLON

OTHER NAMES: Yellow deadnettle, yellow archangel, dummy nettle, weazel snout, dummy nettle

DESCRIPTION: It is similar to the white archangel, but with yellow flowers.

PROPERTIES AND USES: Yellow archangel as well as white archangel are valuable medicinal herbs. A tea is beneficial in abdominal and menstrual complaints, if two cups are sipped during the day. It cleanses the blood and is an effective remedy for sleeplessness and for diverse female troubles. People suffering from continual abdominal complaints

and young girls are said to be benefited by this tea. The leaves and flowers of the yellow archangel are used for similar complaints, but especially for scanty or burning urine, bladder trouble, serious kidney disorders and fluid retention in the heart. The flowers are used for digestive troubles, scrofula and skin rashes when it is recommended that one cup of this tea should be drunk during the morning. For ulcers and varicose veins, compresses made from the infusion are beneficial. Yellow archangel can be recommended for bladder malfunction with older people, as well as for chill in the bladder and nephritis.

RED ARCHANGEL
LAMIUM PURPUREUM

OTHER NAMES: Red deadnettle, bad man's posies, bumble-bee flower, rabbit's meat, red archangel, purple deadnettle, red bee-nettle, badman.

DESCRIPTION: More prostrate and creeping than the above, and more mint-like than nettle-like, with pink/purple/red flowers.

PROPERTIES AND USES:
In Sweden the young leaves used to be boiled and eaten as a vegetable. Medicinally, herbalists used a decoction of the flowering plant to stem haemorrhages, a decoction of the roots was used to treat measles, the bruised leaves were applied to wounds to staunch bleeding, and an infusion of the dried plant offered a remedy for chills. Culpeper noted that for women, white archangel flowers stopped discharges, and red archangel flowers prevented bleeding. Young plants can be stir-fried or used in salads.

ARRACH

ATRIPLEX HORTENSIS formerly *CHENOPODIUM HORTENSIS*
Family Chenopodiaceae, Goosefoot

OTHER NAMES: Culpeper calls this garden arrach, *'called also Orach; and Orage'*. Garden orach, red orach, mountain spinach, red mountain spinach, French spinach, goosefoot, blites, butter leaves. The plant is now classified in the Chenopodiaceae (Goosefoot) subfamily of Amaranthaceae.

DESCRIPTION: With an erect, branching stem, it has small reddish-tinged and yellowish-green flowers, and grows 3–6 feet (90 cm–1.8 m) in height. There are several varieties of arrach of various colourings, with the red, white and green being the most desirable.

PROPERTIES AND USES: John Evelyn wrote *'Orache is cooling, and allays the pituit humors.'* He noted that being set over the fire, neither arrach nor lettuce needs any other water than their own moisture to boil. Heated with vinegar, honey and salt, arrach was applied to cure an attack of gout. The seeds promote vomiting. Culpeper says it is *'under the government of the Moon and in quality cold and moist like her. When eaten it softens and loosens the body of man, and encourages the expulsion of waste. The herb, whether it be bruised and applied to the throat or boiled and applied in like manner, is excellent good for swellings in the throat.'* Garden orache yields a blue dye similar to that obtained from indigo *(Indigofera tinctoria)*.

HISTORY: Pliny writes that Hippocrates prescribed it with beet as a pessary for affections of the uterus; and Lycus of Neapolis recommended it to be taken in drink in cases of poisoning by cantharides (also called *Spanish fly*, caused by blister beetles). He said it could be employed as a liniment for inflammatory swellings, incipient boils, and was good for erysipelas (bacterial skin infection), jaundice and as an emetic. The *Atriplex* genus contains up to 200 species, and is often known as saltbush as it is extremely tolerant of salt content. The plant retains salt in its leaves, so was eaten in prehistoric times, tasting like salty spinach. It was known to be introduced into Britain in 1548. It is still popular in France for its large and succulent leaves, used as a substitute for spinach, for soups, and to correct the acidity of sorrel in salads and cooking. Its use in most of Europe has been overtaken by varieties of spinach. Today saltbush is a preferred plant to prevent soil erosion.

(WILD) ARRACH

ATRIPLEX FOETIDA or *CHENOPODIUM VULVARIA*
Family Chenopodiaceae, Goosefoot

OTHER NAMES: Culpeper names this as '*Vulvaria, from that part of the body upon which it is most used: also Dog's Arrach, Goat's Arrach, and Stinking Motherwort.*' Stinking goosefoot, notchweed, dungweed, stinking arrach

DESCRIPTION: It can be easily identified by its foul smell, caused by its trimethylamine content. Culpeper says: '*It smells like old rotten fish, or something worse.*' The small, insignificant green flowers are borne in spikes and the whole plant is covered with a white, greasy covering, giving it a grey-green appearance, which when touched gives out an enduring odour.

PROPERTIES AND USES: When a plant has a particularly unpleasant smell like the wild arrach, it usually points to a particular purpose, thus stinking arrach was used for foul ulcers. The name stinking motherwort refers to the use of its leaves in cases of 'hysteria' and nervous troubles connected with women's ailments, and it was thought that it could also cure barrenness. It can still be used today, particularly for period problems. Culpeper wrote to a patient: '*To this intent I first commend unto you stinking Arrach, a pattern whereof I have sent you here enclosed; you may find it upon dunghills, especially such as are made of Horse-dung….*' Culpeper describes it as cold and moist, and ruled by Venus in Scorpio. The shape of its leaf was thought to resemble a vulva – hence a common name

for the plant was *Vulvaria*. It typically grew upon dunghills leading to the name 'dungweeds' for the family of plants to which it belongs. Culpeper specifically commends dunghills that '*are made of Horsedung*' because horses are ruled by the Sun, which will enhance the healing potential of the herb. Culpeper writes: '*I commend it for a universal medicine of the womb, and such a medicine as will easily, safely, and speedily cure any disease thereof, as fits of the mother, dislocation, or falling out thereof: it cools the womb being overheated…it cleanseth the womb if it be foul, and strengthens it exceedingly; it provokes the terms if they be stopped, and stops them if they flow immoderately.*'

HISTORY: Pliny said that it had the same uses as garden arrach, but could also be used for dying hair. Only to be used fresh, it was recommended as an antihysteric and antispasmodic herb.

Golden Goose Foot

The genus name *Atriplex* is derived from the Greek *atraphaxis* meaning fast growth. *Chenopodium* literally means goose foot. The name arache, given to this goosefoot and others of the same subfamily, is a corruption of '*aurum*', the Latin word for gold, because its decoction, mixed with wine, was supposed to be a cure for yellow jaundice.

ARSESMART

POLYGONUM HYDROPIPER (syn. *PERSICARIA HYDROPIPER*)
Family Polygonaceae, Knotweed or Smartweed

OTHER NAMES: Culpeper – *'The Hot Arsesmart is also Water-Pepper, and Culrage; the Mild Arsesmart is called Dead Arsesmart, Persicaria, or Peach-Wort, because the leaves are so like the leaves of a peach tree; it is also called Plumbago.'* However, plumbago is leadwort (see below). Smartweed, biting knotweed, marsh-pepper knotweed, red knees, biting pepper, biting persecaria, biting tongue, bloodwort, bog ginger, ciderage, common smartweed, doorweed, marsh pepper, red leaves, redshanks, sickleweed, smartass, water smartweed.

DESCRIPTION: It grows in damp places and shallow water; it is an annual plant with reddish, jointed stems and tiny green flowers with white, pink or yellow edges. The joints in the stem have produced the nickname *red knees*. Although several species possess similar properties, *P. hydropiper* is by far the most powerful in medicine. Most animals avoid the plant because of its burning flavour.

PROPERTIES AND USES:
Arsesmart has long been known for its biting, peppery flavour, and has been used as a seasoning for recorded history. If a piece of smartweed was tucked beneath a horse's saddle, Culpeper said it would keep the horse from feeling hungry or thirsty over a long ride. People used to strew pieces of the plant on the floor of their house to get rid of fleas and drive away flies. Sheets were soaked in water that had smartweed boiled in it to help cholera victims, who were then wrapped in the sheet. Rheumatism sufferers would add the plant to their bath water to get some pain relief. An astringent, diaphoretic and diuretic, it is effective as an extract against coughs and colds. The juice of the plant, mixed with a little water, is effective on sores that have developed pus.

HISTORY: Sir Thomas Browne in *The Garden of Cyrus* (1658) asked: *'Why* [do] *Fenny waters afford the hottest and sweetest plants, as Calamus, Cyperus, and Crowfoot, and mud cast out of ditches most naturally produceth Arsmart?'* In Japan leaves of a cultivar are used as a vegetable. The seeds of the water-pepper are also used in the popular Japanese wasabi sauce and sushi, tempura and sashimi dishes.

Water Pepper

Smartweed is found on stream banks, and the name *hydropiper* is derived from Greek *hydro* (water) and the genus name *piper* (pepper) with reference to both the aquatic habitat and the similarity of the flower-spike to pepper.

ARTICHOKE

CYNARA SCOLYMUS
Family Asteraceae/Compositae, Sunflower/Daisy

OTHER NAMES: Culpeper calls it the *Heartichoke*, and states: '*The Latins call them Cinera, only our college calls them Artichocus.*' Globe artichoke, green artichoke, French artichoke.

DESCRIPTION: A stately plant, it grows 4–5 feet (1.2–1.5 m) tall, with a 3-foot (90-cm) spread, with large, thistle-like, pink-purple flowers. Its head of green buds is edible.

PROPERTIES AND USES:
Culpeper says: '*They are under the dominion of Venus, and therefore it is no marvel if they provoke lust, as indeed they do, being somewhat windy meat; and yet they stay the involuntary course of natural seed in man, which is commonly called nocturnal pollutions…this is certain, that the decoction of the root boiled in wine, or the root bruised and distilled in wine in an alembic, and being drank, purges the urine exceedingly.*' Today artichokes are known to benefit the liver, aiding detoxification. Also a diuretic, it is useful in treating hepatitis and jaundice. Globe artichokes reduce blood sugar and cholesterol levels and help to metabolize fat. Traditionally it was used as both an aphrodisiac and a contraceptive – making it a win-win herb for some people. The plant is named as a *scolymus* (pointed stake) from the Greek island of Kinara *(Cynara)*.

HISTORY: Grown by the Greeks and Romans, they fell out of favour until Catherine de Medici (1519–89) reintroduced them to France in the 16th century, after she married Henri II. Because of its aphrodisiac reputation, French women were often forbidden to eat it, but it was a popular plant for cultivation in monastery gardens. John Evelyn tells us: '*This noble thistle brought from Italy was at first so rare in England that they were commonly sold for crowns apiece.*' King Charles I's French wife, Henrietta Maria (1609–69), had a large garden of artichokes cultivated at her manor house in Wimbledon.

From *Love's Martyr*, 1601

The Father that desires to have a boy,
That may be Heir unto his land and living,
Let his espoused Love drink day by day,
Good Artichocks, who buds in August bring,
Sod in clear running water of the spring;
Wives' natural Conception it doth strengthen,
And their declining life by force doth lengthen.

ASAFOETIDA

FERULA ASSAFOETIDA
Family Apicaeae/Umbelliferae, Carrot/Parsley

OTHER NAMES: Devil's dung, stinking gum, giant fennel, narthex, food of the gods.

DESCRIPTION: A perennial, much like a giant cabbage, growing to 10 feet (3 m) high in its native soil in Iran and Afghanistan, with tiny greenish-yellow flowers. It has a milky juice that exudes from its root and a strong foetid odour. Four- to five-year-old roots of plants that have not flowered are dug up in June, and cut to release the milky juice which solidifies into a brownish resin upon exposure to air.

PROPERTIES AND USES: Research suggests the plant's resin is anticoagulant and lowers blood pressure, and it has been used to treat stomach ailments such as flatulence, bloating and *Candida albicans* fungal infections. It has also been traditionally used for asthma, bronchitis and whooping cough. It was worn round the neck as a protection from infectious diseases, particularly colds. Its effectiveness seems to have been heightened by the fact that its strong smell would keep infectious people away. For some people, the slightest smell of asafoetida has been known to cause vomiting. In 1864, Dr Garrod regarded *'asafoetida as one of the most valuable remedies of the materia medica; far above all other ordinary antispasmodics…the value of the drug is chiefly due to the sulphur oil contained in it.'* In folklore, it was used to repel evil spirits. The gum resin is an important commercial ingredient in the famous Worcestershire (Worcester) Sauce, along with malt vinegar (from barley), spirit vinegar, molasses, sugar, salt, anchovies, tamarind (Indian date) extract, onions, garlic, lemons, cloves, soy sauce, pickles and peppers.

HISTORY: The Romans traditionally used *silphium (laserpitium)* as a condiment, importing it from the former Greek colony of Cyrene in North Africa. This could be purchased at the same price as gold – and it had originally been used as a medicine. It has never been identified and in the middle of the first century it mysteriously disappeared. Asafoetida took its place and was called *'food of the gods'* as it became the favourite Roman condiment. By the Middle Ages it was being used by Arab physicians and across the rest of Europe.

Cursing a Witch

From the website herb-magic.com, we learn that to *'reverse a trick* [witches' spell], *put devil's dung* [asafoetida], *vandal root* [valerian root, also foul-smelling], *black hen feathers, Black Arts powder and a hair of a witch into a bottle. Urinate into the bottle while cursing the witch, cap and seal it with wax from a black candle, and bury it where the witch will walk over it.'*

ASARABACCA

ASARUM EUROPAEUM
Family Aristolochiaceae, Birthwort

OTHER NAMES: European wild ginger, hardy ginger, wild nard, wild spikenard, hazelwort, haslewort cabaret, foal's foot, carn ebol y gerddi (Welsh for lame foal of the gardens), European ginger, European snakeroot, public house plant.

DESCRIPTION: Asarabacca is a creeping evergreen with a very short fleshy stem, bearing two large, dark-green, kidney-shaped evergreen leaves, and a solitary purplish-green drooping flower.

PROPERTIES AND USES: Culpeper says: '*This herb, being drunk, not only provokes vomiting but purges downward… both choler and phlegm. If you add to it some spikenard, with the whey of goat's milk, or honeyed water, it is made more strong; but it purges phlegm more manifestly than choler, and therefore doth much help pains in the hips and other parts; being boiled in whey they wonderfully help the obstructions of the liver and spleen, and are therefore profitable for the dropsy and jaundice: being steeped in wine and drank it helps those continual agues that come by the plenty of stubborn tumours; an oil made thereof by setting in the sun, with some laudanum added to it, provokes sweating (the ridge of the back anointed therewith) and thereby drives away the shaking fits of the ague. It will not abide any long boiling, for it loses its chief strength thereby; nor much beating, for the finer powder doth provoke vomit and urine, and the coarser purges downwards…The leaves and root* being boiled in Iye [a strong alkaline solution from leaching wood ashes], *and the head often washed therewith while it is warm, comforts the head and brain that is ill affected by taking cold, and helps the memory.*' The fresh leaves and roots give an apple-green dye, but if boiled longer the dye is brown.

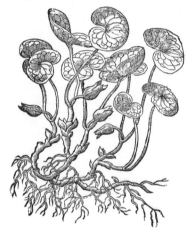

HISTORY: It has been cultivated as a medicinal herb since the 13th century in Britain, but seemed to only grow wild in the Lake District. A traditional use was as an emetic (causing vomiting) after too much alcohol, a practice still pursued in France until recently. The dried leaves when used as snuff will cause sneezing and a copious flow of mucus, so they were one of the ingredients in a tobacconist's 'head-clearing' snuff. Herbalists also recommended asarabacca for treating toothache and eye and throat ailments.

ASH TREE

FRAXINUS EXCELSIOR
Family Oleaceae, Olive

OTHER NAMES: Common ash, bird's tongue, common European ash, English ash, Hampshire weed, husbandman's tree, onnen (Welsh), widow-maker, Venus of the woods (for its beauty).

DESCRIPTION: A tall, very common tree distinguished by its light-grey bark (smooth in younger trees, rough and scaly in older specimens) and by its large, feathery, compound leaves. There is a thick seed-chamber with a long, strap-shaped wing which is known as an ash key (botanically, *samara*). Bunches of 'keys' hang from the twigs in great clusters, at first green and then brown as the seeds ripen. They remain attached to the tree until the succeeding spring, when they are blown off and carried away by the wind. The seedlings are so abundant that it became known to Hampshire foresters as 'Hampshire weed'.

PROPERTIES AND USES: Mrs M. Grieve in *A Modern Herbal* (1931) wrote: '*Both bark and the leaves have medicinal use and fetch prices which should repay the labour of collecting them, especially the bark. Ash bark occurs in commerce in quills [pens] which are grey or greenish-grey externally. Ash bark has been employed as a bitter tonic and astringent, and is said to be valuable as an antiperiodic. On account of its astringency, it has been used, in decoction, extensively in the treatment of intermittent fever and ague...It has been considered useful to remove obstructions of the liver and spleen, and in rheumatism of an arthritic nature. A ley from the ashes of the bark was used formerly to cure scabby and leprous heads. The leaves have diuretic, diaphoretic and purgative properties, and are employed in modern herbal medicine for their laxative action, especially in the treatment of gouty and rheumatic complaints, proving a useful substitute for Senna, having a less griping effect...The distilled water of the leaves, taken every morning, was considered good for dropsy and obesity. A decoction of the leaves in white wine had the reputation of dissolving stone and curing jaundice.*' The spokes of wheels were made from ash, and because of its flexibility it was called '*the husbandman's tree*', being used for every kind of agricultural implement.

HISTORY: The old Latin name for the seeds (ash keys) was *lingua avis* meaning bird's tongue, which they closely resemble. The keys were employed as a remedy for flatulence. They were also preserved with salt and vinegar and eaten as a pickle. John Evelyn wrote: '*Ashen keys have the virtue of capers*', and they were often substituted for them in sauces and salads. Gerard states: '*The leaves and bark of the Ash tree are dry and moderately hot…the seed is hot and dry in the second degree. The juice of the leaves or the leaves themselves being applied or taken with wine cure the bitings of vipers, as Dioscorides says, "The leaves of this tree are of so great virtue against serpents as that they dare not so much as touch the morning and evening shadows of the tree, but shun them afar off as Pliny reports."*' The ash was believed in Britain to provide protection against snakes. Adders could be killed with one fast stroke with an ash stick, and a basking adder could be contained within a circle drawn round it with the same wood. Rockers on a child's cradle were made of ash to protect against snakes.

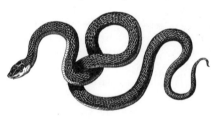

The Tree of Life

The name ash comes from Ask, the first man on earth according to northern European Teutonic mythology. One tradition tells how the ash, called *Yggdrasill* (the Tree of Life), represented the universe. After the universe, the gods and the giants were created, vegetation emerged and the gods then made the first human couple – the man *Ask* from an ash tree *(Fraxinus)* and the woman *Embla* from an elm *(Ulmus)*.

Witches' broomsticks were said to be made from ash to safeguard their riders from drowning, and the wood was used for building boats, including those of the Vikings. A dearth of ash keys portended disaster, and it was a tradition that English ash trees bore no seed in 1648, the year before Charles I (1600–49) was executed. It was known as the widow-maker as a large bough can fall without warning, killing anyone standing under it.

Using Ash to Build Aircraft and Cars

The common ash and the privet are the only British members of the olive family, Oleaceae.

Horticulturalist Maud Grieve in 1931 wrote that '*Ash is the second most important wood used in aeroplanes, and a study of the spacious afforestation scheme now in force over the Crown Lands of the New Forest reveals the fact that especial trouble has been taken to find suitable homes for the Ash. The great bulk of the wood used in aeroplanes is Spruce from the Pacific Coast.*'

Howard Hughes's famous 1947 'Spruce Goose' aircraft was designed using a great deal of birch, not spruce, because of wartime aluminium restrictions, and the Second World War Mosquito combat aircraft was made from laminated plywood. Morgan, the last remaining British car manufacturer, uses ash frames in its sports cars.

ASPARAGUS

ASPARAGUS OFFICINALIS
Family Asparagaceae (formerly Liliaceae), Lily

OTHER NAMES: Culpeper also names it Sparagus and Sperage. Asparagus fern, fern weed, sparrow grass, sparrow weed, white asparagus (normal asparagus that has been shielded from sunlight), wild asparagus.

DESCRIPTION: *Asparagus officinalis*, or wild asparagus, is found on the sea-coasts of most parts of Europe, and from this our garden asparagus has been raised. The 'spears' are eaten when immature shoots before they have a chance to turn woody. The plant has an attractive feathery foliage.

PROPERTIES AND USES: Elizabeth Blackwell, in *A Curious Herbal* (1751) writes: '*The virtues of Asparagus are well known as a diuretic and laxative; and for those of sedentary habits who suffer from symptoms of gravel, it has been found very beneficial, as well as in cases of dropsy. The fresh expressed juice is taken medicinally in tablespoonful doses.*' It is high in potassium and folic acid content. Asparagus contains an excellent supply of the protein called histones, believed to be active in controlling cell growth. Thus some believe asparagus can be a cell growth 'normalizer', helping to control cancer and acting as a general body tonic. Like Jerusalem artichokes, asparagus is one of the few perennial vegetables which do not have to be replanted each year.

HISTORY: The vegetable has been immortalized in the hieroglyphs of Ancient Egypt. Asparagus is derived from a Greek word signifying 'the tearer' in allusion to the spikes of some species; or perhaps from the Persian 'spurgas', a shoot. It was believed that the spears rose from rams' horns buried in the ground. *Asparagus officinalis* has been used from very early times as a culinary vegetable, owing to its delicate flavour and diuretic properties. There is a recipe for cooking asparagus

Not So Sweet Pee

Asparagus has the peculiar property, but only in some people, of making urine take on a distinctive odour. Even stranger, not everyone can detect the asparagus odour in urine. Those people who produce asparagus-smelling urine are not necessarily those who can detect the odour, and those who can detect the odour are not necessarily those who produce it. Both traits appear to be genetically determined.

Dressed to Kill

The brilliant French mathematician Bernard le Bouyer de Fontenelle died a few weeks short of his 100th birthday in 1757. He was a renowned gourmand. A story recounts how one day his friend and colleague the Abbé Terrasson arrived unexpectedly, just as Fontenelle was eagerly awaiting a dish of asparagus which he particularly loved, especially dressed with oil. The abbé, however, preferred his asparagus with butter, so Fontanelle ordered his cook to prepare half the dish with oil, and half with butter. Suddenly, before the dish was served, the abbé fell down dead with apoplexy, whereupon Fontenelle instantly rushed into the kitchen, calling out to his cook *'The whole with oil! The whole with oil, as at first!'*

---

in the oldest surviving book of recipes, the third century CE Roman work *Apicius* or *De Re Coquinaria*. The Greeks and Romans valued it for their tables, and boiled it so quickly that *'velocius quam asparagi coquuntur'* (*'faster than asparagus is cooked'*) was a proverb of the times. The English poet Thomas Tusser wrote in his *Five Hundred Points of Good Husbandry* (1573): *'Sperage let grow two years, and then remove'*. In 1670 forced asparagus was being supplied to the London market. In 2010 the *Worcester News* reported about an *'Asparamancer Jemima Packington'* who predicted the British 'hung parliament' by 'reading' asparagus spears.

PRICKLY ASPARAGUS
ASPARAGUS APHYLLUS
Family Liliaceae, Lily

Culpeper described both types of asparagus as being under the influence of Jupiter: *'The young Bud or branches boiled in ones ordinary broth, makes the Belly soluble and open, and boiled in white Wine, provokes Urine being stopped, and is good against the Strangury, or difficulty of making water; it expels the gravel and stone out of the Kidneys, and helps pains in the Reins: And boiled in white Wine or Vinegar it is prevalent for them that have their Arteries loosened, or are troubled with the Hip-Gout, or Sciatica. The Decoction of the Roots boiled in Wine and taken is good to clear the sight, and being held in the Mouth eases the Toothache: And being taken fasting several mornings together stirs up bodily lust in Man or Woman (whatsoever some have written to the contrary.) The Garden Asparagus nourishes more than the wild; yet hath it the same effects in all the aforementioned Diseases. The Decoction of the Roots in white Wine, and the Back and Belly bathed therewith, or kneeling or lying down in the same, or sitting therein as a Bath, hath been found effectual against pains that happen to the lower parts of the Body; and no less effectual against stiff and benumbed Sinews, or those that are shrunk by Cramps, and Convulsions, and helps the Sciatica.'*

ASTROLOGICAL AND ELEMENTAL GARDENS

These are the major herbs and plants associated with the 12 astrological signs, and the corresponding body parts ruled by the sign and believed to be the cause of illnesses:

Aquarius (Jan 21–Feb 19) *Ankles, circulatory system and shins*: Elderberry, fumitory, mullein, daffodil, sage, comfrey, rosemary, valerian, fennel and mint.

Pisces (Feb 20–Mar 20) *Feet*: Lungwort, meadowsweet, rosehip, sage, lemon balm, basil, lilac, nutmeg, borage, lilies and clove.

Aries (Mar 21–Apr 20) *Head*: Cowslip, garlic, hops, mustard, rosemary, carnation, chervil, basil, nettle, catmint, wormwood, geranium and cypress pine

Taurus (Apr 21–May 21) *Neck and throat*: Coltsfoot, lovage, primrose, mint, thyme, violet, marshmallow, catnip, rose, carnation, saffron, honeysuckle, jasmine, tansy, wormwood, yarrow and soapwort.

Gemini (May 22–Jun 22) *Hands, arms, shoulders and lungs*: Caraway, dill, lavender, parsley, vervain, mint, parsley, anise, marjoram, liquorice, fennel, honeysuckle, horehound and oregano.

Cancer (Jun 23–Jul 23) *Breast and stomach*: Agrimony, balm, daisies, hyssop, jasmine, parsley, sage, aloe, evening primrose, myrtle, cinnamon, lemon balm, hyacinth, bay leaves and water lily.

Leo (Jul 24–Aug 23) *Back, spine and heart*: Bay, borage, chamomile, marigold, poppy, rue, dill, lemon balm, tarragon, clove, sandalwood, frankincense, camphor, eyebright and sunflower.

Virgo (Aug 24–Sep 23) *Intestines and nervous system*: Fennel, savory, southernwood, valerian, chervil, dill, caraway, mint, morning glory, lily, horehound, lavender and marjoram.

Libra (Sep 24–Oct 23) *Buttocks, lower back and kidneys*: Pennyroyal, primrose, violets, yarrow, catnip, thyme, elderberry, iris, lilies, ivy, St John's wort, lemon balm and bergamot.

Scorpio (Oct 24–Nov 22) *Genitals*: Basil, tarragon, wormwood, catmint, sage, catnip, honeysuckle, nettle, onion, coriander, garlic and elder.

Sagittarius (Nov 23–Dec 21) *Liver, thighs and hips*: Feverfew, houseleek, mallow, chervil, saffron, sage, basil, borage, nutmeg and clove.

Capricorn (Dec 22–Jan 20) *Knees, bones and joints*: Comfrey, sorrel, Solomon's seal, dill, tarragon, caraway, rosemary, chamomile, lambs ears and marjoram.

ZODIAC PLANETARY GARDENS

For centuries, people have used the influence of the astrological signs of the Zodiac for direction on planting and harvesting, and now many home owners are building whole gardens around their own Zodiac signs.

Sun: Daisies, chamomile, calendula, celandine, sunflower, and any flower whose petals are arranged to resemble the rays of the sun or associated with the Apollo (Greek sun god).

Moon: White flowering herbs, herbs that are grown in water, and herbs that either decline in moonlight or alternately bloom after dark, or associated with Artemisia (the Moon goddess) or bear her name in their scientific name.

Mars: Any plant with thorns like barberry, nettle, holly, cacti, etc. or herbs with associated with strength such as: coriander, garlic, hops, horseradish, tarragon, mustard, onion and peppers. Also anything associated with the zodiac sign Scorpio.

Mercury: Fennel, parsley, dill, caraway, and lavender or the god of knowledge.

Jupiter: Sage, sweet cicely, camphor, hyssop, houseleek, oak, borage, betony, cannabis and datura, or associated with the god Jupiter.

Venus: Beautiful and delicate flowers, especially primrose, aquilegia, roses, catmint, apple, strawberry and cherries, and, of course, the goddess Venus.

Saturn: Foxglove, Solomon's seal, comfrey, hemlock, monkshood, belladonna and woad or any plant that bears blue flowers.

Bhopal, the scene of the Union Carbide poison gas disaster in India in 1984, has developed a Peace Garden with various plants related to different zodiac signs and planets. These herbs and rare trees represent nine planets, 12 *Rashis* (zodiac signs) and 27 *Nakshatras* (constellations), as mentioned in Hindu scriptures.

ELEMENTAL GARDENS

Owners of a large garden may like to divide it into the Four Elements of the ancients: Fire, Earth, Air and Water, or develop a garden along any of these individual themes.

The **Fire Garden** is south-facing towards warmer winds. The north side of the garden is edged by bushes to serve as a sun trap and shelter from cold winds, to give the garden a climate both for more exotic plants and sun-bathing. The centre is dominated by a large tree and/or place for a fire. A red maple *(Acer rubrum)* would suit, and bushes should have red or orange blossoms or berries.

The **Earth Garden** in its simplest form is a vegetable garden or orchard, often north-facing. If space is available for a large tree, the lime *(Tilia platyphyllos)* will attract bees, and give shade, but in smaller gardens plant fruit trees. Sink part of the garden to create a cooler, calmer atmosphere. Use hedging and grow kitchen and medicinal herbs, and develop a quiet corner for contemplation.

The **Air Garden** is often west-facing. It is open with little protection, a place more for meeting, conversation and playing games than relaxation. Trees like birch and ash give movement and rustle even in the lightest winds, and plants are chosen to attract birds and insects to keep the garden a living, moving experience.

The **Water Garden** can have a large pond with a reed and marsh area, and is west-facing with overgrown labyrinthine paths. There are no straight lines of planting, and transitions between areas are flowing rather than symmetrical. It is a quiet garden like the Earth Garden.

ASTROLOGICAL JUDGEMENT OF DISEASES 1655

Nicholas Culpeper's published books include *The English Physitian* (1652) and the *Compleat Herball* (1653), and their pharmaceutical and herbal information forms a large part of this book. However, *Semeiotica Uranica: or An Astrological Judgement of Diseases* was published in 1651 and *Astrological Judgement of Diseases from the Decumbiture of the Sick* published posthumously in 1655. They are the foundation of his more famous works, and two of the most detailed works on the practice of medical astrology in early modern Europe. Culpeper had been influenced by the notable astrologer William Lilly (1602–81), writing '*Astrology is an art which teaches by the book of creatures what the universal Providence mind and the meaning of God towards man is.*' He quoted Genesis in his support: '*God made the Sun, Moon and Stars to rule over night and day…to be signs of things to come.*'

In the books, Culpeper explains 'decumbiture', the use of astrology to diagnose disease from the time a patient falls ill. He describes the principles of disease and how it should be treated, providing a key to his herbal, *The English Physitian*. The book was largely based upon a translation of a work by Noel Duret, the French royal cosmographer,

and Culpeper admonished his opponents at the Royal College of Physicians: '*Listen to this, O College of Physitians, let me entreat you to learn the principles of your trade, and I beseech you no longer mistake avarice for wit and honesty.*'

The Doctrine of Signatures had naturally led Culpeper and others across Europe to the concept of astrological influence, giving it what was thought to be a more scientific basis – astrology was regarded as a serious science at this time. It also helped normal people to understand their illnesses, and the need for certain types of treatment. Culpeper, as an astrologer himself, believed that only astrologers should be allowed to practise medicine and was in constant conflict with the College of Physicians.

In his *Compleat Herball*, Culpeper set out his theory of the astrological system of diagnosis and treatment:

1. Consider what planet causes the disease; that thou may find it in my aforesaid 'Judgement of Diseases'.

2. Consider what part of the body is affected by the disease and whether it lies in the flesh or blood or bones or ventricles.

3. Consider by what planet the afflicted part of the body is governed; that my 'Judgement of Diseases' will inform you also.

4. *You may oppose diseases by herbs of the planet opposite to the planet that causes them; as diseases of the luminaries by the herbs of Saturn and the contrary; diseases of Mars by the herbs of Venus and the contrary.*

5. *There is a way to cure diseases sometimes by sympathy and so every planet cures its own diseases; as the sun and moon by their herbs cure the eyes, Saturn the spleen, Jupiter the liver, Mars the gall and diseases of the choler, and by Venus diseases in the instruments of generation.*

He notes the basic planetary divisions of the botanic kingdom, based upon the planetary catalogue of Paracelsus:

Sun: Ruled the heart, circulation, and the vertebral column. All plants that 'appeared solar', such as calendula and sunflower fell under its influence, as did those plants that followed the Sun in their growth such as heliotrope. Plants that were heat-producing, such as clove and pepper, and all those having a tonic effect on the heart were classified under the Sun.

Moon: This influenced growth, fertility, breasts, stomach, womb and the menstrual cycle. It also exerted control over the brain and the memory. All body fluids and secretions were under the lunar sway, just like tides. All the plant world was subject to the Moon, as harvesting and planting was performed in accordance with lunar phases. Most especially lunar were those plants with a diaphoretic action, with juicy globular fruits, or moisturizing, cooling or soothing juices.

Mercury: Ruled the nervous system, and organs of speech, hearing and respiration. 'Mercuric plants', such as fennel, dill and carrot, bore finely divided leaves, often produced a sharp and distinctive smell, and often had a mood-elevating, slightly tonic effect.

Venus: She ruled the complexion, sexual organs and the hidden inner workings of the body cells. Venusian plants almost all bore heavily scented, showy blossoms such as the Damascus rose or the apple blossom. The medicinal effects were emollient, anti-nephritic, alterative and often aphrodisiac.

Mars: Mars ruled the muscles, body vitality and libido. It also had influence in the combustion processes of the body and the motor nerves. Its plants affected the blood, being stimulating and in many cases aphrodisiac. Many were hot and acrid in their nature.

Jupiter: Jupiter influenced the liver, abdomen, spleen and kidney. Digestion was governed by this planet as was body growth. Most of Jupiter's plants were edible, many bearing nuts or fruit, such as the chestnut and the apricot. Its medicinal traits were antispasmodic, calmative, hepatic and anthelmintic.

Saturn: Saturn ruled over ageing, bone structure, teeth and all hardening processes. Many of the plants associated with Saturn were poisonous such as hemlock and belladonna. The effects of Saturnian plants were considered to be sedative, pain-relieving, coagulant or bone-forming.

BALSAM TREE

COMMIPHORA OPOBALSAMUM syn. *GILEADENSIS*
Family Burseraceae, Torchwood or Incense Tree

OTHER NAMES: Balm-tree, balsam of Gilead, balsam of Mecca, Mecca myrrh.

DESCRIPTION: This small tree from the Red Sea region grows to 12 feet (3.7 m). It has spreading branches like wands, and a reddish bark which spontaneously exudes sweet-smelling resinous drops in summer. The process is helped by incisions cut into the bark. This is the source of the original *balm of Gilead*, around which many mystical associations have gathered.

PROPERTIES AND USES: Culpeper recommended the liquor as effective against snakes, scorpions, pestilence, obstructions of the liver and spleen, failing memory, falling sickness, earache, film over the eyes, coughs, shortness of breath, consumption, palsy, cramp, urinary infections, diseases of the womb, kidneys and bowels, barrenness, kidney stones, cramp,

infections – in fact virtually anything that could go wrong with the body. The liquor was used by herbalists for throat infections, and as an ointment for the pain and inflammation caused by rheumatism and arthritis. There are pain-relieving substances now known as salicylates in the resin, also present in willow, elder and meadowsweet, which are the basis of the pain relief given by aspirin.

HISTORY: The forces of the Turkish empire destroyed the trees around Jericho and banned its export, growing the trees in guarded gardens at Matarie, near Cairo, where the balsam was valued as a cosmetic by ladies of the court. In the Books of Genesis and Jeremiah in the Bible, and in the works of Theophrastes, Galen and Dioscorides, it is praised. Pliny the Elder states that the tree was first brought to Rome by the generals of Vespasian, while Josephus relates that it was taken from Arabia to Judea by the queen of Sheba as a present for Solomon. There, being cultivated for its juice, particularly on Mount Gilead, it acquired its popular name. Pliny also said that it was one of the ingredients of the 'Royal Perfume' of the Parthians. According to Culpeper, '*the liquor they call Opobalsamum, the berries or fruit of the tree Carpobalsamum, and the sprigs or young branches thereof Zylobalsamum.*'

Rare and Magical

Its rarity and magical properties have caused its name to be adopted for several other plant species. For instance Canary balm *(Cedronella canariensis)* is also known as balm of Gilead, and it has a strong eucalyptus smell similar to many other plants with 'balsam' as part of their name.

BARBERRY

BERBERIS VULGARIS
Family Berberidaceae, Berberis

OTHER NAMES: European barberry, berber, ambarbaris, y Pren Melyn (Welsh for yellow tree), woodsour, woodsower, holy thorn, jaunders tree, jaundice barberry, jaundice berry.

DESCRIPTION: A perennial deciduous shrub with grey, woody stems that can grow up to 10 feet (3 m) tall, with tiny spikes at the base of the leaves, and small yellow flowers that hang in clusters followed by red oblong berries.

PROPERTIES AND USES: The plant has been recommended primarily as a purgative and tonic, and was prescribed for allaying the thirst associated with diabetes. The root has also been used for kidney stones, gall-bladder ailments and painful periods. Culpeper recommended it for choler, yellow jaundice, boils, ringworm, burns, catarrh, diarrhoea etc. The berries have been used to make jams, jellies and syrups, and as the berries contain citric, malic and tartaric acids, they possess medicinal properties as astringents and antiscorbutics. In Wales, honey was added to berry juice to make a medicinal syrup, rich in vitamin C. The roots give a yellow dye used for dyeing wool, cotton and linen and for dyeing wood and polishing leather. The leaves give a black dye and the twigs and young leaves give a red-yellow dye. The hard yellow wood is ideal for turning and for making furniture.

HISTORY: In Egypt the berry juice was taken as a remedy for fever. The generic name may derive from the Phoenician word '*barbar*', which means glossy, referring to the sheen on the leaves. In Italy and parts of Europe, barberry is called *Holy Thorn*, because it is thought to have formed part of the crown of thorns made for our Saviour. Its bitter taste also gave the plant the name *woodsour*. During the medieval period this shrub could be seen growing near churches and monasteries. However farmers from the mid-17th century came to blame the plant for 'blighting' wheat and it was banished to the hedgerows, becoming increasingly scarce. The 'blight' was explained in 1865 by the fact that barberry is actually an intermediate host plant for black rust, a disease of wheat.

Cure For Jaundice

The bark and the yellow wood were part of a cure for yellow jaundice, conforming to the Doctrine of Signatures's principles. It is even today widely and effectively used as a bitter tonic given to jaundice patients several times a day.

THE BARBERS PHYSIC GARDEN

THE BARBER-SURGEONS' HALL, CITY OF LONDON

The Barbers Company, founded in 1308, had a hall near the current site in 1445. In 1500 there were 26 halls of Livery Companies, and by 1600 there were 46 halls of which 24 had gardens. The Drapers had a large garden which was open to the public, and the Grocers also had a big garden, while that of the Parish Clerks in Bishopsgate was of modest size, being only 72 by 21 feet (22 by 6.4 m). The livery gardens were valued for recreation, as well as for growing fruit, herbs and flowers, and several had bowling alleys. In 1605 the Gardeners' Company was founded. Today just ten companies still have gardens in the City, and although of necessity a few are small, it is good to find that the tradition of Livery Company gardens lives on. The companies are the Barbers, Drapers, Girdlers, Goldsmiths, Grocers, Merchant Taylors, Plaisterers, Salters, Stationers, and Tallow Chandlers. In 1540 the company amalgamated with the Surgeons' Guild to form the Barber-Surgeons' Company, hence the name of the Hall today. However, in 1745 the surgeons left and it is now again the Worshipful Company of Barbers of London. John Gerard (1545–1612) was a surgeon and also a renowned plantsman, author and gardener. His famous *Herbal* was published in 1597,

and he became Master of the Barber Surgeons in 1607.

It is likely that the Company had a garden when their hall was built in 1445 but the first written record of it was in 1555. It was not a herb or medicine garden. In 1630, we know that the Company bought 100 '*sweete briars*' (*Rosa rubiginosa* or eglantine), probably to form a stout hedge and for the rosehips, and also rosemary, strawberry, violets and vines. In 1666 the garden prevented the Great Fire of London from reaching the Anatomical Theatre, though the rest of the Hall was lost. The succeeding Hall was destroyed by bombing in 1940, and the splendid new Barber-Surgeons' Hall was opened in 1969. The site of the present garden is on one of the 21 bastions built in 300 CE for Emperor Hadrian's stone fort, itself built in 122 CE. Thus it was necessary to get Scheduled Monument Consent to create the new Physic Garden from 1987 onwards. It was constructed on a derelict bomb site by the Parks and Gardens Department of the Corporation of London, who manage the garden. The Company wanted to present a broad view of the way in which plants have been used from the earliest times to the present day in the practice of medicine and surgery. It is cared for by the Corporation, and Liveryman Arthur Hollman. The garden is open to the public and is approached from Wood Street via St Giles Church. The Company had no garden from 1666 to 1987 and the present one is its first medicinal or herbal garden.

Plants are the origin of over 30 major medicines (drugs) whose value has been proven by scientifically controlled therapeutic trials and which are used worldwide to day, and the aim of the new Physic Garden was to present a broad view of the way in which plants had been used from the earliest times to the present day, in relation both to the practice of medicine and surgery and to the use of plants in domestic and civic environments. To show the relationship of plant use to the Barber-Surgeons' Company, plants were selected which were especially mentioned by its former Master, the celebrated John Gerard. The plants fall into four main categories:

A. 'Gerard' plants related to surgery, dentistry, wounds and burns: e.g. parsley, spurge, daisy, lady's mantle, comfrey, selfheal, henbane.

B. Plants used traditionally for their pleasant smells, for strewing on the ground, for nosegays, for their use against insects and for dyeing: meadowsweet, chamomile, marjoram, apothecary's rose, lavender, sweet woodruff, cotton lavender, dyer's woodruff.

C. Medicinal plants, now discarded, which were formerly in the official pharmacopoeia: lily of the valley, rhubarb, aconite, pulmonaria (lungwort), valerian.

D. Plants which yield modern pharmaceutical medicines with confirmed efficacy: camellia, sweet clover, meadowsweet, meadow saffron, mandrake, may apple, foxglove, liquorice, yew, Madagascar periwinkle, henbane, feverfew, opium poppy, willow, barley.

In the 13th and 14th centuries the City had important royal, religious and lay residences and most of them had gardens, some of them quite large, such as that of the bishop of Ely with a perimeter of over 600 yards (550 m). These medieval gardens contained fruit trees, vines and herbs for the kitchen or for strewing on the floor. Vegetables were less important because this was an age principally of meat eating but lettuce, spinach, cucumber and cabbage were used for flavouring and sauces. Some gardens also had bee hives, because sugar was a rare commodity. Leisure use was important too and there were fine lawns with flowers such as violets, roses and lilies. However, by the early 1600s the City's population had rapidly increased to 200,000, and the demand for housing led to a considerable loss of gardens. The example of the renewal of this urban Physic Garden has led to others being created, e.g. within the 12th-century town walls of Cowbridge, in the Vale of Glamorgan.

BARTRAM'S BOTANIC GARDEN

PHILADELPHIA

The Pilgrim Fathers explored the local countryside before settling at Plymouth Colony, Massachusetts in 1620, and Edward Winslow noted that onions, leeks, vines, strawberry leaves, sorrel, yarrow, brooklime, watercress, liverwort and flax were growing wild. These and other early American settlers took with them the great 17th-century herbals of Parkinson and Gerard, along with a selection of seeds and rootstocks for nearly all the recommended medicinal herbs. European plants taken to, and cultivated in, America included anise, apple, bedstraw, beet, bloody cranesbill, bugleweed, currant, raspberry, strawberry, carrot, cowslip, cotton lavender, Canterbury bells, creeping bellflower, dandelion, English ivy, fennel, feverfew, cottage pink/dianthus, garlic, gillyflower, heartsease, hop, lavender, leek, lesser periwinkle, lettuce, lily of the valley, meadowsweet, meadow rue, mint, onion, parsley, parsnip, pea, pot marigold, radish, rose, sweet flag, sneezewort, sea holly and Solomon's seal. Ships returned to England with native North American plants to be cultivated in home soil. The properties of many of these plants were learned from the Native Americans, which led to the 1672 publication of John Josselyn's book, *'New England's Rarities Discovered'*. The book included *'The Physical and Chyrurgical Remedies Wherewith the Natives Constantly Use to Cure Their Distempers, Wounds and Sores'*.

In 1728, the Quaker John Bartram (1699–1777) founded North America's first botanic garden near Philadelphia. Bartram travelled extensively in the eastern American colonies collecting plants. Many of his acquisitions were transported to wealthy collectors and gardens in Europe, and in return they supplied him with books and apparatus. From about 1733, Bartram collaborated with the English merchant Peter Collinson, regularly sending *'Bartram's Boxes'* to Collinson every autumn for distribution in England to a wide list of clients. Each box generally contained 100 or more new varieties of seeds, and sometimes also included dried plant specimens and natural history curiosities. Live plants were more difficult and expensive to send, being reserved for Collinson and a few special correspondents. Word of Bartram's collecting quickly spread in Europe, and soon Collinson was acting as Bartram's agent for a variety of other important patrons. These included Philip Miller, who wrote the popular *Gardener's Dictionary*; Sir Hans Sloane, whose collections helped to form the British Museum; Lord Petre, a noted plant collector; the earls of Bute, Leicester and Lincoln; the dukes of Argyle, Richmond, Norfolk, Marlborough and Bedford; Queen Ulrica of Sweden; and Peter Kalm, the Swedish plant explorer and student of Linnaeus.

In 1743 Bartram visited Lake Ontario in the north, describing his expedition in 'Observations on the Inhabitants, Climate, Soil, Rivers, Productions, Animals, and other Matters Worthy of Notice, made by Mr. John Bartram in his Travels from Pennsylvania to Onondaga, Oswego, and the Lake Ontario, in Canada' (London, 1751). During the winter of 1765/6 he visited East Florida in the south, and an account of this trip was published with his journal in London in 1766. He also visited the Ohio River in the west, and in 1765, King George III commissioned him 'Botanizer Royal for America', on a pension of £50 a year. Bartram and his son William are credited with identifying and introducing into cultivation more than 200 American native plants.

Bartram's Garden (46 acres/18.6 ha) is the oldest surviving botanic garden in North America, and includes an historic botanical garden and arboretum (established c.1728), located on the west bank of the Schuylkill River, Philadelphia, Pennsylvania. Three generations of the Bartram family continued to maintain the garden as the premier collection of North American plant species in the world. Bartram's house still stands in the garden, and he was visited by notable figures such as George Washington, Thomas Jefferson and Benjamin Franklin.

Carl Linnaeus (1707–78), the Swedish taxonomist responsible for developing the basis of scientific classification used today and himself a recipient of many Bartram specimens, called Bartram 'the greatest natural botanist in the world'. His death in 1777 was said to be precipitated by the threat to his garden of advancing British troops. In Bartram's Botanic Garden we can still see the following plants listed as being grown by him there:

OLD WORLD PLANTS

Pennyroyal	Spice bush
Agrimony	Clove pink (Carnation)
Peony	St John's wort
Apothecary's rose	Comfrey
Periwinkle	Sweet basil
Bay laurel	Dill
Pomegranate	Sweet flag
Blackberry	English holly
Pot marigold	Sweet woodruff
Borage	Fennel
Rosemary	Tansy
Cassia (Alexandrian senna)	Foxglove
	Thyme
Rue	French tarragon
Catnip	Woodbine honeysuckle
Saffron crocus	Fuller's teasel
Chamomile	Yarrow
Sage	Germander
Chives	Horehound

NEW WORLD PLANTS

Horseradish
Balm of Gilead
Hyssop
Bee balm
Lavender
Black cohosh
Lemon balm
Boneset
Lovage
Dogwood
Lungwort
Great lobelia
Madonna lily
Sassafras
Mint
Wild ginger
Mullein
Wintergreen
Myrtle
Witch hazel

BASIL

OCIMUM BASILICUM
Family Lamiaceae/Labiatae, Mint

OTHER NAMES: Sweet basil, French basil, Genovese basil, common basil, American dittany, our herb, St Joseph's wort, witches' herb, king of herbs, holy basil.

DESCRIPTION: A tender aromatic annual which grows to 18 inches (46 cm) high with a 12 inch (30 cm) spread, the leaves have the stimulating flavour of a cross between anise and mint, but are slightly hotter. There are now about 160 varieties of basil throughout the world. What we call 'wild basil' is also named cushion calamint, and is *Clinopodium vulgare*. It does not smell of basil, but of thyme, and looks more like mint. It was carried in posies to ward off the smells which were thought to carry infection.

PROPERTIES AND USES: Basil is more than just a culinary herb, being used to improve appetite and also taken as a restorative, stimulant and nerve tonic. Like other herbs in the mint family it is carminative and disinfectant. Nicholas Culpeper wrote: *'This is the herb which all authors are together by the ears about, and rail at one another (like lawyers). Galen and Dioscorides hold it not fitting to be taken inwardly; and Chrysippus rails at it with downright Billingsgate rhetoric; but Pliny, and the Arabian physicians,* defend it…an herb of Mars, and under the scorpion, and, perhaps therefore called basilicon, and it is no marvel if it carry a kind of virulent quality with it. Being applied to the place bitten by venomous beasts, or stung by a wasp or hornet, it speedily draws the poison to it. Every like draws its like.' Culpeper adds that if grown in horse-dung, basil will 'breed venomous beasts' and that a French physician who 'by smelling it had a scorpion bred in his brain.' He tells us that basil and rue will not grow together, because 'rue is as great an enemy to poison as any that grows'. He believed that basil 'expels both birth and after-birth'. The fresh picked leaves make a stimulating and refreshing tea. If basil oil is burned while working or reading, it helps one to concentrate and uplifts the mood. It is the basis of pesto sauce, and fresh, torn leaves added to pasta, salad and tomato dishes will aid digestion. Scientific studies have established that compounds in basil oil have potent antioxidant, anticancer, antiviral and anti-microbial properties. Basil essential oil is now used in aromatherapy to alleviate tiredness and depression, and also makes an excellent skin tonic and assists hair growth. It reduces inflammation from insect bites.

HISTORY: Basil has been used to relieve melancholy, fatigue, anxiety and depression, and even as an aphrodisiac, over the centuries. In India, where the herb originated, a basil leaf was placed on the tongue of the dead to assist their passage to heaven. However, the Greeks disliked basil, believing that scorpions would breed under the pots in which it grew. To the ancient Romans, basil was a symbol of hatred, yet later became a token of love in Italy. In Elizabethan times it was used to clear the brain, as a snuff for colds and to cure headaches. Young girls would wear a sprig of basil in their hair to show that they were not engaged, and in Romania if a boy accepted a sprig of basil from a girl, it meant that they were engaged. Basil is said to bring wealth to those people that carry it on their person, and brings good luck to a new home. It has been used to purify and protect, and to guard a person from evil.

Insect Repellent

The juice of the leaves, crushed on the skin, repels mosquitoes, as has been proven by recent scientific studies. The Greek form was placed in pots on tables at mealtimes to repel flies. Place a sweet basil leaf by a window or just outside a kitchen door to repel flies. If they are persistent, crush a leaf to release a stronger aroma. The strong clove scent of sweet basil comes from eugenol, the same chemical as found in cloves. Eugenol has antiseptic properties and kills bacteria.

A Cure For the Bite of a Basilisk

Basil supposedly derives its name from the terrifying basilisk, a half-lizard, half-dragon, fire-breathing creature in Greek mythology with a fatal piercing stare. The wild basil plant was considered to be a magical cure against the look, breath or even the bite of the basilisk when a leaf was medicinally applied. Throughout history, basil was considered a medicinal cure for venomous bites. Because of its hostile status, Greeks and Romans believed that the most potent basil could only be grown if one sowed the seed while ranting and raving. Another source of its name is from *basileus*, the Greek for king, as it was found where St Constantine and Helen found the True Cross.

BAY

LAURUS NOBILIS
Family Lauraceae, Laurel

OTHER NAMES: Sweet bay, true laurel, bay laurel, daphne, Grecian laurel, noble laurel, Roman laurel.

DESCRIPTION: Bay trees grow up to 50–60 feet (15–18 m) high in warm climates. The bay is a perennial glossy evergreen with small yellow flowers followed by black berries.

PROPERTIES AND USES:
The leaves are used to flavour savoury dishes, soups and stews in Mediterranean cuisine, and to aid digestion. They are an essential ingredient of a bouquet garni. An infused oil of bay has been used as a pain reliever for arthritic aches and pains, lower back pain, earaches, and sore muscles and sprains. With analgesic, antiseptic and antispasmodic properties, bay is used for treating dandruff, boosting hair growth, rheumatism, sprains, bruises, ulcers and scabies. Placing a couple of leaves of bay in a storage jar of rice or flour will deter weevils.

HISTORY: Bay was a symbol of both wisdom and glory to the Greeks and Romans, and laurel wreaths were placed on the heads and necks of victorious leaders and athletes. Culpeper wrote: '*The Delphic priestesses are said to have made use of the leaves. That it is a tree of the Sun, and under the celestial sign Leo, and resists witchcraft very potently, as also all the evils old Saturn can do to the body of man, and they are not a few, for it is the speech of one, and I am mistaken if it were not Mizaldus, that neither witch nor devil, thunder nor lightning, will hurt a man in the place where a bay-tree is.*'

Wreath of Bay Leaves

The sun god Apollo was also the god of music, poetry, archery, prophecy and healing. When he tried to seduce the nymph Daphne, she ran away and to protect her her father, the river god Peneus, turned her into a bay tree. Consumed by guilt, Apollo then always wore a wreath of bay leaves on his head. As Apollo was the god of the arts of music and poetry, in medieval times successful students were crowned with a wreath, a '*bacca laurea*' (laurel berry) made from bay leaves. Accepted history is that the important French examination, the Baccalaureate, takes its name from this wreath. However, its etymology may derive from the Latin word '*bachelarius*' (bachelor), referred to a junior knight, and then by extension to the holder of a university degree inferior to that of a Master or Doctor. This was later re-spelled baccalaureus to reflect a false derivation from *bacca laurea*, alluding to the possible laurel crown of a poet, artist or conqueror.

BEET

BETA VULGARIS subsp. *VULGARIS*
Family Amaranthaceae (formerly Chenopodiaceae), Amaranth

OTHER NAMES: Beetroot, garden beet, table beet, blood turnip

DESCRIPTION: All beets, such as sugar beet, spinach beet (leaf beet), chard, mangel-wurzel and beetroot are descended from sea beet, *Beta vulgaris* subsp. *maritima*, which has long fleshy roots and nutritious leaves and grows near the coast. Culpeper also describes the *white beet* in the same entry, which is the white turnip (*Brassica rapa* var. *rapa*).

PROPERTIES AND USES: Culpeper says that the root is '*red, spongy, and is not used to be eaten*'. However, the white beet (white turnip) may be eaten. Romans used beetroot to treat fevers and constipation, with Apicius giving recipes for three soups which include beetroot to be given as a laxative. Hippocrates recommended the use of beet leaves as binding for wounds. Culpeper advocated the 'red beet' to '*stay the bloody diarrhoea, women's menses, and discharges, and to help the yellow jaundice. The juice of the root put into the nostrils purges the head, helps the noise in the ears, and the toothache; the juice stuffed up the nose helps a stinking breath, if the cause lies that way.*' He believed the 'white beet' or turnip to be far more efficacious as it: '*much loosens the belly, and is of a cleansing digesting quality, and provokes urine: the juice of it opens obstructions, both of the liver and spleen, and is good for the headache and swimmings therein, and turnings of the brain; and is effectual also against all venomous creatures; and applied to the temples, stays inflammations in the eyes; it helps burnings, being used without oil, and with a little alum put to it, is good for St. Anthony's fire* [ergot poisoning or erysipelas]. Beetroots are boiled and eaten as a cooked vegetable, or served cold with salads after adding oil and vinegar. Beet soup, borscht, is extremely popular in Eastern Europe. Betanins from the roots are used as red food colorants. For many people, including this author, the consumption of beets causes pink urine.

HISTORY: Beet has been cultivated since the second century BCE, but leafy varieties lost their popularity following the introduction of spinach.

Juicy Aphrodisiac

Beetroot juice boosts stamina and lowers blood pressure. It increases perfusion, or blood flow, to the white matter of the front lobes of the brain, helping fight dementia. Since Roman times, beetroot juice has been considered an aphrodisiac.

BERGAMOT
MONARDA DIDYMA
Family Lamiaceae/Labiatae, Mint

OTHER NAMES: Scarlet mondara, horsebalm, bee balm, crimson beebalm, Oswego tea. Not mentioned in Culpeper, but was brought from the United States in the late 17th century.

DESCRIPTION: This hardy perennial grows 2–3 feet (60–90 cm) in height, with the stems square in cross-section. It has ragged, bright red tubular flowers over an inch (2.5 cm) long, on showy heads of about 30 blossoms, with reddish bracts. Bees love the flowers, earning the herb the name '*bee balm*'.

PROPERTIES AND USES: As with most mints, bee balm is helpful with digestive disorders. It also has excellent antibacterial qualities that make it useful for treating infections. Native Americans such as the Blackfeet and Winnebago recognized its strong antiseptic action, and used poultices of the plant for skin infections and minor wounds. A tea made from the herb was also used to treat mouth and throat infections. Bergamot is the natural source of the antiseptic thymol, the primary active ingredient in commercial mouthwashes. The Winnebago Indians used a tea made from bee balm as a general stimulant, and it was also used as a carminative herb to treat excessive flatulence. The flowers and leaves are excellent ingredients for pot-pourris. The name Oswego tea comes from the Oswego Indians who taught the American colonists how to use it for tea after the Boston Tea Party of 1773.

HISTORY: Its name is derived from its odour which is considered similar to the bergamot orange (*Citrus bergamia*, used to flavour Earl Grey tea). The scientific name comes from Nicolás Monardes (1493–1588) who described the first American flora in 1574. The Spaniard Monardes believed that tobacco smoke was the infallible cure for all ills, and lived to be 95.

WILD BERGAMOT
MONARDA FISTULOSA

This has varied coloured flowers, including purple, lavender, magenta, rose, pink, yellowish pink, whitish and dotted. It is also known as bee balm, like bergamot, and as horsemint. There is a strong fragrance, and it was used by Native Americans to treat colds as it increases mucus flow. It was also used for headaches, burns and warts. Wild bergamot kills bacteria, fungus growth and intestinal worms. Very high in vitamins A and C, it can be eaten in salads or made into tea like *Monarda didyma*.

Slowing Alzheimer's

The US Food and Drug Administration (FDA) approved tacrine hydrochloride (Cognex), a medication derived from bergamot, that seems to slow the progression of Alzheimer's disease by preserving acetylcholine in the brain.

BIRCH TREE

BETULA PENDULA (formerly *ALBA*)
Family Betulaceae, Birch

OTHER NAMES: Silver birch, white birch, weeping birch, European weeping birch, lady of the woods.

DESCRIPTION: The young branches are rich red-brown or orange-brown, and the trunks usually white. The leaves are small, giving a dappled shade effect. Coleridge called it the *'lady of the woods'*. It is noted for its lightness and elegance, and after rain it has a fragrant odour. It is the national tree of Finland.

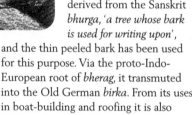

PROPERTIES AND USES: Culpeper tells us: *'It is a tree of Venus, the juice of the leaves, while they are young, or the distilled water of them, or the water that comes from the tree being bored with an auger, and distilled afterwards; any of these being drank for some days together, is available to break the stone in the kidneys and bladder and is good also to wash sore mouths.'* The leaves have an aromatic, agreeable odour and a bitter taste, and have been employed in birch tea as a tonic for sufferers of gout, rheumatism and dropsy. It is also recommended as a reliable solvent of stone in the kidneys. A decoction of leaves has been used for bathing skin problems such as eczema, as the oil is astringent. It is known to keep away insects and prevent gnat bites when smeared on the hands. The wood is soft and not very durable, but is cheap, and the tree is prolific in any situation and soil. It has thus been used for thread bobbins, herring-barrel staves, broom handles and various fancy articles. In country districts the birch has very many uses, the lighter twigs being employed for thatching and wattles. The twigs were also used in broom-making and in the manufacture of cloth.

HISTORY: The word birch is probably anciently derived from the Sanskrit *bhurga*, *'a tree whose bark is used for writing upon'*, and the thin peeled bark has been used for this purpose. Via the proto-Indo-European root of *bherag*, it transmuted into the Old German *birka*. From its uses in boat-building and roofing it is also connected with the Anglo-Saxon *beorgan*, *'to protect or shelter'*. Bunches of birch sticks, or 'fasces', incorporating an axe were used as a symbol by Italian Fascists, supporters of Benito Mussolini.

Fairy Folklore

Birch trees have spiritual importance in many historical religions and are associated with elves in Gaelic folklore. As such, birches frequently appear in Scottish, Irish and English folklore in association with death or fairies, or returning from the grave.

BISHOP'S WEED

AMMI MAJUS
Family Apiaceae, Carrot

OTHER NAMES: Culpeper notes '... *it is usually known by the Greek name, ammi and ammios, some call it Aethiopian cummin-seed, and others Cummin-royal, as also Herb William, and Bulwort.*' Bishop's flower, snow flakes, bullwort, greater ammi, lady's lace, laceflower, Queen of Africa, false Queen Anne's lace (*Daucus carota*, an invasive weed, is known as Queen Anne's lace). Note that in the United States bishop's weed is another name for goutweed, the invasive perennial *Aegopodium podagraria* which is known as ground elder in Britain.

DESCRIPTION: The annual grows to 3–4 feet (90–120 cm), and has feathery dill-like leaves and elegant umbels of white lace-like flowers followed by tiny, hot parsley-like seeds.

PROPERTIES AND USES: Culpeper notes: '*It is hot and dry in the third degree, of a bitter taste, and somewhat sharp withal; it provokes lust to purpose; I suppose Venus owns it. It digests humours, provokes urine and women's menses, dissolves wind, and being taken in wine it eases pain and griping in the bowels, and is good against the biting of serpents; it is used to good effect in those medicines which are given to hinder the poisonous operation of Cantharides upon the passage of the urine; being mixed with honey and applied to black and blue marks coming of blows or bruises, it takes* them away; and being drank or outwardly applied, it abates a high colour, and makes it pale; and the fumes thereof taken with rosin or raisins, cleanses the womb.*'

The plant is used as a diuretic and has antispasmodic properties. It is commonly used as a cardiac tonic for the treatment of angina and palpitations. Medical research labs are testing *Ammi majus*, as it is showing promise in cancer and AIDS therapy. The flowers are used in floristry to add a lacy delicate look to bouquets. However, be careful handling any plants in the genus *Ammi*, as the sap may bring about a skin rash or irritation. Its photoactive compounds can cause blistering to normal skin when exposed to the sun.

HISTORY: The herb originated in the Nile River valley, and in Egypt was used to treat skin diseases. Culpeper noted that it grew wild across England and Wales.

Asthma Treatment

Bishop's weed has traditionally been used in the treatment of wheezing or coughs. The seeds are now used to synthesize the prescription drug sodium cromoglycate (Intal), which is used in inhalers to prevent asthma attacks.

BISTORT

POLYGONUM/PERSICARIA BISTORTA
Family Polygonaceae or Persicaria, Knotweed

OTHER NAMES: Culpeper says *'It is also called Snakeweed, English Serpentary, Dragon-wort, Osterich, and Passions.'* Common bistort, English serpentaria, snakeroot, adderwort, serpentary dragonwort, dracunculus, Easter giant, Easter ledger, Easter ledges, Easter mangiant, gentle dock, great bistort, osterick, oysterloit, passion dock, patient dock, pink pokers, pudding grass, pudding dock, red legs, twice-writhen, water ledges.

DESCRIPTION: Found wild in moist areas, it has an erect pink flower spike and grows to 3 feet (90 cm) tall. *'Bistorta'* means twice-twisted, and refers to the appearance of its snake-like rhizomes. Twice-writhen is a literal translation of the Latin, writhing meaning twisting. The rootstock resembles a letter S, about 2 inches (5 cm) long and 3–5 inches (7.5–13 cm) broad.

PROPERTIES AND USES: The leaves were eaten formerly as a vegetable. It removed inflammation of the eyes. The roots contain much starch, and can be nutritious boiled or made into bread. It is now used for poultices for wounds, as a gargle for oral infections and as a tea for diarrhoea. The name Easter mangiant is a corruption of the French mangeant (eating), signifying that it was a plant to be eaten at Easter, often in a herb pudding. The name passions also has an Easter link.

HISTORY: Culpeper says that a decoction in wine, made from the powder, was drunk freely *'to stay internal bleedings and fluxes'*, being considered *'available against ruptures, burstings and bruises from falls and blows.'* It could also *'help jaundice, expel the venom of the plague, smallpox, measles or other infectious disease, driving it out by sweating.'* A distilled water of the leaves and roots was used to wash any part stung or bitten by a venomous creature, or to wash running sores or ulcers. It was also used as a gargle in sore throats and to harden spongy gums, attended with looseness of teeth and soreness of the mouth. Gerard stated that the root would have this effect, *'being holden in the mouth for a certaine space and at sundry times'*. He also states that *'the juice of Bistort put into the nose prevaileth much against the disease called Polybus [polyps]'*.

Dock Pudding

Bistort leaves are the principal ingredient of dock pudding, formerly a north of England delicacy. Recipes differ, but oatmeal, nettles, onion and seasoning are also used to create this dish. Traditionally the pudding is cooked in a frying pan along with bacon.

BITTERSWEET

SOLANUM DULCAMARA
Family Solanaceae, Nightshade

OTHER NAMES: Culpeper prefers to call it Amara-Dulcis, and says that it is called different names across the land, such as mortal, bitter-sweet, woody nightshade and felon-wort. Felonwood, nightshade, woody nightshade, bittersweet nightshade, bitter nightshade, blue nightshade, fever twig, garden nightshade, nightshade vine, scarlet berry, staff vine, violet bloom. The species name of the bittersweet herb, *dulcamara*, is a reference to the taste of the berries. They initially have a bitter taste and then become unpleasantly sweet as they ripen. In the Middle Ages the name dulcamara was written more properly as Amaradulcis, and literally means bittersweet.

DESCRIPTION: It is a perennial woody vine found in moist areas, among hedges and thickets and the climbing sterns can reach a length of up to 10 feet (3 m). The pinkish-purple, star-shaped flowers with yellow stamens are followed by a green, then deep red, bitter berry that hangs on the vine for months after the leaves have fallen. Bittersweet berries are red, rather than black like those of deadly nightshade.

PROPERTIES AND USES: Herbalists used the root and twig for purifying blood, treating ailments of the liver, pancreas, spleen, glandular organs, piles, jaundice, gout, herpes, bruises, sprains, corns, burns and fever. A weak poison, it is used almost always externally. It is being researched for anticarcinogenic properties.

HISTORY: Gerard wrote: '*The juice is good for those that have fallen from high places, and have been thereby bruised or beaten, for it is thought to dissolve blood congealed or cluttered anywhere in the entrails and to heal the hurt places.*' The herb was used in treating all kinds of sores and swellings, especially to lower the level of inflammation affecting the region around the nails. Its names of felonwood and felonwort do not refer to criminals, but rather to the old name for whitlow, which is inflammation of the toe or finger around the nail. The plant was used to dissolve blood clots (in bruises), for rheumatism, fever and as a restorative. Farmers used it as a charm around the necks of animals they thought to be under the evil eye.

Aiding the Oversexed

The bittersweet was reputed to be an antaphrodisiac, '*beneficial in the reduction of mania accompanied by powerful excitement of the venereal functions; it can depress the libido in oversexed individuals*'. Possibly sex-addiction clinics could be significant customers for this herb.

BLACKBERRY

RUBUS FRUTICOSUS
Family Rosaceae, Rose

OTHER NAMES: Bramble (Culpeper), bly, fingerberry, bumble-kite, bramble-kite, blackbide, moocher, blackbutter, brummel, thimbleberry, brambleberry, brameberry, scaldhead, scaldberry, gouthead.

DESCRIPTION: The blackberry name derives from *brambel,* or *brymbyl*, which means 'prickly'. The Anglo-Saxon name for the blackberry was the bramble-apple. The prickly stems, or brambles, were known as '*lawyers*', as '*once they get their hands into you, it's not easy to get shot of them*'. It grows up to 10 feet (3 m) and comprises a mass of arched thorny stems, which often grow down to the ground to root and form new plants. The white to pink flowers have five petals and are followed by the familiar 'blackberry' fruits.

PROPERTIES AND USES: The leaves have been used for cleaning wounds and for staunching blood flow, are also useful as a tonic and have astringent properties. They have been used to help treat dysentery, diarrhoea and piles, and are an excellent source of tannin, flavonoids and gallic acid. The berries are a good source of vitamin C and are excellent for tea, wine and jam making. Culpeper advised the use of buds, leaves and branches of the blackberry for treating putrid sores in the mouth and throat. Blackberry vinegar has long been a remedy for treating feverish colds. The juicy berries are traditionally made into jam, pies, crumbles, wine and vinegar. The fruit when mordanted (set) with alum gives a slate blue natural dye while the roots yield an orange colour that can be used as a dye for wool and cotton.

HISTORY: The Greek physician Pedanius Dioscorides (*c.*40–90 CE) advocated using the berries when made in to a gargle for treating sore throats and chewing the fresh raw leaves to stop gums bleeding, advice followed by Culpeper. It was believed that the blackberry bush helped to protect the dead from the devil, so they were often found planted on graves to guard the deceased.

Scald Head

The name *scaldhead* comes from the belief that children who ate too many blackberries suffered with a disease of the scalp called scald head. In Robinson's *New Family Herbal* the leaves are boiled in a lye solution for washing a head that is itchy, although it is noted that doing this tended to make the hair go black.

BLACKTHORN OR SLOE

PRUNUS SPINOSA
Family Rosaceae, Rose

OTHER NAMES: Mother of the wood, wishing thorn, wild plum, winter-picks (winter-picks wine used to be drunk instead of port). Culpeper calls it the '*Black-Thorn, or Sloe-Bush.*' (The whitethorn is the hawthorn).

DESCRIPTION: This tree grows to 12 feet (3.7 m) and has small, serrated, oval leaves on dark, thorny branches with creamy-white blooms and purplish-black fruit. The English botanist Willam Withering reported: '*I have repeatedly observed to follow a wound from the thorns, I find reason for believing that there is something poisonous in their nature, particularly in the autumn*', and it seems that stock animals can be easily infected from sloe thorn pricks.

PROPERTIES AND USES: Culpeper tells us: '*The fruit is chiefly used, being restringent and binding, and good for all kind of fluxes and hæmorrhages. It is likewise of service in gargarisms for sore mouths and gums, and to fasten loose teeth. The juice of sloes being boiled to a consistence, is the acacia germanica, of the shops, which is now-a-days made use of instead of the true, and put into all the great compositions…It is the juice of this berry that makes the famous marking ink to write upon linen; it being so strong an acid that no other acid known will discharge it. An handful of the flowers infused, is a safe and easy purge; and taken in wine and water, is excellent to dispel the windy cholic. The bark reduced to power, and taken in doses of two drachms, has cured some agues. The juice expressed from the unripe fruit is a very good remedy for fluxes of the bowels; it may be reduced by a gentle boiling to a solid consistence, in which state it will keep the whole year round.*' The flowers and fruit can make a tonic for diarrhoea, and sloe syrup has antirheumatic properties and can help fight influenza. The plant is also used for nosebleeds, constipation and eye pain. Sloes can also be made into a paste for whitening teeth and removing tartar, and the leaves can make a mouthwash. The thin-fleshed astringent fruits make sloe gin, a red liqueur based on gin or vodka and flavoured with pricked sloe berries. Sugar is required to ensure that the sloe juices are extracted from the fruit. The sharp thorns have been used for centuries as awls. Traditionally the wood was used to make clubs, such as the traditional Irish shillelagh or cudgel. The wood also is used for marquetry and walking sticks.

HISTORY: The berries taste better and not so bitter if harvested after a few frosts. The sloes used to be buried in straw-lined pits for a few months to ripen them and make them sweeter. A Neolithic lake village in Glastonbury was found to have such a pit, full of sloe stones. The word sloe comes from Old English slāh: a similar word is noted in all the Germanic/Slavic languages. The term sloe, or *sla/slāh*, means not the fruit but the hard trunk, being connected with a verb signifying to slay, or strike, probably because the wood of this tree was used as a flail, and now makes a bludgeon. It was believed that Christ's Crown of Thorns was made from blackthorn, and to bring blackthorn blossom into the home meant a certain death would follow. Blackthorn in bloom is considered an emblem of life and death together as the flowers appear when the tree has no leaves. It is said that a hawthorn will destroy any blackthorn near it. It is believed that if the blackthorn and the hawthorn have many berries then the ensuing winter will be severe. In Irish folklore it was believed that '*the little people*' lived in blackthorn bushes. Fairy tribes, called *Lunantishees*, are said

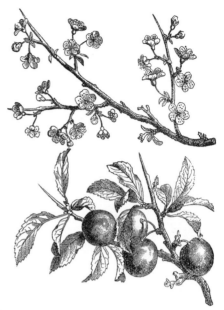

to guard blackthorn trees and will not let you cut branches off it on 11 November or 11 May. If you do you will be cursed with bad luck. It was also bad luck to wear the flowers in your buttonhole.

Blackthorn Winter

On 13 March 2008, 'Geoff F' posted a report on the *Wild about Britain* website: '*Today I noticed some Blackthorn bushes were just starting to flower. Snapes Point, Salcombe Harbour, S. Devon close to the sea. Local tradition is that we will have a touch of cold and unsettled weather with strong easterly winds now; known in this area as the Blackthorn Winter…I did know somebody who would try to shake off the blackthorn flowers at the bottom of his garden in the hope that the weather* would improve then.' On 30 March 2010 *The Times* reported '*only two years ago the Easter weekend in late March was marked by a hefty snowfall that produced a winter wonderland. This cold spell was so common in the past that it used to be called the "blackthorn winter", when ancient folklore described how the blossom of blackthorn bushes appeared during mild weather, only to be destroyed by a cold snap at the end of March.*' Thus the 2008 forecast proved accurate that year.

BLADDERWRACK

FUCUS VESICULOSUS
Family Fucaceae, Brown Algae

OTHER NAMES: Maud Grieve, in *A Modern Herbal* (1931) notes '*Sea-Wrack. Kelp-Ware. Black-Tang. Quercus marina. Cutweed. Bladder Fucus. Fucus (Varech) vesiculeux. Blasentang. Seetang. Meeriche.*' Rockweed, sea oak, black tany, dyers fucus, rock wrack.

DESCRIPTION: The perennial frond or *thallus* is light yellow or brownish-green in colour, from 2 to 3 feet (60–90 cm) in length and attaches itself to rocks by branched, root-like extremities. The air vesicles, or bladders, are about half an inch (13 mm) in diameter and allow this common seaweed to float upright when the sea covers it.

PROPERTIES AND USES: Bladderwrack is commonly found as a component of kelp tablets or powders used as nutritional supplements. It is sometimes loosely called kelp, but that term refers to a different variety, a larger seaweed. The consumption of seaweeds has been associated with lower cancer rates. It is a concentrated source of minerals, including iodine, potassium, magnesium, calcium, and iron. For vegans, seaweeds such as kelp and bladderwrack supply vital vitamin B12, which is otherwise found almost exclusively in animal products. Bladderwrack is used as an additive and flavouring in various food products in Europe.

HISTORY: Dried bladderwrack, *Fucus vesiculosus*, was the original source of iodine, being discovered as such by French chemist Bernard Courtois in 1812. It thus assists in the production of thyroid hormones, which are necessary for maintaining healthy

---

Welshman's Caviar

There are many edible seaweeds; red, green and brown algae have featured in Japanese, Chinese and Korean diets since prehistoric times. *Sushi* is wrapped in *nori* seaweed, and a similar type of seaweed, *laver*, has been traditionally used in northern Europe for centuries. Laver is unique among seaweeds, being only one cell thick, and it still popular in Wales in the form of '*laverbread*', described by the actor Richard Burton as '*the Welshman's caviar*'. Laver has many uses in traditional and modern cuisine, and the delicious laverbread is made by being cleansed in fresh water (to get rid of any sand), boiled and puréed. It is then often rolled in oatmeal to make small cakes, fried in bacon fat and served with bacon and cockles to make a gourmet's breakfast.

Shoreline Sheep

The semi-feral North Ronaldsay sheep exists on the northernmost of the Orkney Islands in Scotland, an area of just 2.7 square miles (7 km²). Along with the Shetland sheep, it is the only survivor of a type of short-tailed sheep formerly found across the islands of Orkney and Shetland. They are most notable for living almost entirely on seaweed for several months of the year, except for a short lambing season. This is the only food source available to them, as they are confined to the shoreline by a high dry-stone wall which encloses the whole island. The wall was built to preserve the limited grazing inland. The sheep have evolved a somewhat different physiology from other sheep, and their digestive system has adapted to extract the sugars in seaweeds more efficiently. Also, instead of grazing during the day and ruminating at night as other sheep do, North Ronaldsays graze as the tide reveals the shore (twice in 24 hours), and ruminate on the thin strip of shoreline left at high water. The sheep's source of fresh water is limited to the few freshwater lakes and ponds along the seashore.

metabolism in all cells of the body. This increases the rate at which the body uses energy and, as a consequence, decreases fat deposits. Both kelp and bladderwrack can stimulate weight loss when used as part of a low-calorie diet. In 1862 Dr Godfroy Duchesne-Duparc found, while experimenting with bladderwrack in cases of chronic psoriasis, that weight was reduced without injuring health, and used the drug with success. He experimented on himself, losing 5¼ pounds (2.4 kg) in a week, after taking a bladderwrack extract made into pills before his three meals a day. It was used extensively to treat goitre, a swelling of the thyroid gland related to iodine efficiency. Maud Grieve (1858–1941) recommended bladderwrack for rheumatism (as a liniment), for arthritis inflammation (as a poultice), but its main herbal use is now to 'remineralize' the body. Bladderwrack has been a source of valuable manure for potatoes and other crops, being gathered for this purpose all along European coastlines. Fresh seaweed contains 20–40 pounds (9 to 18 kg) of potash to the ton, and dried seaweed 60–230 pounds (27–104 kg), so its collection and use were recommended to farmers when the Second World War caused a shortage of artificial fertilizers. It may be spread on the land and left for some time before ploughing in, but should not be left in heaps, as rotting liberates the potash which may thus be wasted. All seaweed may be dried and burnt to ashes, then sprinkled on the ground as 'kelp'. Kelp-burning was a major source of iodine, but a cheaper process of obtaining it from the purification of Chile saltpetre destroyed the industry. Kelp was also used as a source of impure carbonate of soda, containing sulphate and chloride of sodium and a little charcoal, for soap and glass manufacture. It use was rendered obsolete by the process of obtaining carbonate of soda more cheaply from common salt.

BLUEBELL

HYACINTHOIDES NON-SCRIPTA
Family Hyacinthaceae, formerly Roseaceae, Rose

OTHER NAMES: Culpeper calls it the jacinth, or wild hyacinth. Nodding squill, common bluebell, auld man's bell, calverkeys, culverkeys, English bluebell, ring-o'-bells, wood bells.

DESCRIPTION: The flowers are lavender-blue, pendulous, tubular with the petals recurved only at the end, and borne on one side of the flowering stem only. The flower stem bends over at the top. Note that the bluebell of Scotland is a different plant, what we call the harebell elsewhere, *Campanula rotundifolia*.

PROPERTIES AND USES: Culpeper: '*It abounds in a slimy juice, but it is to be dried, and this must be done carefully; the decoction of it operates well by urine, and the powder is balsamic, and somewhat styptic. It is not enough known: there is hardly a more powerful remedy for the whites* [discharges or leucorrhoea].' The bulbs of bluebells are poisonous in the fresh state and have diuretic and styptic properties. The abundant mucilage (gluey substance produced by most plants) was used as a substitute for starch when stiff ruffs were worn. It was also used for fixing feathers onto the shafts of arrows, instead of glue, and as bookbinders' gum for the covers of books.

HISTORY: The *non-scripta* or *non-scriptum* part of the botanical name means 'unlettered' or 'unmarked', to distinguish it from the classical hyacinth of Greek mythology. Tennyson speaks of bluebell juice being used to cure snake-bite. To the 19th century Romantic poets the bluebell symbolized solitude and regret.

Spanish Invasion in the Woods

In spring bluebells cover woodland floors and are often used as an indicator species to identify ancient woodlands. It is estimated that 70 per cent of all common bluebells are found in Great Britain. However, there has been extensive hybridization with the recently introduced, and more vigorous, Spanish bluebell, *Hyacinthoides hispanica*. As the hybrids can thrive in a wider range of environmental conditions, they are frequently outcompeting native bluebells. The easiest ways to identify the Spanish bluebell or one of its offspring are that the stems are upright and not nodding, and the flowers are borne on more than one side of the flowering stem. Real bluebell woods have a remarkable fragrance, whereas the scent of other bluebells is less strong and less sweet.

BONESET

EUPATORIUM PERFOLIATUM
Family Asteraceae, Daisy

OTHER NAMES: Common boneset, thoroughwort, agueweed, crosswort, feverwort, Indian sage, sweating plant, vegetable antimony, wood boneset.

DESCRIPTION: Common in North America, it was not known by Culpeper. It grows around 2–4 feet (60–120 cm) tall and has large leaves and a white flower head. The leaves distinguish the species, and the stems appear to pierce, or go through, the leaf. The words *through* and *thorough* used to be interchangeable, so the name *thoroughwort* alludes to this distinction. (We see the same thing happening in the word *thoroughfare* today.)

PROPERTIES AND USES: Grieve and others tell us it is a stimulant, febrifuge and laxative, acting slowly and persistently, with its greatest effect in illnesses of the stomach, liver, bowels and uterus. In large doses it is emetic and purgative. In moderate doses it was regarded as a mild tonic, and was also used as a diaphoretic, especially when taken as a warm infusion, for attacks of muscular rheumatism and general cold. As a remedy in catarrh and in influenza, it was extensively used, given in doses of a warm wineglassful every half hour, the patient remaining in bed. After four or five doses, heavy perspiration occurred and relief was obtained. Boneset stimulates resistance to viral and bacterial infections, and reduces fever by encouraging sweating. It also acts as an expectorant for catarrh.

This species of *Eupatorium* was also employed in cutaneous diseases, and in the expulsion of tapeworms from the gut.

HISTORY: The plant was a favourite medicine of Native North Americans, who called it ague weed. Some writers described it as a diuretic, useful in dropsy, but this property was possessed by the purple-flowered *Eupatorium purpureum*, known as gravel root or Joe Pye weed, named after a famous Native American 'medicine man' who used to cure typhus.

Break Bone Fever

Native North Americans used boneset to cause profuse perspiration and to treat fevers associated with a number of illnesses. They introduced the use of boneset leaves and flowering tops to the early settlers for the treatment of colds, catarrh, influenza, rheumatism, and all kinds of fevers, including *break bone fever* (dengue), *intermittent fever* (malaria), and *lake fever* (typhoid). The pain of dengue fever feels like one has broken bones, and it is from this association that boneset gets its name, not from any capacity to mend broken bones.

BORAGE

BORAGO OFFICINALIS
Family Boraginaceae, Borage

OTHER NAMES: Star flower, starflower, beeplant (bees love it), talewort, cool tankard, bugloss, burrage, llawenlys (Welsh, meaning herb of gladness), tafod y fuwch or tafor yr ych (Welsh, meaning buck's tongue or ox tongue), bronwerth (Welsh, meaning breastherb).

DESCRIPTION: Pretty flowering herb with blue star-shaped flowers, around 2–3 feet (60–90 cm) in height and spread. The leaves are covered in bristly hairs and may cause dermatitis. The brilliant blue colour of the petals is believed to have been the inspiration for the colour of the Madonna's robes in many Renaissance paintings, in which the expensive pigment ultramarine was used.

PROPERTIES AND USES: The young leaves, which taste faintly of cucumber, and flowers can be used in salads and the flowers in drinks. An infusion of the leaves was said to aid kidney function and help with feverish catarrh. It is diuretic, demulcent and emollient, and externally it can be used as a poultice to reduce inflammation. Culpeper: *'They are all three* [borage species] *herbs of Jupiter, and under Leo, all great cordials and strengtheners of nature. The leaves or roots are to very good purpose used in putrid and pestilential fevers, to defend the heart, and help to resist and expel the poison or the venom of other creatures: the seed is of the like effect; and the seed and leaves are good to increase milk in women's breasts:*

Saucy Ingredient

Borage is one of the main ingredients of the superb Hessian green sauce popular in Frankfurt am Main, along with hard-boiled eggs, oil, vinegar, salt and six other herbs – sorrel, cress, chervil, chives, parsley and salad burnet. Green sauce is a popular accompaniment to many local dishes in the *apfelwein* house (cider pub) which I used to frequent, Adolf's in Sachsenhausen, Frankfurt, Germany.

Adolf Wagner's wine-press hall is full of wooden benches and serves a traditional appetiser or snack with *apfelwein* (apple wine = cider), called *'Handkäse mit Musik'* (Handmade Cheese with Music). The small cheese is topped with chopped pickled onions, and its unusual name comes from the idea that one makes music via flatulence from eating onions. It is delicious, as is the *apfelwein*.

the leaves, flowers, and seed, all or any of them, are good to expel pensiveness and melancholy; to clarify the blood, and mitigate heat in fevers.' According to Gerard and Culpeper, borage and bugloss *(Anchusa arvensis)* could be used interchangeably. As a companion plant to tomatoes, it is believed that it deters tomato worm, but borage is highly attractive to blackfly. However, this can be turned to advantage by planting it as a decoy close to fruit and vegetables, to prevent them from being blighted by pests.

HISTORY: The name *burrage* seems to come from the Gaelic *borrach*, meaning 'courage'. Others believe that its name is derived from the French *bourrache*, which means 'hairy' or 'rough'. The Welsh name 'buck's tongue' indicates the roughness of the leaves. Historically it was considered a plant that would raise the spirits and drive away melancholy. According to Dioscorides, borage can *'cheer the heart and lift the depressed spirits.'* Both Dioscorides and Pliny thought that borage was the famous *'Nepenthe'* of Homer's

Odyssey which, when drunk steeped in wine, brought absolute forgetfulness. Nepenthe, however, may have been a blend of wine and either mint or opium. Borage was given to young Roman soldiers for courage and comfort, and borage flowers were floated in stirrup cups to give to Crusaders. Gerard repeated the claim of Pliny *'Ego borago gaudia simper ago'* – *'I, borage, always bring courage'*. Gerard wrote that its flowers were used in salads *'to exhilarate and make the minde glad'* while cooks used them *'for the comfort of the heart, to drive away sorrow, and increase the joy of the minde'*. An old English saying is: *'To enliven the sad with a joy of a joke, / Give the wine with the borage put in to soak.'* Bacon told us *'The leaf of burrage hath an excellent spirit to repress the fuliginous vapour of dusky melancholia'* and Salmon wrote that *'Borage is one of the four cordial flowers; it comforts the heart, cheers melancholy, and recovers the fainting spirits'*. The leaves and flowers were originally used in Pimms before it was replaced by mint, but the flowers still make a pretty ingredient.

Symbol of Hope

Borage seed oil has the highest concentration of gamma linolenic acid (GLA) naturally found, twice that of the *evening primrose*, which is used to treat pre-menstrual syndrome (PMS). GLA is an omega-6 polyunsaturated fatty acid, which is active against various cancers, including breast, brain and prostate. It prevents the spread of malignant tumours by restricting blood vessel growth. For these reasons, borage has been adopted as the symbol of National Cancer Day, as promoted by Cancer Research UK. Borage seed oil *(starflower oil)* is known to be very beneficial for skin disorders such as psoriasis and eczema, and sun-damaged or ageing skin.

BOUQUET GARNI

This 'garnished bouquet' is a bundle of herbs tied together with string or wrapped in a muslin or cheesecloth bag, used to prepare soup, stock and casseroles. There is no generic recipe, but most formulations include bruised bay leaves, thyme and parsley or marjoram. Depending on the recipe, the bouquet garni can include a combination of basil, burnet, celeriac, chervil, coriander seeds, garlic, lemon zest, lime zest, marjoram, orange peel, peppercorns, rosemary, savory and tarragon. Vegetables such as carrot, celery (leaves or stem), celeriac, leek, onion and parsley root can also be included. The choice of ingredients is often dependent upon what is at hand and in season. If sage is added, use only a small piece as it could swamp the other flavours. An interesting twist to add flavour is to use a strip of cleaned leek leaf to tie the ingredients together. The bouquet should be left in the pot for at least two hours from the start of cooking, and be removed prior to consumption. (Also see the entry on *Fines Herbes* and *Herbes de Provence*.)

A simple basic recipe for dried ingredients, if one is using a muslin bag in cooking, is to combine ¼ cup dried parsley, 2 tablespoons dried thyme, 2 tablespoons dried bay leaf and 2 tablespoons dried rosemary. The mixture can be placed in an airtight container, and stored in a cool, dark place for up to six months.

If using fresh ingredients, tie together a bunch of parsley, 3 sprigs of thyme, a peeled clove of garlic and 2–3 bay leaves, using a long piece of string so that you can easily remove the bouquet. Another simple recipe using fresh and dried ingredients is 2 sprigs fresh thyme, 2 dried bay leaves, leafy greens from 2 celery stalks and 6 sprigs fresh parsley. Many chefs prefer the herbs to be tied with string rather than be in a muslin bag, for better flavour.

Some cookery writers divide the ingredients into *liaison* herbs, *mild* herbs, *robust* herbs and other flavours like this:

Liaison herbs: 1 cup parsley and ½ cup chives.
Mild herbs: 1 cup total – basil, coriander leaves, lemon thyme, marjoram.
Robust herbs: ½ cup total – oregano, sage, thyme, winter savory, rosemary, spearmint.

Other flavours: ¼ cup total – herbal seeds, spices, garlic, onion, citrus peel. You can choose as many ingredients as you wish from each category, removing woody stems and experimenting with your own favourite flavouring for different dishes. Chop or food process the ingredients, and use immediately. Alternatively, coat the herbs with extra virgin olive oil and store in an airtight container in a refrigerator.

BROOM

CYTISUS SCOPARIUS
Family Fabaceae/Leguminosae, Pea

OTHER NAMES: Besom, bizzon, brum, Irish tops, common broom, Scotch broom, green broom, butcher's broom, Jew's myrtle, sweet broom.

DESCRIPTION: A perennial, leguminous shrub growing to 9 feet (2.75 m) tall with thin stems, covered with profuse golden-yellow flowers which turn into black seedpods.

PROPERTIES AND USES: Broom buds were a delicacy and an appetizer, being served at the Coronation feast of King James II. The blossoms were used for making a salve to cure gout, and King Henry VIII drank flower-water to counteract 'surfeit' – excessive eating and drinking. Gerard tells us: *'The decoction of the twigs and tops of Broom doth cleanse and open the liver, milt* [spleen] *and kidneys.'* Culpeper considered its decoction to be good for dropsy, *'black jaundice* [Weil's disease]*'*, ague, gout, sciatica and various pains of the hips and joints.

HISTORY: The names of besom and broom refer to its use in the making of brushes from the earliest times. Its medicinal use under the name *Genista*, is mentioned in the *Herbarius Latinus* of 1485, the *Hortus Sanitatis* of 1491, the *Grete Herball* of 1516, and the *London Pharmacopeia* of 1618 It was used in Anglo-Saxon medicine, and the 13th century Physicians of Myddfai in Wales recommended a mixture of broom tops and boys' urine to cure pain caused by a thorn. They said that *'The fat of a wild cat is also good.'*

Heraldic Broom

Geoffrey of Anjou (1113–51) thrust a sprig of broom flowers into his helmet before a battle, that his troops might see and follow him. The Latin name for the plant was *planta genista* [greenweed plant], and it became the heraldic symbol of Geoffrey. He married a daughter of Henry I, and their son Henry II was the first of the 'Plantagenet kings' of England, a dynasty that lasted from 1154 to 1485. A representation of the plant may be seen on the Great Seal of Richard I (1157–99).

(WHITE) BRYONY

BRYONIA ALBA
Family Cucurbitaceae, Cucumber

OTHER NAMES: Briony, devil's turnip, navet du diable (devil's turnip also in France), English mandrake, wild vine, wood vine, white vine, wild hops, wild nep (wild parsnip), ladies' seal, tetterbury.

DESCRIPTION: The single representative of the cucumber family native to Britain, with small greenish-white flowers, its tendrils help a single plant to spread and cover over several yards of hedgerow. Culpeper also notes the black bryony or black vine having the same uses, but this is a plant in another family, *Dioscorea communis*, one of the Dioscoreaceae, or yam family.

PROPERTIES AND USES: Culpeper says it is a *'furious martial plant'*, but good for many complaints such as *'stitches in the side, palsies, cramps, convulsions…The root cleanseth the skin wonderfully from all black and blue spots, freckles, morphew, leprosy, foul scars, or other deformity whatsoever: as also all running scabs and manginess.'* The root is acrid and cathartic and the berries poisonous. The root was given for dropsy, sciatica, rheumatism, lumbago, gout, pleurisy, influenza, bronchitis and whooping cough. If applied to the skin, the root produces redness and even blisters. Withering noted that a decoction made by boiling one pound of the fresh root in water is *'the best purge for horned cattle'*.

HISTORY: Bartholomew's *Anglicus* tells us that Augustus Caesar wore wear a wreath of bryony during a thunderstorm to protect himself from lightning. The nauseous and bitter root juice was prescribed by Galen and Dioscorides as a violent purgative. Called wild nep, it was valued in the 14th century as an antidote to leprosy.

Moulded into 'Mandrakes'

The root used to be seen suspended in herb shops, sometimes trimmed into a rude human form. In Green's *Universal Herbal* of 1832 we read: *'The roots of Bryony grow to a vast size and have been formerly by imposters brought into a human shape, carried about the country and shown for Mandrakes to the common people. The method which these knaves practised was to open the earth round a young, thriving Bryony plant, being careful not to disturb the lower fibres of the root; to fix a mould, such as is used by those who make plaster figures, close to the root, and then to fill in the earth about the root, leaving it to grow to the shape of the mould, which is effected in one summer.'*

BUGLE

AJUGA REPTANS
Family Lamiaceae/Labiatae, Mint

OTHER NAMES: Bugleweed, blue bugle, bugleherb, creeping bugleweed, creeping carpet bugle, carpetweed, middle comfrey, middle consound, brown bugle, common bugle, sicklewort (as is a woundwort), herb carpenter, carpenter's herb, thunder and lightning.

DESCRIPTION: This common perennial is found in damp woods and grassy pastures. It is a low-growing plant on creeping runners with stems up to 6 inches (15 cm) in length. Purplish-blue flowers appear above its rosettes of leaves, and creeping runners produce more leafy rosettes so that the whole plant eventually forms a carpet-like mat, often used as a ground cover. The species name of the bugle, *reptans*, alludes to the snake-like creeping runners, which make it a nuisance in lawns.

PROPERTIES AND USES:
Culpeper says that the similar white bugle *(Ajuga reptans alba)* has the same properties, and there is also a pink variety. Remedies made from bugle have been used for treating persistent coughs, ulcers, rheumatism and all kinds of liver disorders. In its action, it resembles digitalis, lowering the pulse and equalizing the circulation, being called *'one of the mildest and best narcotics in the world'* (Green's *Universal Herbal* 1832). Culpeper is enthusiastic about many medicinal uses, such as a wash *'for such ulcers and sores as happen in the secret parts of men or women'*.

HISTORY: Bugle was used by Charles V of Spain to cure his gout in the 15th century. It is called *carpenter's herb* as it can staunch bleeding and possibly heal cuts, because of its tannin content. Herbalists used bugle remedies to stop internal bleeding in the lungs as well as to staunch other kinds of internal haemorrhaging. In addition, bugle has also been used to prevent hallucinations following the consumption of excessive amounts of alcohol. Bugle is also seen by some herbalists as possessing mildly · narcotic and sedative effects and its use is believed to possibly have a lowering effect on the heart rate similar to the action of the foxglove *(Digitalis)*.

Relieving Pain

Recent research seems to support bugle's use in hyperthyroid conditions and to ease breast pain (mastodynia). The lithospermic acid in bugleweed is believed to decrease levels of certain hormones, especially the thyroid hormone thyroxine, and also keeps antibodies from binding to and 'burning out' cells in an overactive thyroid gland. By moderating oestrogen levels, bugleweed possibly relieves breast pain. Bugle's nerve-calming action makes it useful in pain relief for those with sensitivities to salicylates such as aspirin.

BURDOCK

ARCTIUM LAPPA formerly *LAPPA MAJOR*
Family Asteraceae/Compositae, Sunflower

OTHER NAMES: Greater burdock, edible burdock, great burdoak, thorny burr, beggar's buttons, sticky bobs, love leaves, turkey burrseed, hardock, hare burr, cockle buttons, fox's clote. Culpeper calls it also '*Personata, Bardona, Lappa Major, Great Burdock and Clotbur*'. Happy-major is a folk-name derived from *Lappa major.*

DESCRIPTION: The light-brown sturdy taproot may weigh up to 2–4 pounds (0.9–1.8kg). It is a large-leaved hardy biennial that grows to 7 feet (2.1 m), with thistle-like purple flowers and many hooked seed-bearing burrs. *Lappa* means burr. Its leaves are like those of dock, thus the name *burr-dock*, burdock.

PROPERTIES AND USES: Culpeper recommends it for many illnesses, e.g.: '*the juice of the leaves, or rather the roots themselves, given to drink with old wine, doth wonderfully help the bitings of serpents: and the root beaten with a little salt, and laid on the place, suddenly eases the pain thereof, and helps those that are bit by a mad dog: the juice of the leaves, taken with honey, provokes urine, and remedies the pain of the bladder: the seed being drunk in wine forty days together, doth wonderfully help the sciatica…*' Burdock leaves were recommended to relieve sores, and the juice soothed burns and was an antidote to snakebite. A decoction of the roots or leaves was a blood purifier and helpful for skin problems. It will help with constipation, liver problems and balances the helpful bacteria in the bowel. It enhances immunity, reduces fluid retention and is anti-inflammatory. Burdock roots and leaves can also be used to treat rheumatism and gout because they encourage the elimination of uric acid via the kidneys. Burdock root oil extract *(Bur oil)* has traditionally been

---

Burry Man

Since at least 1687 a man has dressed himself from head to toe in burrs, and paraded the streets of South Queensferry in Scotland, being rewarded for his pains with tots of whisky drunk through a straw in local pubs. During August's 'Ferry Fair', the '*Burry Man*' dresses in a full body costume made of flannel, then completely covers himself with the hooked fruits of *Arctium lappa* and *Arctium minus* (wood burdock), the greater and lesser burdock. After nine or so hours of slow walking, in a heavy costume, this spirit of vegetation and fertility will have had a considerable amount to drink and will be truly exhausted.

popular in Europe as a scalp treatment applied to improve hair strength, shine and body, and to combat hair loss. Indeed, modern studies indicate that burdock root oil extract is rich in phytosterols and essential fatty acids required for healthy scalp and natural hair growth. The root of burdock contains up to 45 per cent insulin, a non-nutritious fibre. The insulin makes burdock valuable in treating diabetes, because the insulin grabs sugars from the digestive tract, which prevents the sugar from entering the bloodstream. Roots can be roasted and young shoots peeled and eaten raw or used in soups. Rich in minerals, this plant has been used as a food by many cultures.

HISTORY: North American herbalists particularly valued the seeds to treat skin problems, while in China the seeds are used to treat measles, sore throats, tonsillitis, colds, and flu. Burdock was considered to be sacred by the Celts and the Germanic peoples held it sacred to the god Thor. Since Thor reigned over the summer storms, the plant was gathered in midsummer. It was placed on the gables of buildings to protect against lightning. In the late Middle Ages burdock was still being strung over doors or braided into hair to ward off evil. Burdock has an ancient reputation as a nutritive liver tonic that helps to clean and build the blood, while its diuretic action helps in the elimination of toxins. Taken internally, this root promotes sweating and urination. In the second half of the 20th century, burdock achieved recognition for its culinary use, owing to the increasing popularity of macrobiotic diets which advocate its consumption.

Inventing Velcro

After an Alpine walk in 1941, a Swiss engineer noticed burdock burrs attached to his clothes and his dog's fur. Under a microscope, George de Mestral looked closely at the hook-and-loop system that the seeds use to hitchhike on passing animals, aiding seed dispersal. He realized that the same approach could be used to join other things together, and the resulting invention was *Velcro*, named after the French words *velour* (a plush knitted fabric) and *crochet* (hook).

The hundreds of 'hooks' on each burr catch on anything with a loop, such as clothing or animal fur. Developing the idea, he discovered that cotton wore out quickly on his prototypes, so de Mestral turned his attention to synthetic fibres, settling on the newly invented nylon as an ideal material. An American article dated 1958 reads: '*A "zipperless zipper" has been invented – finally. The new fastening device is in many ways potentially more revolutionary than was the zipper a quarter century ago.*'

BUTCHER'S BROOM

RUSCUS ACULEATUS
Family Ruscaceae (formerly Liliaceae), Ruscus

OTHER NAMES: Kneeholy, knee holly, kneeholm, kneehulver (hulver is an old name for holly), Jew's myrtle, sweet broom, pettigree, bruscus.

DESCRIPTION: There is no similar British plant. Its tough, erect stems have no bark, but very rigid leaves, each terminating in a single sharp spine. There are small greenish-white flowers.

PROPERTIES AND USES: According to Culpeper, *'It is a plant of Mars, being of a gallant cleansing and opening quality: the decoction of the roots, made with wine, opens obstructions, provokes urine, helps to expel gravel, and the stone, the stranguary, and women's courses, as also the yellow jaundice, and the head-ache; and, with some honey or sugar put therein cleanses the breast of phlegm, and the chest of much clammy humours gathered therein; the decoction of the root drunk, and a poultice made of the berries and leaves being applied, are effectual in knitting and consolidating broken bones, or parts out of joint. The common way of using it, is to boil the root of it and parsley, and fennel, and smallage, in white wine, and drink the decoction, adding the like quantity of grass roots to them; the more of the roots you boil, the stronger will the decoction be…'* A decoction was commonly used for jaundice and gravel stones. Sweetened with honey, it was said to clear the chest of phlegm and relieve difficult breathing.

HISTORY: The plant was recommended by Dioscorides and others as an aperient and diuretic in cases of dropsy, urinary obstructions and nephritis. Parkinson related that butcher's broom was used to preserve *'hanged meate'* from being eaten by mice, and also for the making of brooms, *'but the King's Chamber is by revolution of time turned to the Butcher's stall, for that a bundle of the stalkes tied together serveth them to cleanse their stalls and from thence have we our English name of Butcher's broom.'* The matured branches were bound into bundles and sold to butchers for sweeping their blocks, hence the name. Research has shown that the plant enhances blood flow to the brain, hands and legs. It improves circulation, and relieves constipation and water retention. It is used to treat varicose veins and haemorrhoids, as it tightens blood vessels and capillaries.

Knee Holly

Butcher's broom was also called 'knee holly' because it rises to about the height of a man's knee and from its having prickly evergreen leaves. Its other name 'Jew's myrtle' occurred because it was used for service during the Feast of Tabernacles.

BUTTERBUR

PETASITES VULGARIS (syn. *HYBRIDUS* or *OFFICINALIS*)
Family Asteraceae/Compositae, Sunflower

OTHER NAMES: Common butterwort, langwort, umbrella plant, bog rhubarb, flapperdock, blatterdock, capdockin, bogshorns, butter-dock, pestilence wort, plague flower, devil's hat.

DESCRIPTION: A herbaceous perennial with pale pink inflorescenses, before the leaves appear. The leaves are round with a diameter of up to 27 inches (69 cm), borne on stout tall stems up to 4 feet (1.2 m) high.

PROPERTIES AND USES:
Culpeper was certain '*that this root, beyond all things else cures pestilential fevers, and is by long experience found to be very available against the plague, by provoking sweat; if the powder thereof, be taken in wine, it also resists the force of any other poison…away all spots and blemishes of the skin It is a great strengthener of the heart and cheerer of the vital spirits…the decoction of the root in wine is singularly good for those that wheeze much or are short-winded…The powder of the root takes.*' The root has been used traditionally since the Middle Ages, and in North America during colonial times as a heart stimulant, acting as a cardiac tonic and also as a diuretic, to treat fevers, wheezing and colds. Modern research supports the opinion that butterbur root extract is effective for treatment of seasonal allergies, asthma and migraines. In Germany, butterbur extract is approved for the treatment of spasmodic urinary pain, particularly when there are stones present. Butterbur is thought to work by reducing spasms in muscle tissues, including blood vessels.

HISTORY: '*The name of the genus, Petasites, is derived from the Greek word for the felt hats worn by shepherds, like that of depictions of Mercury, in reference to the large leaves of the plant which block out light and air and prevent other plants from growing*' (Maud Grieve, *Modern Herbal* 1931). Henry Lyte, in his *Herbal* of 1578, calls it '*a sovereigne medicine against the plague*', and remarks of its leaves that '*one of them is large enough to cover a small table, as with a carpet*'. Gerard recommends its use '*against the plague and pestilent fevers, because it provokes sweat and drives from the heart all venom and evil heat; it kills worms. The powder of the roots cures all naughty filthy ulcers, if it be strewed therein.*'

Plague Flower

The name butterbur comes from the old practice of wrapping up butter in the large leaves of this herb during warm weather. It was called *plague flower* in old herbals, because of its value as a remedy in times of disaster.

CABBAGES and COLEWORTS

BRASSICA OLERACEA
Family Brassicaceae/Cruciferae, Cabbage or Mustard

OTHER NAMES: Sea cabbage, wild mustard, wild cabbage – its descendants include garden cabbages, broccoli, sprouts, seakale, kale and cauliflower. It is unsure which varieties Culpeper is describing. Colewort is now used to describe a cabbage which does not form a compact head.

DESCRIPTION: The wild plant, *Brassica oleracea* var. *oleracea*, called colewort or field cabbage, has a group of basal leaves (a basal 'rosette') and an open stalk (panicle) of flowers.

PROPERTIES AND USES: Culpeper tells us: 'The Cabbages or Coleworts boiled gently in broth, and eaten, do open the body, but the second decoction doth bind the body. The juice thereof drank in wine, helps those that are bitten by an adder, and the decoction of the flowers brings down women's courses. Being taken with honey, it recovers hoarseness, or loss of the voice…The often eating of them well boiled, helps those that are entering into a consumption. The pulp of the middle ribs of Coleworts boiled in almond milk, and made up into an electuary with honey, being taken often, is very profitable for those that are puffy and short winded. Being boiled twice, an old cock boiled in the broth and drank, it helps the pains and the obstructions of the liver and spleen, and the stone in the kidneys …*

The juice boiled with honey, and dropped into the corner of the eyes, clears the sight, by consuming any film or clouds beginning to dim it; it also consumes the cankers growing therein. They are much commended, being eaten before meat to keep one from surfeiting, as also from being drunk with too much wine, or quickly to make a man sober again that was drunk before… The decoction of Coleworts takes away the pain and ache, and allays the swelling of sores and gouty legs and knees, wherein many gross and watery humours are fallen, the place being bathed therewith warm. It helps also old and filthy sores, being bathed therewith, and heals all small scabs, pushes, and wheals, that break out in the

A Family of Cabbages

The 1935 Triangle of U theory about the evolution of relationships within the cabbage family has been proved recently. Three separate ancestral species of Brassica – *Brassica rapa* (turnip, Chinese cabbage); *Brassica nigra* (black mustard); and *Brassica oleracea* (cabbage) – combined to create the three new separate species known as Indian mustard; Ethiopian mustard; and rapeseed and rutabaga.

Varieties Developed Include:

Cabbage (*Brassica oleracea* var. *capitata*) was developed by the 12th century. It has a large head on a stout stem. Fleshy leaves are folded into a head, or leaves are somewhat open. There are now more than 200 cultivars of cabbage.

Kohlrabi or 'cabbage turnip' (var. *caulorapa*) in its primitive form was used in Charlemagne's gardens. It is now widely used as animal fodder, being nutritious and easily stored.

Kale and collards (var. *acephala*) were developed for their leaves.

Broccoli (var. *botrytis*, formerly var. *italica*) has edible stems and flower buds, and was favoured by Romans.

Cauliflower (var. *botrytis*) We eat the white inflorescence, which lacks chlorophyll. There is a condensed, much branched thickened stem supporting tightly closed flower buds, developed in Italy from broccoli before the 1600s.

Brussel sprouts (var. *gemmifera*). The plants that have a main stem on which the axillary buds develop into small, edible heads (like baby cabbages).

skin. *The ashes of Colewort stalks mixed with old hog's-grease, are very effectual to anoint the sides of those that have had long pains therein, or any other place pained with melancholy and windy humours… this I am sure, Cabbages are extremely windy, whether you take them as meat or as medicine: yea, as windy meat as can be eaten, unless you eat bag-pipes or bellows, and they are but seldom eaten in our days; and Colewort flowers are something more tolerable, and the wholesomer food of the two.'* Recent research into the unpleasant smell associated with cooking cabbage has proved that it is caused by over-cooking. The odour doubles when cooking is prolonged from five to seven minutes; for best results cabbage should be sliced thinly and cooked for four minutes. Sauerkraut (Germany) and Kimchi (Korea) were developed because cabbage

could not be stored for long periods. Cabbage is an excellent source of vitamins A and C. It also contains significant amounts of glutamine, an amino acid that has anti-inflammatory properties. Cabbage is often included in dieting plans, such as the 'cabbage soup diet', as it is a low calorie food.

HISTORY: Forms of *Brassica oleracea* have been chosen for cultivation from earliest times. There is evidence of this plant growing at the Neolithic dwellings at Robenhausen, near Lake Pfäffikon, Switzerland. Plants were selectively bred over the years for the following features: loss of the strong, pungent flavours produced by the irritant mustard oils (sulphur-containing glucosinolates); enlargement of certain parts for eating; loss of toughness; and growth in cool climates with long, cool growing seasons.

CARAWAY

CARUM CARVI
Family Apiaceae/Umbelliferae, Carrot

OTHER NAMES: Persian cumin, meridian fennel.

DESCRIPTION: Hardy biennial, growing to two feet (60 cm) tall with a 12-inch (30-cm) spread and bearing delicate white flowers. Its feathery leaves resemble those of carrots, and its leaves and hollow stem taste of aniseed. Each 'seed' is half of a caraway fruit, used whole or ground in cooking and herbal medicine.

PROPERTIES AND USES:

All parts of the plant are edible: roots, leaves and seeds. The leaves are used in soups and salads. The roots may be boiled and treated like cooked parsnips or carrots. The liquorice-flavoured seeds give rye bread its characteristic taste and are also used in potato soup, cheese spreads, sauerkraut and salad dressings. It is one of the ingredients in kümmel liqueur. Culpeper wrote: '*Caraway Seed has a moderate sharp quality whereby it breaks Wind and provokes Urine…and helpeth to sharpen the Eye-sight. The Powder of the Seed put into a Poultice, takes away black and blue spots of Blows or Bruises. The Herb it self, or with some of the Seed bruised and fryed, laid hot in a bag or double cloth to the lower part of the Belly, easeth the pains of the wind Chollick. Caraway Comfits, once only dipped in Sugar, and half a spoonful of them eaten in the morning fasting, and as many* after each meal is a most admirable *Remedy for such as are troubled with Wind.*' In Elizabethan times, eating the seeds ended a banquet to aid digestion and sweeten the breath.

HISTORY: Caraway seeds have been found in prehistoric food remains from 3500 BCE and Dioscorides mentioned that the seeds aided digestion. It was offered at the caravan stops on the Silk Road and is found in Egyptian tombs. Throughout history, caraway was a favourite addition to laxative herbs because it tempered their often violent effects. It was also used for menstrual cramps, menstruation promotion and milk promotion in nursing mothers.

A Burglar Alarm

Caraway was thought to confer the gift of retention, preventing the theft of any object which contained it, and holding the thief in custody within the broken-into house. Similarly, it was used to keep lovers from straying, forming an ingredient of Elizabethan love potions, and also to prevent fowls and pigeons from straying. '*It is an undoubted fact that tame pigeons, who are particularly fond of the seeds, will never stray if they are given a piece of baked Caraway dough in their cote.*' (Maud Grieve, 1931)

CARNATION

DIANTHUS CARYOPHYLLUS
Caryophyllaceae, Carnation

OTHER NAMES: Culpeper calls this the '*Clove Gillyflower*'. Gilliflower, July flower, pink, clove pink, gillie, Jove's flower, scaffold flower, sops-in-wine.

DESCRIPTION: Probably native to the Mediterranean, its exact range is unknown due to extensive cultivation for the last 2000 years. It is the wild ancestor of the garden carnation, a herbaceous perennial plant growing to 2 feet (60 cm) tall. The leaves are slender, up to 6 inches (15 cm) long, and the flowers are sweetly scented. The original natural flower colour is bright pinkish-purple, but cultivars of other colours, including red, white, yellow and green, have been developed. Pinks are not named for their colour, but because their petals appear to be 'pinked' or ragged. The term is still used in 'pinking shears' or scissors.

PROPERTIES AND USES: In the Renaissance, white wine infused with the petals (until they are pale, then strain) was drunk as a nerve tonic: '*They are great strengtheners of the brain and heart, and will therefore make an excellent cordial for family purposes. Either the conserve or syrup of these flowers taken at intervals, is good to help those whose constitution is inclinable to be consumptive. It is good to expel poison and help hot pestilent fevers.*' The pestilence referred to is the bubonic plague, prevalent in Europe at this time. Gerard says: '*A water distilled from Pinks has been commended as excellent for curing epilepsy.*' The largest world producer is now Colombia, as part of a US-financed programme to replace drug cultivation.

HISTORY: *Dianthus caryophyllus* is so named after *anthos* (flower), *dios* (of Jupiter, Io), and *caryophylli* (cloves). Crusaders brought them back to Europe, where they were grown in medieval gardens and in pots indoors in great houses. In the Middle Ages, the petals were used as a substitute for cloves, which were more expensive and had to be imported. The petals were also steeped in rosewater and used as a hair perfume. Culpeper's 'gillyflower' may be a stock, a wallflower or carnation. The word is often regarded as a modification of *July flower*, or of the French *giroflee*, or the Old English *gilofre*, clove.

Carnations were thought to have a rejuvenating effect on the body and spirit. In Elizabethan times, the highly fragrant flowers were steeped in wine and ale to make a delightful drink. Sops, small pieces of toast or stale bread, were offered as solid food for dipping in the tasty liquid of '*soppes in wine*'.

(WILD) CARROT

DAUCUS CAROTA
Family Apiaceae/Umbelliferae, Carrot

OTHER NAMES: Queen Anne's lace, bird's-nest (as the seeds ripen, the umbels contract to form a cup-like shape).

DESCRIPTION: Unlike our modern carrot, the wild carrot has a white, woody taproot, rather than the orange, fleshy one we are familiar with after hundreds of years of development for the table. It has small white flowers, grows to 3 feet (90 cm) tall and has a deep, fleshy, conical root.

PROPERTIES AND USES:
Culpeper wrote: *'Wild carrots belong to Mercury, and therefore expel wind, and remove stitches in the sides, provoke urine and women's menses, and help to break and expel the stone; the seed also of the same work the like effect, and is good for the dropsy, and those whose bellies are swollen with wind ...'* Its seeds were used by sufferers of flatulence and coughs, something some older people sometimes suffer simultaneously. Carrot roots, the part that we eat, contain 89 per cent water and about 4.5 per cent sugar, making them a good snack food for dieters. These domesticated carrots are not the same species as the wild carrot, commonly known as *Queen Anne's lace*, the seed of which is the part used medicinally. The best-known use for the seeds has been as a natural morning-after contraceptive. Today, as it is rich in vitamin A, wild carrot is used in antiwrinkle creams.

HISTORY: The carrot was well known to Greek and Latin writers under various names, and the name *Carota* for the garden carrot is found first in the writings of Athenaeus (200 CE). From the time of Dioscorides and Pliny to the present day, the carrot has been in constant use by all nations. In the 16th and 17th centuries, the feathery leaves decorated ladies' head-dresses. In *Love's Martyr* (1601) we read: *'This Root procured in Maids a perfect love'*, but it seems that young women these days require more than a carrot as a token of affection.

Orange Carrots

Until 400 years ago, carrots were always white, cream and purple. There was no orange carrot, but the Dutch wanted to create a vegetable in their national colour, and so bred the carrot that we now recognize today. We can now buy pale cream carrots again in supermarkets, such as *Crème de Lite*. New fruit and vegetables are constantly being developed, such as *Tiny Tangerines*, *Black Velvet Apricots* and *Baby Lemons* (chop one in half for two gin and tonics).

CATMINT

NEPETA CATARIA
Family Lamiaceae, Mint

OTHER NAMES: Catnip, catnep, cat's wort, cat, catrup, field balm. Culpeper calls this nep.

DESCRIPTION: A hardy perennial which grows to 3 feet (90 cm) with a spread of 2 feet (60 cm), with clusters of pinkish-white flowers and downy heart-shaped leaves. It has an aromatic odour, which resembles both mint and pennyroyal. The scent has a strange fascination for cats, which according to Grieve *'will destroy any plant of it that may happen to be bruised'*.

PROPERTIES AND USES: Young minty leaves can be used in soups and sauces. It has been used for children's coughs and colic, and its leaves can be made into an ointment to relieve haemorrhoids. Catmint leaves contain the antioxidant vitamins C and E, and its primary phytochemicals are mild sedatives. It induces sleep and soothes the nervous system. Catnip teas have long been used in traditional herbal medicine to quell digestive disturbances, and help stimulate menstruation. Researchers have discovered that the essential oil in catnip that gives the plant its characteristic odour is ten times more effective at repelling mosquitoes than the modern formulation DEET.

HISTORY: Nicholas Culpeper wrote: *'Nep is generally used for women to procure their courses, being taken inwardly or outwardly, either alone, or with other convenient herbs in a decoction to bathe them, or sit over the hot fumes thereof; and by the frequent use thereof it takes away barrenness, and the wind, and pains of the mother. It is also used in pains of the head coming of any cold cause; catarrhs, rheums, or any swimming and giddiness thereof, and is of special use for the windiness of the stomach and belly. It is effectual for any cramp, or cold aches, to dissolve cold and wind that affects the place; and is used for colds, coughs, and shortness of breath. The juice thereof drank in wine, is profitable for those that are bruised by an accident. The green herb bruised and applied to the fundament, and lying there for two or three hours, eases the pains of the piles; the juice also being made up into an ointment, is effectual for the same purpose. The head washed with a decoction thereof, it taketh away scabs, and may be effectual for other parts of the body also.'*

Cool For Cats

Catnip acts as a mild sedative and digestive aid for most animals, making it very useful to treat high-strung animals with nervous stomach upsets. Cats seemingly become intoxicated when they sniff the bruised leaves of this plant. Some people, noticing the effect upon cats, have taken to smoking catmint as a milder substitute for cannabis.

(GREATER) CELANDINE

CHELIDONIUM MAJUS
Family Papaveraceae, Poppy

OTHER NAMES: Celandine, common celandine, garden celandine, kill wart, wart flower, wart weed, devil's milk, swallow wort, tetter wort, dilwydd.

DESCRIPTION: This upright, widely branching perennial grows to a height of between 1 to 2 feet (30–60 cm) and bears flowers with four yellow petals. Like the yellow Welsh poppy, the greater celandine has yellow sap or latex rather than the white sap of other poppies. It can blister the skin, being caustic, and is poisonous, leading to the common name of 'devil's milk'. The seeds are small and black, borne in a long fleshy capsule. This attracts ants to disperse the seeds in suitable habitats (a type of seed dispersal known scientifically as myrmecochory).

PROPERTIES AND USES: Greater celandine acts as a mild sedative and has been used historically to treat asthma, bronchitis, and whooping cough. Its antispasmodic effect improves bile flow in the gallbladder and it has been reputed to treat gallstones and gallbladder pain. Modern herbalists value its purgative properties. Culpeper recommended it for yellow jaundice, dropsy, itch, old sores, toothache and *'griping pains in the bowels'*.

HISTORY: As far back as Pliny the Elder and Dioscorides, the herb has been recognized as a detoxifying agent. The root has been chewed to relieve toothache. It was formerly used by gypsies as a foot refresher, and across Europe as a herbal aid in removing warts, papillomas and other skin malformations, hence the name kill wart. A yellow juice pervades the plant's root, stem and leaves. Its resemblance to bile in colour led those who practised the Doctrine of Signatures to use the drug in hepatic disorders. In the Middle Ages, this acrid juice was used to remove filming from the cornea of the eye, *'for the juice cleanseth and consumeth away slimy things that cleaves about the ball of the eye and hinder the sight.'* Culpeper recommended this course of action rather than a needle to clean the eye, mixing the celandine latex with breast-milk to allay the *'sharpness of the juice'*.

Hard to Swallow

This plant is said to derive its name *Chelidonium* from the Greek *chelidon*, swallow, as it comes into flower when these birds arrive and fades at their departure. Celandine is a corruption of the Greek. It was also thought that swallows used the juice of the celandine to feed their young and improve their eyesight.

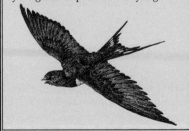

(LESSER) CELANDINE

RANUNCULUS FICARIA
Family Ranunculaceae, Buttercup

OTHER NAMES: Small celandine, figwort, pilewort, smallwort, brighteye, butter and cheese.

DESCRIPTION: This is a low-growing, hairless perennial plant, with fleshy, dark green, heart-shaped leaves, and yellow buttercup-like flowers with eight to 12 petals. It is one of the earliest spring flowers. It was loved by Wordsworth and its flowers were carved on his tomb, but like all the buttercup family, it is toxic. The blossoms shut up before rain, and even in fine weather do not open before 9 a.m. By 5 p.m. they have already closed for the night. It derives its species name *ficaria* from *ficus*, the Latin word for the fig, and this relates to the appearance of the root tubers of the plant.

PROPERTIES AND USES: Culpeper wrote: *'It is certain by good experience that the decoction of the leaves and roots doth wonderfully help piles and haemorrhoids; also kernels by the ears and throat called the King's Evil, or any other hard wens or tumours…The very herb borne about one's body next the skin helps in such diseases though it never touch the place grieved.'* The plant used to be known as pilewort, as it was used to treat haemorrhoids. Supposedly the knobbly tubers resemble piles, and according to the Doctrine of Signatures this resemblance suggests that pilewort could be used to cure piles. Its saponins are fungicidal and locally antihaemorrhoidal, an action enhanced by its astringent tannins, and protoanemonin in the fresh plant is antibacterial.

HISTORY: In the Western Isles of Scotland they were believed to resemble a cow's udder, and they were hung in cow byres to encourage high milk yields. Boiled with white wine and sweetened with honey then drunk before bed, lesser celandine was believed to induce pleasant dreams. It was used as a visionary herb to increase psychic abilities and as a wash in divination, to consecrate a divinatory tool or to bathe the body. The German name *Scharbockskraut* (scurvywort) derives from the use of the early leaves, which are high in vitamin C, to prevent scurvy. The Russian name for it is *chistotel* (clean body) and it is brewed and used in baths to help cure dermatitis and other skin irritations such as rosacea. It was believed that beggars would use lesser celandine juice to create sores on their bodies to encourage people to give them alms.

(WILD) CELERY

APIUM GRAVEOLENS
Family Apiaceae/Umbelliferae, Carrot/Parsley

OTHER NAMES: Culpeper calls it *Smallage.* Smallage is the wild variety of celery. The two domestic cultivars cultivated from it are what we now call celery (*Apium graveolens* var. *dulce*) and celeriac (*Apium graveolens* var. *rapaceum.*)

DESCRIPTION: A plant growing 1–3 feet (30–90 cm) tall, this is the ancestor of our garden celery, with thin hollow stalks and a marked smell of celery. It blossoms with flat, umbrella-like masses of tiny white blooms. Italian farmers developed what we now call celery in the 17th century.

PROPERTIES AND USES: Culpeper noted '*It is under the dominion of the Sun, as are all celeries. The root, in its wild state, is of an acrid, noxious nature, but culture takes away those properties, and renders the plant mild and succulent.*' Celery has been promoted as a stimulant, diuretic and tonic, promoting restfulness and sleep. In France, smallage is often used in soups and stews, as the French feel it gives more concentrated flavour than domesticated celery. One French name for smallage, '*celeri à couper*' (celery to cut), tells us that it can be treated as a cut-and-come-again plant. However, celery is among a small group of foods, such as peanuts, that can cause severe allergic reactions. Wild celery seeds are those sold as 'Celery Seed' in health food shops. It is drunk as tea to reduce blood pressure and lower cholesterol levels as it contains chemical compounds called coumarins that thin the blood. Celery seed also helps rid the body of uric acid that often causes pain and inflammation in gout and arthritis. The plant compound luteolin reduces inflammation in the brain, and benefits cognitive health.

HISTORY: Traditionally it was used in Indian medicine to treat flatulence, asthma and hiccups, and remains of it was found in Tutankhamen's tomb – as was chervil. Smallage is one of the oldest vegetables in recorded history. Ancient Egyptians were known to gather wild celery from marshy seaside areas for food, and Greeks crowned their athletes with celery leaves to honour them.

Attractive to Bees

Apium graveolens is a member of the Apiaceae (parsley) family and a relative of dill and carrots. The genus name is derived from the Latin, *apis* (bee), as bees are attracted to its small white flowers. The species name *graveolens* means 'heavy scented'. Our English word celery is possibly from the Latin *celer*, meaing swift, as celery is considered a fast-acting remedy.

CENTAURY (CENTAURIUM)

CENTAURIUM ERYTHRAEA
Family Gentianaceae, Gentian

OTHER NAMES: Bitterherb, centaury gentium, common centaury, European centaury, '*Ordinary Smaller Centaury*' (Culpeper).

DESCRIPTION: An erect biennial herb growing to 18 inches (46 cm) from a small basal rosette, and bearing many pinkish-lavender inflorescences

PROPERTIES AND USES: '*Of all the bitter appetizing wild herbs which serve as excellent simple tonics, the Centaury is the most efficacious, sharing the antiseptic virtues of the Field Gentian and the Buckbean.*' (Grieve 1931). It is a gentle laxative, and an excellent remedy for heartburn. Like other bitter tonics, centaury is effective in reducing fever and has been used in place of quinine. Culpeper recommended centaury for sciatica, colic, jaundice, obstructions of the liver, spleen and gall, ague, dropsy, '*worms in the belly*', childbirth, joint pains, snake bites, gout, cramp, convulsions, dimness of sight, ulcers, wounds, scabs etc.

HISTORY: It is one of the '*nine sacred herbs*' of the Anglo-Saxons, the others being fennel, chervil, crab apple, nettle, betony, watercress, plantain and mugwort.

Centaur Chiron's Herbal Cure

The name of the species to which centaury is at present assigned, *Erythraea*, is derived from the Greek *erythros* (red), referring to the colour of the flowers. The genus was formerly called *Chironia*, from the centaur Chiron, who was famous in Greek mythology for his skill in using medicinal herbs, and who is supposed to have cured himself with it from a wound he had accidentally received from an arrow belonging to Heracles. The arrow's tip had been poisoned with the blood of the Hydra.

...A mighty arrow not for him to wield,
The wound being deep, and with a
venomed point,
To Deaths arrestment he began to yield,
And there with sundry Balms they did
anoint,
His wounded foot being stricken through
the joint:
All would not serve till that an old man
brought,
This Centaurie that ease to him hath
wrought...

Robert Chester, *Love's Martyr*, 1601

CHAMOMILE

ANTHEMIS NOBILIS (SYN. *CHAMAEMELUM NOBILE*)
Family Asteraceae/Compositae, Sunflower

OTHER NAMES: Camomile, chamomel, maythen (Saxon), whig plant, earth apple, English chamomile, garden chamomile, lawn chamomile, low chamomile, Roman chamomile, manzanilla (Spanish, 'little apple'), noble chamomile, ground apple. In Greek, chamaimelon means earth-apple and refers to the strong apple-like scent when walked upon. Its Welsh name is *camri*, meaning footsteps or walk. It is also called the physician's plant, as when planted next to sick plants, it helps them revive.

DESCRIPTION: A hardy low-growing herb, with profuse white daisy-like flowers with yellow centres.

PROPERTIES AND USES: It makes an excellent calming tea, helping with stress and insomnia, and has a soothing effect on the digestion. It is a good herb to give to hyperactive children or children with colic. It can relieve the pain of arthritis and gout, and also period pains, PMT and thrush. It also helps with colds, catarrh, hay fever and asthma. Used as an oil, chamomile is anti-inflammatory, cooling and calming. It is good for allergies and inflamed itchy skin conditions. Culpeper wrote: '*A decoction made of Camomile, and drank, taketh away all pains and stitches in the side...The flowers of Camomile beaten, and made up into*

balls with oil, drive away all sorts of agues, if the part grieved be anointed with that oil, taken from the flowers, from the crown of the head to the sole of the foot, and afterwards laid to sweat in his bed, and that he sweats well.' Chamomile is also used commercially in a number of personal care products including cosmetics, hair colourings, mouthwash, sunscreen, shampoos and conditioners to bring out the highlights in blonde hair, and as a moisturiser for dry hair.

HISTORY: Chamomile has been accepted as an herbal remedy for stress and restlessness since the time of ancient Egypt. It was worshiped by Egyptians and dedicated to their Sun god Ra because of its gold-centred disc, and because it was well known for its power to cure chills and fevers. It was also prescribed by Greek doctors and is celebrated as one of the most sacred herbs in the Anglo-Saxons' collection of medical remedies, the manuscript known as *Lacnunga*. Chamomile was often used to create a lawn instead of grass, and was employed as a strewing herb and to scent herb seats in medieval gardens. '*Though the camomile, the more it is trodden upon, the faster it grows...*' William Shakespeare, *Henry IV Part I*. Before the invention of refrigeration, meat was immersed in a camomile infusion to prevent spoilage.

CHASTE TREE
VITEX AGNUS-CASTUS
Family Lamiaceae (formerly Verbenaceae), Verbena

OTHER NAMES: Chasteberry, monk's pepper, Abraham's balm, chaste lamb-tree, safe tree. It is not mentioned in Culpeper, although it was known in his time.

DESCRIPTION: A deciduous shrub native to the Mediterranean region with lance-like leaves, fragrant flowers and grey or purple berries

PROPERTIES AND USES: The herb has had a history as an effective treatment for menstrual disorders for at least 2500 years. The Greek physician Hippocrates (460-377 BCE) wrote, *'If blood flows from the womb, let the woman drink dark wine in which the leaves of the chaste tree have been steeped.'*

HISTORY: Pliny and Dioscorides (first century CE), and Theophrastus (third century CE) recommended its use. Athenian matrons in the sacred rites of Ceres used to string their couches with the leaves of the chaste tree, because of the seed's reputation for securing chastity. Dioscorides recommended the fruit for inflammations of the womb and to stimulate milk flow in nursing mothers. Gerard (1633) recommended chaste tree for those *'willing to live chaste'* and for treating inflammation of the uterus. In Rome, vestal virgins carried twigs of chaste tree as a symbol of chastity. Later ceremonial uses include the strewing of flowers along the entrances of monasteries as a symbol of celibacy.

From *Love's Martyr,* 1601

[Phoenix] *Here need they not of aches to complain,*
For Physics' skill grows here without compare:
All herbs and plants within this Region are,
But by the way sweet Nature as you go,
Of Agnus Castus speak a word or two.
[Nature] *That shall I briefly;*
it is the very handmaid
To Vesta, or to perfect Chastity,
The hot inflamed spirit is allayed

By this sweet herb that bends to Luxury,
It drieth up the seed of Venerie:
The leaves being laid upon the sleepers bed,
With chasteness, cleanness, pureness he is fed.
Burn me the leaves, and straw then on the ground,
Whereas foul venomous Serpents use to haunt:
And by this virtue here they are not found...

Robert Chester

CHERRY TREE

PRUNUS AVIUM
Family Rosaceae, Rose

OTHER NAMES: Wild cherry, sweet cherry, gean, mazzard, massard.

DESCRIPTION: Masses of showy white or pink flowers, the tree can grow over 50 feet (15 m) in height, and bears fleshy fruits which vary from red to purple in colour.

PROPERTIES AND USES: The vast majority of eating cherries are derived from either *Prunus avium*, the wild cherry or from *Prunus cerasus*, the sour cherry. Culpeper: '*Cherries, as they are of different tastes, so they are of different qualities. The sweet pass through the stomach and the belly more speedily, but are of little nourishment; the tart or sour are more pleasing to an hot stomach, procure appetite to meat, and help to cut tough phlegm and gross humours; but when these are dried, they are more binding to the belly than when they are fresh, being cooling in hot diseases, and welcome to the stomach, and provoke urine. The gum of the cherry-tree, dissolved in wine, is good for a cold, cough, and hoarseness of the throat; mends the colour in the face, sharpens the eyesight, provokes appetite, and helps to break and expel the stone; the black cherries bruised with the stone, and dissolved, the water thereof is much used to break the stone, and to expel gravel and wind.*' Compounds in cherry juice significantly reduce the chemicals in the body that cause joint inflammation. The hard, reddish-brown wood is valued as a hardwood for turnery, musical instruments and cabinet-making.

HISTORY: Wild cherry stones have been found in Bronze Age settlements throughout Europe, carbon dated to 2000 BCE. By 800 BCE, cherries were being cultivated in Asia Minor, and soon after in Greece. As the main ancestor of the cultivated sweet cherry, the wild cherry is one of the two cherry species which supply most of the world's commercial cultivars of edible cherry. The other is the sour cherry *Prunus cerasus*, also known as Morello cherry, which is mainly used for cooking.

Bird Cherry

The wild cherry's scientific name *Prunus avium* literally means 'bird cherry'. However, the bird cherry species is actually *Prunus padus*. The English name refers to the berries, which are astringent and bitter-sweet. They are seldom used in Western Europe but readily eaten by birds, which do not taste astringency as unpleasant. It was used medicinally during the Middle Ages, and the bark, placed at the door, was supposed to ward off plague. Another name for *Prunus padus* is the *Hagberry*, and the fruit can be known as hags.

CHERVIL

ANTHRISCUS CEREFOLIUM
Family Umbelliferae/Apiaceaea, Umbillifers

OTHER NAMES: Garden chervil, gourmet's parsley, French parsley, anise parsley. Culpeper says '*It is called cerefolium, mirrhis, and mirrha, chervel, sweet chervil, and sweet cicely.*' (However, for Culpeper's sweet chervil see sweet cicely, and for his wild chervil see cow parsley).

DESCRIPTION: Hardy biennial, growing up to 2 feet (60 cm) tall with fern-like leaves and tiny white flowers. The leaves taste slightly of aniseed, resembling a mixture of sweet cicely and parsley.

PROPERTIES AND USES: Chervil is a traditional remedy for bad dreams, burns and stomach upsets. It is an excellent source of antioxidants that stabilize cell membranes and reduce inflammation associated with headache, sinusitis, peptic ulcers and infections. It is a good source of vitamin C, magnesium and carotene. Chervil infusions are used to lower blood pressure. It is used as a digestive aid, diuretic, stimulant and for menstrual cramps. Chervil is particularly popular in France, where it is added to omelettes, salads and soups. The root can be eaten as a vegetable. More delicate than parsley, it has a faint taste of liquorice. Cooking destroys the colour and flavour of this delicate herb, so add last to soups and stews. Leaves infused in water act as a skin freshener and to treat eczema. '*The garden chervil being eaten, doth moderately warm the stomach, and is a certain remedy (saith Tragus) to dissolve congealed or clotted blood in the body, or that which is clotted by bruises, falls, &c. The juice or distilled water thereof being drank, and the bruised leaves laid to the place, being taken either in meat or drink, it is good to help to provoke urine, or expel the stone in the kidneys, to send down women's courses, and to help the pleurisy and pricking of the sides*' (Culpeper).

HISTORY: The herb was found in Tutankhamen's tomb. It was a popular herb at Lent, being eaten on Maundy Thursday for its blood-cleansing properties – a 'Spring cleansing' tonic for the body.

The name is derived via Latin from the Greek *chairephyllon*, a compound of *chairein* ('to delight in') and *phyllon* ('leaf'), a reference to the plant's pleasing scent. Chervil was one of the nine sacred herbs of the Anglo-Saxons, along with betony, mugwort, plantain, watercress, chamomile, crab apple, nettle and fennel.

Gather With Care

It is not advisable to collect chervil from the wild as it resembles hemlock, which is poisonous. It is one of the traditional '*fines herbes*' of French cuisine along with parsley, chives and tarragon, and is used in *ravigote* and *Béarnaise* sauces.

(SWEET) CHESTNUT

CASTANEA SATIVA
Family Fagaceae, Beech

OTHER NAMES: Culpeper calls it a '*chesnut tree*'. Marron, Sardian nut, Jupiter's nut, husked nut, Spanish chestnut, Portuguese chestnut, European chestnut.

DESCRIPTION: This tree can reach a huge size – up to 115 feet (35 m) in height – and is used for landscaping.

PROPERTIES AND USES: Culpeper: '*The tree is abundantly under the dominion of Jupiter, and therefore the fruit must needs breed good blood, and yield commendable nourishment to the body; yet if eaten over-much, they make the blood thick, procure head-ach, and bind the body; the inner skin, that covereth the nut, is of so binding a quality, that a scruple of it taken by a man, or ten grains by a child, soon stops any flux whatsoever: The whole nut being dried and beaten into powder, and a dram taken at a time, is a good remedy to stop the terms in women. If you dry chesnuts, (only the kernels I mean) both the barks being taken away, beat them into powder, and make the powder into an electuary with honey, so have you an admirable remedy for the cough and spitting of blood.*' Easy to peel, unlike their spiky 'conker' cousins, horse chestnuts, sweet chestnuts can be eaten raw but are usually roasted. They also make an excellent stuffing for turkey and pheasant. Chestnut leaves were chewed or made into tea as a popular remedy in fever and ague, for their tonic and astringent properties. Chestnut powder was sold for paroxysmal and convulsive coughs. The candied nuts are sold as *marron glacés*.

HISTORY: It was introduced into Europe from Sardis in Asia Minor, thus the fruit was called the 'Sardian nut'. Theophrastus called it the 'Euboean nut' from the large Greek island in the Adriatic, where it was abundant. Roman soldiers were given chestnut porridge before entering battle. Evelyn spoke of chestnuts as '*delicacies for princes and a lusty and masculine food for rusticks, and able to make women well-complexioned*', and then complained that in England they were chiefly given to pigs. In many European countries, they are sold, freshly roasted, by street vendors as a snack. Chestnut wood is more durable than oak for woodwork that has to be partially sunk in the ground, such as stakes and fenceposts. Because of this, it was used for making pit-props, wine barrels, house building and household furniture. In hop-growing areas it was in great demand for hop poles.

CHICKWEED

STELLARIA MEDIA
Family Carophylaceae, Pink

OTHER NAMES: Starweed, star chickweed, common chickweeds, adder's mouth chickweed, Indian chickweed, satinflower, scarweed, scarwort, starwort, stitchwort, tongue grass, white bird's-eye, winterweed (as it is found year-round), little star lady, bird herb, chick whittle, chicken's meat, cluckweed (chickens love it, as do most birds).

DESCRIPTION: This small creeping plant is found everywhere, throughout the year; it has small white starry flowers on weak stems.

PROPERTIES AND USES: '*It is a fine soft pleasing herb under the dominion of the Moon. The herb bruised or the juice applied with cloths or sponges dipped therein to the region of the liver, and as they dry to have it fresh applied, doth wonderfully temperate the heat of the liver*', Nicholas Culpeper. Chickweed is best known for its ability to cool inflammation and speed healing for internal or external flare-ups. Herbalists often recommend it as a poultice or ointment for minor burns, insect bites, skin irritations, skin abscesses and boils. Chickweed's use as a wound herb is probably due to its saponin content. It can cool inflammation and speed healing. It is used for rashes, particularly when associated with dryness and itching. Chickweed is an effective and gentle laxative. Chickweed water is an old remedy for obesity, which may have been associated with its laxative properties. The juice was once taken to combat scurvy. Fresh chickweed can be eaten in summer salads and can be fed to pets to assist in the expulsion of hair balls, and sooth the digestive tract.

HISTORY: It can be used both internally and externally for healing and has been used throughout history to stop bleeding in the stomach and bowels. Chickweed has been used as a culinary herb in Britain since at least the Middle Ages. Paracelsus in 1530 described it as '*The Elixir of Life...one of the supreme healers*'.

Chicken Feed

Chickweed is a favourite source of food for chickens kept outdoors, hence its name. 'Scarwort' alludes to its healing properties for skin abrasions, and 'stitchwort' probably applies to chickweed lotion being used when wounds have been stitched. All varieties of chickweed share the interesting practice termed the *Sleep of Plants*, when every night (and when the weather is cloudy) the leaves fold over the tender buds and the new shoots.

CHICORY

CICHORIUM INTYBUS
Family Asteraceae/Compositae, Daisy

OTHER NAMES: Culpeper calls it succory or garden succory. Leaf chicory, Italian chicory, witloof, Belgian endive, French endive, red endive, sugar loaf chicory, radicchio, barbe de capucin (blanched), blue sailors, coffeeweed.

DESCRIPTION: A hardy perennial which grows 2–3 feet (60–90 cm) high, with dandelion-like leaves and edible bright pale blue/lavender (sometimes white) flowers which can colour a salad or rice dish.

PROPERTIES AND USES: Culpeper: '*Garden Succory, as it is more dry and less cold than endive, so it opens more. An handful of the leaves, or roots boiled in wine or water, and a draught thereof drank fasting, drives forth choleric and phlegmatic humours, opens obstructions of the liver, gall and spleen; helps the yellow jaundice, the heat of the reins, and of the urine; the dropsy also; and those that have an evil disposition in their bodies, by reason of long sickness, evil diet, &c. which the Greeks call Cachexia* [a loss of body mass, caused by chronic illness, that cannot be reversed nutritionally]. *A decoction thereof made with wine, and drank, is very effectual against long lingering agues; and a dram of the seed in powder, drank in wine, before the fit of the ague, helps to drive it away. The distilled water of the herb and flowers*

(if you can take them in time) hath the like properties, and is especially good for hot stomachs, and in agues, either pestilential or of long continuance; for swoonings and passions of the heart, for the heat and headache in children, and for the blood and liver. The said water, or the juice, or the bruised leaves applied outwardly, allay swellings, inflammations, St. Anthony's fire, pushes, wheals, and pimples, especially used with a little vinegar; as also to wash pestiferous sores. The said water is very effectual for sore eyes that are inflamed with redness, for nurses' breasts that are pained by the abundance of milk. The Wild Succory, as it is more bitter, so it is more strengthening to the stomach and liver.'

A tonic was made, to increase the flow of bile, and a tea made from the leaves was used to aid the liver and digestion. A decoction of the bitter root was recommended for jaundice, liver enlargements, gout and rheumatic complaints. Syrup of succory was a popular laxative for children, and the leaves when bruised made a good poultice for swellings, inflammations and inflamed eyes. The flowers were also used to make a distillation to help cure inflammation of the eyes, and chicory leaves can make a blue dye. The leaves are used in salads, generally blanched, as unblanched leaves

Regular Hours

When fully opened, the blooms are large and shaded a delicate tint of blue, blossoming from July to September. However, even on a sunny day, by the early afternoon every bloom is closed, the petal-rays drawing together. Linnaeus used the chicory as one of the flowers in his *Floral Clock* (see pages 152–153) at Uppsala, in Sweden because of its regularity in opening at 5 a.m. and closing at 10 a.m. at that latitude. In Britain, it opens between 6 and 7 a.m. and closes just after midday.

'Non-forcing' chicories produce large-hearted lettuce-like heads in the autumn and are known as *Sugarloaf* varieties. Red chicory *(radicchio)* includes older cultivars which respond to lower temperatures and daylight hours by turning an attractive red colour.

HISTORY: Chicory was used by the Egyptians, Greeks and Romans as a salad plant, vegetable and medicinal plant. In 1573, Thomas Tusser thought that chicory, together with endive, was a remedy for ague. The botanist and apothecary to King James I and Charles I, John Parkinson (1567–1650), pronounced succory a *'fine, cleansing, jovial plant.'* With violets, chicory was used to make the sweet, *'violet plates'* (tablets), in the time of Charles II. The confections used sweet violets and chicory flowers, being *'most pleasant and wholesome, and especially it comforteth the heart, and inward parts'*. The tablets were also added to soups and stews. Used as a fodder plant in Europe, the young and tender roots or blanched heads are also boiled and eaten with butter like parsnips.

are bitter. This forced foliage is termed by the French *barbe de capucin* and forms a favourite winter salad, much eaten in France and Belgium. Chicory is becoming increasingly popular, and is an excellent winter crop for salads. There are three main types, all with slightly bitter leaves. 'Forcing' chicories such as *Witloof* (white leaf) give leafy plump heads known as *chicons* when blanched.

Bitter Coffee

Chicory roots were roasted and ground as a coffee substitute in France during Napoleonic times, when the naval blockade cut off coffee supplies. It is extensively cultivated in Europe to supply ground chicory which forms an ingredient or addition to some coffees. When infused, chicory gives to coffee a more bitter taste and a darker colour. The French believe it to be a *'contra-stimulante'*, correcting the

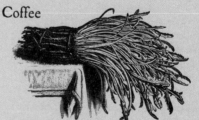

excessively stimulative effects caused by coffee, and think that such a drink suits bilious subjects who suffer from habitual constipation.

CHILLI PEPPER

CAPSICUM FRUTESCENS
Family Solanaceae, Nightshade or Potato

OTHER NAMES: Culpeper calls it guinea pepper, cayenne pepper and bird pepper. Red pepper, pimento.

DESCRIPTION: A small shrub, whose white flowers become green, yellow and bright red, with hot-tasting seed pods.

PROPERTIES AND USES: Culpeper: *'...All kinds of guinea pepper are under Mars, and are of a fiery, sharp, biting taste, and of a temperature hot and dry, to the end of the fourth degree; they burn and inflame the mouth and throat so extremely that it is hard to be endured, and if it be outwardly applied to the skin in any part of the body, it will exulcerate and raise it as if it had been burnt with fire, or scalded with hot water. The vapours that arise from the husks or pods, while a person opens them to take out the seed, (especially if he beats them into powder, or bruises them) will so pierce the brain by flying up into the head through the nostrils, as to produce violent sneezings, and draw down abundance of thin rheum, forcing tears from the eyes, and will pass into the throat, and provoke a sharp coughing, and cause violent vomiting; and if any shall with their hands touch their face or eyes, it will cause so great an inflammation that it will not be remedied in a long time by all the bathing thereof with wine or cold water that can be used, but yet will pass away without further harm. If any of it be caste into fire, it raises grievous strong and noisome vapours, occasions sneezing, coughing, and strong vomiting to all that be near it; if it should be taken simply of itself (though in very small*

quantity, either in powders or decoction) it would be hard to be endured, and might prove dangerous to life. Such are the dangers attending the immoderate use of these violent plants and fruits; yet, when corrected of their evil qualities, they are of considerable service...' He recommends making a powder to season meat or sauces, then: *'It is of singular service to be used with flatulent or windy diet, and such as breeds moisture and crudities; one scruple of the said powder, taken in a little broth of veal or of a chicken, gives great relief and comfort to a cold stomach, causing phlegm and such viscous humours as lie low in the bottom thereof, to be voiced: it helps digestion, for it occasions an appetite to meat, provokes urine, and taken with saxifrage water expels the stone in the kidneys, and the phlegm that breeds it, and takes away dimness or mistiness in the sight, being used in meats...it helps the dropsy...expels the dead birth...will ease all the pains of the mother...it helps the*

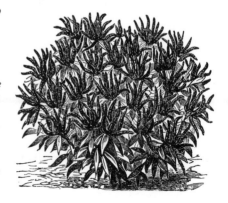

quinsy…it takes away the morphew and all freckles, spots, marks, and discolourings of the skin…dissolves all cold imposthumes and carbuncles, and mixed with sharp vinegar dissolves the hardness of the skin…The decoction of the husks themselves, made with water, and the mouth gargled therewith, helps the tooth-ach, and preserves the teeth from rottenness; the ashes of them being rubbed on the teeth, will cleanse them, and make them look white…A little of the pulpy part of the fruit, held in the mouth, cures the tooth-ache…' Its name possibly comes from Greek *kapso* to bite, and cayenne and tabasco are obtained from varieties of chilli pepper. The world's hottest chilli, the *Dorset Naga*, measures 1.6 million SHUs (Scoville heat units), compared to the 2500–5000 rating of tabasco sauce. Capsaicin, the essential ingredient, has antibiotic qualities and can be detected by taste buds at a level of 1 in 15,000,000 parts. Capsaicin clears mucus and aids nasal and lung decongestion. It eases pain, prevents stomach ulcers, lessens the risk of blood clots and lowers cholesterol.

HISTORY: Chilli was a common folk remedy for flatulence, and for centuries red pepper was rubbed into inflamed and painful joints. It now gives relief from lumbago, arthritis, rheumatism and neuralgia when applied in an ointment. For reasons still not completely understood, capsaicin interferes with the action of *substance P*, a nerve chemical that sends pain messages to the brain. It is also used to help cure cluster headaches.

Why Is A Chilli Pepper Hot?

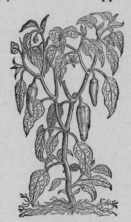

The areas of the tongue that normally sense heat and pain are stimulated by capsaicin, which also increases perspiration and raises the heart rate. Most of the heat-causing capsaicin is found in the white pith of the chilli pepper, not in the seeds as most celebrity chefs inform us. The burning sensation causes the release of endorphins, natural painkillers in the body that also give us a feeling of happiness. Some people build up their tolerance of chilli peppers over time. If a curry containing excessive chilli is too hot, the Indian cucumber- and yoghurt-based side dish, *raita*, seems to dissolve the capsaicin and relieve the burning sensation. Also the proteins in a drink of milk help to wash away capsaicin.

CHIVES
ALLIUM SCHOENOPRASUM
Family Alliaceae, Onion

OTHER NAMES: Culpeper calls these '*Cives, Rush-Leeks, Civet and Sweth*'. Rush leek is a translation of its Latin name.

DESCRIPTION: Hardy perennial with a 12-inch (30-cm) height and spread, with pink or purple globe-shaped flowers. Will multiply rapidly and form clumps.

PROPERTIES AND USES:
The flowers are edible, with a mild onion flavour, to decorate salads, and can be infused in white wine vinegar to make fine-tasting pink vinegar. Leaves are best used fresh and go well with cheese, eggs, pasta and potatoes or with anything that does not overpower their delicate taste. Cooking takes away a lot of their flavour so add them last to a dish that is cooking. Chives can be useful in fighting infection and anaemia and provide antibacterial, antiviral and antifungal actions. Culpeper states: '*They are indeed a kind of leeks, hot and dry in the forth degree, and so under the dominion of Mars. If they be eaten raw (I do not mean raw opposite to roasted or boiled, but raw opposite to chemical preparation) they send up very hurtful vapours to the brain, causing troublesome sleep and spoiling the eyesight; yet of them, prepared by the act of the alchemist, may be made an excellent remedy for the stoppage of urine.*' The rhyme '*chives next to rosies creates posies*' denoted that the plant kept black spot away from the flowers.

HISTORY: Chives were used as far back as 3000 BCE as a remedy to staunch blood flow and as an antidote to poison. Having a bunch of chives in the house was thought to ward off evil spirits and disease. In Ancient Rome chives were used to relieve the pain from sunburn or a sore throat, increase blood pressure and encourage urination. It is said that during the approach of Alexander the Great (356–23 BCE) the people of the Persian province of Bactria appealed to him (in honour of his upcoming marriage to their Princess Roxana) with their only treasure, chives, because it was believed to be an aphrodisiac. The belief that chives was an aphrodisiac remained part of folklore until into the 19th century.

Aiding Digestion

Whenever serving a dish that is high in fats, consider also serving a salad that has fresh chives added. Even chewing one fresh stalk will aid the digestion of a fatty meal, and the scent on one's breath does not last as long as onion or garlic. '*He who bears chives on his breath / Is safe from being kissed to death.*' (*Epigrams* of Marcus Valerius Martialis, *c.*100 CE.)

CINNAMON

CINNAMOMUM VERUM
Family Lauraceae, Laurel

OTHER NAMES: Sweet wood, true cinnamon.

DESCRIPTION: A medium sized evergreen tree, of which the former name was *Cinnamomum zeylanicum*, named after the island of Ceylon. Ninety per cent of the world's production comes from Ceylon (now Sri Lanka). It is harvested by growing the tree for two years and then coppicing it. The following year, about a dozen shoots will form from the roots. The outer bark is scraped off, and the inner bark is beaten out in long lengths. These curl into rolls ('quills') on drying, then the bark is sold either cut into 2–4 inch (5–10 cm) lengths, or powdered.

PROPERTIES AND USES:
Cinnamon bark is widely used as a culinary spice, often in desserts, such as apple pie, doughnuts and pastries, as well as used in spicy sweets, tea and liqueurs. This is true cinnamon, rather than the stronger cassia *(Cinnamon aromaticum)*. In medicine its antimicrobial oil acts like other volatile oils and was once used as a cure for colds. It has also been used to treat diarrhoea and other problems of the digestive system. According to Maud Grieve, *'It stops vomiting, relieves flatulence, and given with chalk and astringents is useful for diarrhoea and haemorrhage of the womb.'* Cinnamon is high in antioxidants. Half a teaspoon of cinnamon a day reduces blood sugar levels in diabetics.

HISTORY: Cinnamon was one of the first known spices. Moses was commanded to use it as an anointing oil, and in the Book of Proverbs the lover's bed is perfumed with aloe, myrrh and cinnamon The Romans believed cinnamon's fragrance was sacred and Nero is said to have burned a year's worth of the city's supply for his wife Poppaea Sabina, in remorse for having murdered her in 65 CE. At that time, Pliny the Elder wrote of 350 grams of cinnamon as being equal in value to over five kilograms of silver, about 15 times the value of silver per weight. Throughout the Middle Ages, the source of cinnamon was a mystery to the Western world. Arab traders brought the spice via overland trade routes to Alexandria in Egypt, where it was bought by Venetian traders who held a monopoly on the spice trade in Europe.

Safe Harvest

Herodotus wrote of the huge Phoenix bird gathering the priceless cinnamon spice sticks. Gatherers would lure the bird with heavy pieces of meat which the bird would laboriously haul to its nest. In legend, the weight of the meat would cause the nest to fall, allowing the valuable sticks to be harvested safely.

(WILD) CLARY

SALVIA VERBENACA
Family Lamiaceae, Mint

OTHER NAMES: Culpeper writes: *'Wild Clary is often, though I think imprudently, called Christ's Eye, because it cures the diseases of the eyes.'* Wild sage, wild clear-eye, vervain sage, vervain salvia, wild English clary, Christ's eye, oculus Christi, eyeseeds.

DESCRIPTION: A perennial herb about 18 inches (46 cm) high, smaller than clary sage, with hairy stems and branches, with soft purple to violet lipped flowers. To protect the honey from the rain and flies, the tube of the corolla is lined with hairs. A bee inserting its head in the mouth of the flower touches the inner end of the anther, and raising it acts as a lever and causes the outer surface to rub on its back and so deposit pollen.

PROPERTIES AND USES: Culpeper: *'It is something hotter and drier than the garden clary, yet nevertheless under the dominion of the Moon, as well as that the seeds of it being beaten in powder and drunk in wine is an admirable help to provoke lust; a decoction of the leaves being drunk warms the stomach, and it is a wonder if it should not, the stomach being under Cancer in the house of the Moon. It helps digestion, scatters congealed blood in any part of the body, and helps dimness of the sight; The distilled water thereof cleans the eyes of redness,*

wateriness and heat: it is a gallant remedy for dimness of sight, to take one of the seeds of it and put it into the eyes, and there let it remain till it drops out of itself, the pain will be nothing to speak on: it will cleanse the eyes of all filthy and putrid matter; and in often repeating, will take off a film which covers the sight. It is a great deal handsomer, safer and easier remedy than to tear it off with a needle.'

HISTORY: This aromatic sage was used as flavouring in foods and to make tea. The flowers can be added to salads. Eyeseeds was a name given because it was *'a plant whose seeds if blown into the eye are said to remove bits of dust, cinders, or insects that may be lodged there'*.

Clearing the Eyes

This type of clary was thought to be more beneficial to the eye than the garden clary variety, clary sage. The seeds, like those of the garden clary, produce a great quantity of soft, tasteless mucilage when moistened. If seeds were inserted under the eyelids for a few moments, the tears dissolved the mucilage, which then enveloped any dust or motes and brought irritating matter out safely.

CLEAVERS

GALIUM APARINE
Family Rubiaceae, Madder

OTHER NAMES: According to Culpeper: '*Aparine, Sticky Weed, Grip Grass, Goose-Share and Goosegrass*'. Clivers, catchweed, beggar lice, goose-grass, goosebill, sticky willy, stickyweed, catchweed bedstraw, Robin-run-the-hedge, bedstraw, coachweed, cleaverwort, goose's hair, gosling weed, hedge-burrs, clabber grass, milk sweet, poor Robin, stick-a-back, sweethearts, scratchweed, barweed, hedgeheriff, hariff, hayriffe, hayruff, hay reve, eriff, scratweed, mutton chops, Robin-run-in-the-grass, everlasting friendship, loveman.

DESCRIPTION: The long stems of this climbing plant sprawl over the ground and other plants, reaching heights of 4–6 feet (1.2–1.8 m). Both leaves and stem have fine hairs tipped with tiny hooks, making them cling to clothes and fur. The bristle-covered fruit (burrs) will latch on (cleave) to animals who brush past, hence its names *cleavers* and *catchweed*.

PROPERTIES AND USES: Use leaves for an infusion to treat sunburn and a tea for insomnia. In France, the plant is crushed and used as a poultice for blisters and sores. Herbalists have long regarded cleavers as a valuable lymphatic tonic and diuretic. A tea made from cleavers can be used as a skin wash to improve the complexion and to treat skin disorders, minor cuts and scrapes. The tea can also be put to good use as a hair rinse to help combat dandruff.

HISTORY: Seeds have been found in Neolithic settlements, and in times past the herb was used to curdle milk into cheese. Over the centuries used for skin conditions, internal and external ulcers, wounds and as a diuretic for bladder problems. Culpeper noted, '*It is under the dominion of the Moon. The juice of the herb and the seed together taken in wine, help those bitten with an adder, by preserving the heart from the venom. It is familiarly taken in broth, to keep them lean and lank that are apt to grow fat.*'

Making Cheese

Galium is derived from the Greek word for milk, relating to the fact that the plant has the ability to curdle milk, which was beneficial in the making of cheese. The specific name of the plant, *aparine*, also refers to its habit of 'catching', being derived from the Latin *aparare*. Loveman and everlasting friendship are Anglicized versions of *philanthropon*, its Greek name. It was often collected for feeding to poultry, and horses, cows and sheep will also eat it with relish.

CLOWN'S WOUNDWORT

STACHYS PALUSTRIS
Family Lamiaceae/Labiatae, Mint

OTHER NAMES: Also known as woundwort, marsh woundwort, clown heal, hedge nettle, downy woundwort, swine's beads, swine's arnit, marsh betony.

DESCRIPTION: An invasive perennial, it reaches 22–32 inches (56–81 cm) in height. It has velvety leaves and there are spikes of pink/purple hooded flowers.

PROPERTIES AND USES:
The green parts have been used in poultices to stem bleeding for centuries. The young shoots can be cooked like asparagus, and the tubers are also edible when cooked. The bulb-like swellings at the ends of the rhizomes were boiled, dried and used in making bread.

HISTORY: Culpeper noted: '*It is singularly effectual in fresh and green wounds, and therefore bears not the name for nought: And is very available in staunching of blood, to dry up the fluxes of humours in old fretting ulcers, cancers, &c. that hinder the healing of them. A syrup made of the juice of it is inferior to none for inward wounds, ruptures of veins, bloody flux, vessel broken, spitting, pissing, or vomiting blood: rupture are excellently and speedily, even to admiration, cure by taking now and then a little of the syrup, and applying an ointment or plaster of the same to the place; and also if any vein be swelled, or muscle cut, apply a plaster of this herb to it, and, if you add a little comfrey to it, it will not do amiss: I assure you this herb deserves commendation, though it have gotten but a clownish name; and whoever reads this, if he try it as I have done, will commend it as well as me, it is of an earthly nature.*' Pigs love the roots, thus the names swine's beads and arnit (earth-nut).

Curing Grievous Wounds

John Gerard, in his 1597 *Great Herbal*, tells us that he was in Kent, visiting a patient, when he heard of a farm worker who had cut himself severely with a scythe. The labourer had bound all-heal, bruised with grease and '*laid upon in manner of a poultice*', over the wound, which healed in a week, though it would '*have required forty days with balsam itself…I saw the wound and offered to heal the same for charity, which he refused, saying I could not heal it so well as himself – a clownish answer, I confess, without any thanks for my good-will: whereupon I have named it "Clown's Woundwort."'* Gerard himself realized the herb's use and according to his own account, afterwards '*cured many grievous wounds, and some mortal with the same herb*'.

CLUBMOSS

LYCOPODIUM CLAVATUM
Family Lycopodiaceae, Clubmoss

COMMON NAMES: Wolf's claw, wolfpaw clubmoss, stag's horn moss, stagshorn clubmoss, vegetable sulphur, selago, foxtail clubmoss, foxtail, common clubmoss, running clubmoss, running ground-pine, groundpine, running pine, running moss, princess pine, *muscus terrestris repens* (Grieve).

DESCRIPTION: Clubmoss is usually ground-creeping, and often inhabits moist places, with stems up to 10 feet (3 m) long. The stems are much branched, and densely clothed with small spirally-arranged leaves. The stems superficially resemble small seedlings of coniferous trees. Evolutionarily, it is more advanced than other mosses.

PROPERTIES AND USES:
Traditionally, herbal healers employed the entire plant to relieve muscle cramping, and as a diuretic in kidney and liver complaints. It may have analgesic and antiseptic properties. Today, the only part of the plant used medicinally are the powdered spores by which it reproduces. It promotes healing in wounds, stops bleeding and helps drain tissues of excess fluids. The leaves and stems contain two poisons, lycopodine and clavadine, but the spores are completely non-toxic.

HISTORY: Maud Grieve says: '*the whole plant was used, dried, by ancient physicians as a stomachic and diuretic, mainly in calculous and other kidney complaints; the spores do not appear to have been used alone until the seventeenth century*' for dropsy, diarrhoea, suppression of urine, spasms, hydrophobia, gout, scurvy, rheumatism and as an application to wounds. Native North Americans used the spores as a drying agent for wounds and rashes. It is such a powerful water-repellent that when a hand is coated with the spore powder, it will not become wet when dipped in water, so it has also been used to coat medicine tablets and to dress moulds in iron foundries. Clubmoss is an ingredient in traditional Chinese medicine to treat fever and inflammation. Recently it has been found to contain a substance which appears to shield brain cells from injury and it may be useful in treating strokes, epilepsy and Alzheimer's disease.

Explosive Dust

Its oily, yellow spore dust was known as '*druid's flour*', and was said to be used by the druids and holy men over the centuries. It explodes with a bright flash when thrown onto flames, this effect impressing onlookers, and was used even by 19th-century theatre directors as a stage effect. These reproductive spores, also known as '*vegetable sulphur*' and '*lycopodium powder*', can be explosive if present in the air in sufficient density, and they were used for fireworks and as flash powder in early photography.

COFFEE

COFFEA ARABICA
Family Rubiceae, Madder or Coffee

OTHER NAMES: *Coffea arabica* is a species of coffee indigenous to the mountains of Yemen in the Arabian Peninsula (hence its name), Ethiopia and Sudan. It is also known as the coffee shrub of Arabia, mountain coffee or arabica coffee, and has much less caffeine than other coffee species. It is considered to produce better coffee than the other major commercially grown coffee species, *Coffea canephora* (syn. *robusta*), and is the coffee referred to, and much hated by, Culpeper. Seventy-five per cent of the world's coffee production is of the arabica species.

DESCRIPTION: In the wild, plants grow up to 36 feet (11 m), with open branches and broad, glossy leaves. The white flowers are followed by fruits technically known as drupes, but which are commonly called coffee berries. These bright red to purple drupes each contain two seeds, wrongly called coffee 'beans'.

PROPERTIES AND USES: Global consumption of caffeine has been estimated at 120,000 tonnes per year, making it the world's most popular psychoactive substance. This amounts to one serving of a caffeinated beverage, usually coffee, for every person on Earth every day. Caffeine is a central nervous system and metabolic stimulant, and is used both recreationally and medically to reduce physical fatigue and restore mental alertness when unusual weakness or drowsiness occurs. Research is contradictory on health benefits, but some studies suggest that coffee consumption

Coffeehouse Culture

A coffeehouse or coffee shop is called a *café* in France or Portugal, and a *cafeteria* or *café* in Spain. In Italy they are *caffetterias*, and *Kaffeehausen* in Germany. They first spread across the Ottoman Empire, but in Mecca they were banned (along with coffee) by the imams between 1512 and 1524 because they became a centre for political gatherings. In 1530 the first coffee house was opened in Damascus, Syria and soon after coffeehouses had spread to Cairo. The Turkish chronicler Ibrahim Peçevi reported the opening of the first known coffeehouse in Istanbul in 1555. In the 17th century, coffee appeared for the first time in Europe outside the Ottoman Empire, and coffeehouses were rapidly established. The first coffeehouse in England was set up in Oxford in 1650 in a building now known as 'The Grand Café'. In Germany women were allowed to frequent *Kaffeehausen*, but in England and France they were banned from using them.

There's an Awful Lot of Coffee...

Brazil is the world's largest producer of coffee beans with an estimated 2.6 million tonnes being produced per annum (2006 figures). Thousands of square miles of rainforest have been lost for its cultivation. It is surprisingly followed by Vietnam (0.85mmt), then more predictably comes Colombia (0.70mmt) and Indonesia (0.65mmt). Finland is the highest per capita consumer of coffee in the world, with a yearly average of 26.5 pounds (12 kg) per person. It is followed by eight other Northern European countries: Norway, Iceland, Denmark, Netherlands, Sweden, Switzerland, Belgium and Luxembourg. The UK lies in 47th place with 6.2 pounds (2.8 kg) per year, probably because tea is the more common drink. The USA is surprisingly only in 26th place, despite the preponderance of coffee shops, with 9.3 pounds (4.2 kg). However, it is the greatest consumer by nation, with each coffee drinker consuming an average 3.2 cups per day.

---

reduces the risk of being affected by Alzheimer's disease, Parkinson's disease, heart disease, diabetes mellitus type 2, cirrhosis of the liver, and gout. The presence of antioxidants in coffee has been shown to prevent free radicals from causing cell damage.

HISTORY : *Coffea arabica* was probably the first species of coffee to be cultivated, having been grown in southwest Arabia for well over 1000 years. In legend, human cultivation of coffee began after goats in Ethiopia were seen mounting each other, after eating the leaves and fruits of the coffee tree. The first written record of coffee made from roasted coffee beans comes from Arabian scholars who wrote that it was useful in prolonging their working hours. Culpeper described coffee: '*It is said of itself to be insipid, having neither scent nor taste, but being pounded and baked, as they do prepare it to make the coffee-liquor with it then stinks most loathsomely...the proponents for this filthy drink affirm that it causes watchfulness...they also say that it makes them sober when they are drunk; yet they would always be accounted sober persons, or at least think themselves so, when they can but once sit down in a coffee-house. If there had been any worth in it, some of the ancient Arab physicians, or others near those parts, would have recorded it; but there is no mention made of any medicinal use thereof; neither can it be endowed with any such properties as the indulgers of it feed their fancies with...*'

The first coffeehouse in London opened in 1652 in St Michael's Alley, Cornhill, and by 1675 there were more than 3000 coffeehouses in England. Culpeper's *Herbal* was published in 1653, and he died on 10 January 1654, so we can see the astonishing speed of their growth.

COLTSFOOT

TUSSILAGO FARFARA
Family Asteraceae/Compositae, Sunflower/Daisy

OTHER NAMES: Horsehoof, horsefoot, foal's foot, ass's foot, bullsfoot, hallfoot, fieldhove, coughwort.

DESCRIPTION: The name coltsfoot refers to its hoof-shaped round leaves. The hardy perennial does not flower while it is in leaf, as its large yellow dandelion-like flowers come in early spring.

PROPERTIES AND USES:
'The plant is under Venus. The fresh leaves, or juice, or a syrup made thereof, is good for a hot dry cough, for wheezings and shortness of breath' (Nicholas Culpeper). It has been used to treat asthma and as an expectorant and cough suppressant for thousands of years. Maud Grieve noted that there was a fine coating of hairs on the leaves: *'This felty covering easily rubs off and before the introduction of matches, wrapped in a rag dipped in a solution of saltpetre and dried in the sun, used to be considered an excellent tinder.'*

HISTORY: Pliny recommended that the dried leaves and roots of coltsfoot should be burned and the smoke drawn into the mouth through a reed and swallowed, as a remedy for an obstinate cough, the patient sipping a little wine between each inhalation. To derive the full benefit from it, it had to be burned on cypress charcoal. In 1931, Grieve wrote: *'Coltsfoot has justly been termed "nature's best herb for the lungs and her most eminent thoracic"*...

The leaves are the basis of the British Herb Tobacco, in which Coltsfoot predominates, the other ingredients being Buckbean, Eyebright, Betony, Rosemary, Thyme, Lavender, and Chamomile flowers. This relieves asthma and also the difficult breathing of old bronchitis. Those suffering from asthma, catarrh and other lung troubles derive much benefit from smoking this Herbal Tobacco, the use of which does not entail any of the injurious effects of ordinary tobacco.' A replica of the coltsfoot flower was placed above the door of pharmacies in Paris as an emblem of the effectiveness of their medicine.

Dispelling Coughs

The botanical name *Tussilago* means 'cough dispeller', and the leaf was dried and smoked as a herbal tobacco to ease coughs and asthma, hence the name coughwort. Mrs Grieve writes: *'The specific name of the plant is derived from Farfarus, an ancient name of the White Poplar, the leaves of which present some resemblance in form and colour to those of this plant. An old name for Coltsfoot was Filius ante patrem (the son before the father), because the star-like, golden flowers appear and wither before the broad, sea-green leaves are produced.'*

COMFREY

SYMPHYTUM OFFICINALE
Family Boraginaceae, Borage

OTHER NAMES: Knitbone, boneset, slippery root, blackwort, bruisewort, consound, healing herb, gum plant, knitback, ass ear, miracle herb, wallwort, blackwort, Welsh llysiau'r cwlwm (knot herb).

DESCRIPTION: A hardy perennial which can grow up to 3–4 feet (90–120 cm), with a 3-foot (90-cm) spread, it has hairy, lance-shaped, broad leaves and clusters of white, cream, pink or purple bell-shaped flowers. Its black, turnip-like root is responsible for its folk name of *blackwort*, and the shape of its leaves for the name *ass ear*.

PROPERTIES AND USES: Young leaves were eaten like spinach, and it has been used as a compress for cuts, for varicose veins and for sores on animals. '*Comfrey roots, together with chicory and dandelion roots, are used to make a well-known vegetation "Coffee", that tastes practically the same as ordinary coffee, with none of its injurious effects*' (Grieve). However, internal consumption, such as in the form of herbal tea, is now discouraged for fear of possible liver damage. Comfrey relieves pain and inflammation caused by injuries and degeneration, especially the symptoms of rheumatoid arthritis and osteoarthritis. Comfrey creams and oils can be used in arthritic pain-relieving massages. Research is ongoing into its allantoin content, which stimulates the growth of new cells. This cell proliferant repairs damaged tissue, so comfrey is the best of all herbs for applying to bruises, sprains and fractures. Adding comfrey to the bath water is said to promote a youthful skin.

HISTORY: Dioscorides in *Materia Medica* (*c*.50 CE) prescribed the plant to heal wounds and broken bones. Comfrey has been used for centuries for its bone-mending qualities, for its healing effects on ulcers, and for its general soothing effect on the mucous membranes, making it invaluable in soothing sore throats and coughs. *Symphytum* comes from the Greek word *symphyo* meaning to unite, and comfrey is believed to come from Latin *confera* – knitting together. Comfrey is believed to have been brought to Europe by the Crusaders. '*This is an herb of Saturn, and I suppose under the sign Capricorn, cold, dry, and earthy in quality... the root boiled in water or wine, and the decoction drunk, helpeth all inward hurts, bruises, and wounds, and the ulcers of the lungs, causing the phlegm that oppresseth them to be easily spit forth*' (Culpeper). Carrying the herb, especially if it was placed in the shoe, was supposed to ensure safety while travelling.

COMPANION HERBS

COMPANION PLANTING PRINCIPLES

Beneficial Habitats: Some plants provide a beneficial environment for predatory and parasitic species of insect which help to keep pest populations in check. Predators include ladybirds, lacewings, hoverflies, spiders and predatory mites.

Biochemical Pest Suppression: Some plants exude chemicals from roots or aerial parts that suppress or repel pests, protecting neighbouring plants. For example, the African marigold releases *thiophene* – a nematode repellent – which makes it a good companion for certain garden crops. Also, if you use rye as mulch, its leached allelochemicals prevent weed germination but do not harm transplanted tomatoes, broccoli, or many other vegetables.

Nurse Cropping: Tall or densely canopied plants can protect more vulnerable species through shading or by forming a windbreak. 'Nurse crops', for example oats, are used to help establish alfalfa and other forage plants by supplanting the more competitive weeds that would otherwise grow in their place.

Security Through Diversity: A greater mixture of various crops and varieties provides some security to the grower. If pests or adverse conditions reduce or destroy a single crop or cultivar, others remain to produce a level of yield.

Spatial Interactions: Tall-growing, sun-loving plants may share space with lower-growing, shade-tolerant species, resulting in higher total production. This type of planting can also yield pest control benefits.

Symbiotic Nitrogen Fixation: Legumes, such as peas, beans and clover, have the ability to 'fix' atmospheric nitrogen for their own use and for the benefit of neighbouring plants, via a symbiotic relationship with *Rhizobium* bacteria. Forage legumes are commonly seeded with grasses to reduce the need for nitrogen fertilizer. Similarly, beans are sometimes interplanted with corn.

Trap Cropping: A neighbouring crop may be selected because it is more attractive to pests, distracting them from attacking the main crop.

COMPANION HERBS

Anise: Grows well with coriander, and together they are a good deterrent for snails and slugs.

Basil: Improves growth and flavour of tomatoes. Indoors it repels houseflies. Do not plant near rue and they do not do well when grown together.

Beebalm: Companion to tomatoes, improves growth and flavour.

Borage: Companion to tomatoes, squash and strawberries; deters tomato worms; attracts bees.

Caraway: Improves the growth and flavour of peas, and loosens heavy soil.

Catnip: Plant in borders; deters flea beetles.

Chamomile: Companion to cabbage and onions, improving growth and flavour.

Repels flying insects. Chamomile tea is good for plants as well as people.

Chervil: Companion to radishes, making them hotter and crisper.

Chives: Plant near carrots, roses and apples to make them grow and taste better, preventing scab and black spot.

Comfrey: 'Plant healer' – an excellent garden barrier plant.

Coriander: General and anise, attracting bees and improving flavour.

Dill: Helps corn, lettuce, cucumber, carrots and tomatoes. Attracts hoverflies.

Fennel: General, and attracts hoverflies.

Flax: Protects potatoes against Colorado potato beetle, and improves clay or heavy soil.

French marigold: Plant near tomatoes to repel whitefly.

Garlic: Plant near roses and raspberries, and throughout the garden or vegetable plot to deter beetles.

Horehound: Repels grasshoppers. Improves fruit yield on tomatoes.

Horseradish: Plant at corner of potato patch to deter potato pests.

Hyssop: Companion to cabbage and grapes, deters cabbage moth, but keep away from radishes. Improves the yield from grape crops.

Lavender: Attracts butterflies and bees love it, repels rabbits, mice, ticks, moths and mosquitoes.

Lemon balm: Plant with cucumbers and tomatoes.

Lemon verbena: Repels midges, flies and other pests.

Lovage: Improves the health of all nearby plants, especially beans and sweet peppers.

Marjoram: Companion to sweet peppers and sage.

Mint: Companion to tomatoes and cabbage, deters cabbage moths, grubs, mice and flies.

Nasturtium: Companion to radishes, brassicas, apple, broad beans, tomatoes and cucumbers. Repels aphids, whitefly and ants, and attracts blackfly to itself.

Nettle: Plant with angelica to control blackfly and improve soil content.

Parsley: Good for chives, tomatoes, carrots, roses and asparagus.

Pennyroyal: General planting as it repels ants.

Rosemary: Plant near cabbage, beans, carrots, sage. It deters cabbage moths, bean beetles, carrot flies,

Rue: Good with roses and raspberries. Disliked by cats and dogs, it is incompatible with sage, basil and cabbage.

Sage: Good with tomatoes, carrots, vines, cabbage, cabbage and rosemary, repelling cabbage white butterfly and many other flying insects.

Santolina: Good with roses.

Southernwood: Companion to cabbage and deters cabbage moth.

Summer savory: Companion to onions and beans, attracts bees and deters bean beetles.

Thyme: Good for most other herbs and vegetables, particularly aubergines and cabbage.

Valerian: Stimulates growth of all other plants and vegetables in the vicinity; it attracts earthworms.

Yarrow: Invigorating to cucumbers, corn and other herbs, enhances essential oil production.

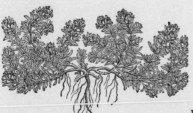

CORIANDER

CORIANDRUM SATIVUM
Family Apiaceae/Umbelliferae, Carrot

OTHER NAMES: Cilantro, Chinese parsley, Greek parsley, Japanese parsley, Arab parsley.

DESCRIPTION: It grows to a height of around 24 inches (60 cm) and a spread of 9 inches (23 cm), and has pale mauve to white flowers followed by round seeds which have a spicy orange flavour. The leaves are finely cut, aromatic with a unique spicy taste, extremely popular in Indian cuisine.

PROPERTIES AND USES: Coriander is a digestive stimulant, helping with the absorption of nutrients, and has recently been studied for its cholesterol-lowering effects and use in type-2 diabetes. Health disorders such as Alzheimer's disease, diabetes and fibromyalgia have been linked to high levels of heavy metals such as mercury, lead and aluminium in the body. Scientific studies and anecdotal evidence support coriander's reputation as a purifying purgative. A New York doctor reported that after finding he had been heavily exposed to mercury, he discovered that when taken in a lightly cooked form it causes a massive excretion of mercury via his urine. Herbalists such as Culpeper recommended the seeds as a remedy for worms and in the treatment of sickness and sluggish digestion. They were also used to disguise unpleasant tastes and chewed to counter bad breath. Coriander was employed in poultices to treat inflammation and swellings. The small ball-shaped seeds are used to flavour gin and wheat beers. Seeds lose flavour quickly when ground, so grind just before using. They lose their disagreeable scent on drying and become fragrant, being used in pot-pourris. Culpeper wrote: *'The green herb coriander being boiled with crumbs of white bread, or barley meal, consumes and drives away hot tumours, swellings, and inflammations; and with bean-meal, it dissolves the King's Evil* [scrofula, tuberculosis of the neck], *hard knobs, and worms; the juice applied with ceruse* [a poisonous white pigment containing lead], *litharge of silver* [a form

---

Drunken Plant

This author was puzzling why the old Welsh word for coriander, *brwysgedlys*, meant drunken plant. However, coriander seeds can have a narcotic effect when consumed in quantity, which is probably how it became to be known as *'dizzycorn'* among early American colonists. Perhaps that is the answer.

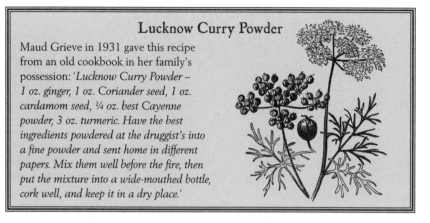

Lucknow Curry Powder

Maud Grieve in 1931 gave this recipe from an old cookbook in her family's possession: *'Lucknow Curry Powder – 1 oz. ginger, 1 oz. Coriander seed, 1 oz. cardamom seed, ¼ oz. best Cayenne powder, 3 oz. turmeric. Have the best ingredients powdered at the druggist's into a fine powder and sent home in different papers. Mix them well before the fire, then put the mixture into a wide-mouthed bottle, cork well, and keep it in a dry place.'*

of lead oxide which is a by-product when separating silver from lead], *vinegar, and oil of roses, cures St Anthony's Fire* [ergotism or erysipelas], *and assuages and eases the pains of all inflammations.'* Thai research has shown that coriander has an excellent antibacterial effect against the food-poisoning bacteria *Campylobacter*.

HISTORY: Hippocrates and other Greek physicians recommended it, and its name *Coriandrum* is derived from *koriannon* (a bug or bedbug), in reference to the foetid smell of the leaves. Culpeper calls it a *'stinking plant'*. It has been found in Neolithic settlements in Israel. Five thousand years ago, coriander seeds from the Mediterranean were being carried along the Silk Road in the caravanserai to enrich the cuisine of China. Cilantro is mentioned in the *Medical Papyrus of Thebes* (1552 BCE) and is one of the plants which grew in the Hanging Gardens of Babylon. The Hebrews used coriander to flavour cakes and it plays a role in Jewish ritual as one of the *'bitter herbs'* prescribed at the Feast of the Passover. It is often mentioned in the Bible: *'And the house of Israel called the name thereof Manna: and it was like Coriander seed, white'* (Exodus, 16:31). Egyptian mourners placed jars of coriander in Tutankhamen's tomb to accompany his spirit to the Land of the Dead. Roman soldiers used coriander as a meat preservative and to flavour food. Chinese dined on the plant in the hope of making themselves immortal. Coriander was thought to have been brought to Britain by the Romans, but seeds imported from the Mediterranean have been found in Bronze Age huts. In medieval times it became an aphrodisiac ingredient in love potions, being referred to as such in *The Arabian Nights*. The herb is believed to have been one of the earliest plantings in North America, in 1670 in Massachusetts. Coated in sugar, coriander seeds were eaten as a pink and white sweet, known as *'coriander comfit'* and later referred to as 'sugarplums', as in the famous 19th-century poem 'The Night Before Christmas' *'…The children were nestled all snug in their beds, While visions of sugarplums danced in their heads'*. The confection offered a sweet start and then a spicy burst of flavour.

CORNFLOWER

CENTAUREA CYANUS
Family Asteraceae, Daisy

OTHER NAMES: Culpeper calls it *Blue-Bottle:* '*It is also called Cyanus, I suppose from the colour of it; Hurt-Sickle, because it turns the edge of the sickles that reap the corn; Blue-Blow, Corn-Flower and Blue-Bottle.*' Bachelor's buttons, ragged sailor, corn bluebottle, sultan's flower.

DESCRIPTION: A hardy annual, growing to 2 feet (60 cm), with pretty single and double blue flowers and lanced leaves.

PROPERTIES AND USES:
Flowers are edible as a tonic and stimulant, and can be dried. It has been used for conjunctivitis and corneal ulcers. Culpeper wrote: '*As they are naturally cold, dry, and binding, so they are under the dominion of Saturn. The powder or dried leaves of the Blue-bottle, or Corn-flower, is given with good success to those that are bruised by a fall, or have broken a vein inwardly, and void much blood at the mouth; being taken in the water of Plantain, Horsetail, or the greater Comfrey, it is a remedy against the poison of the Scorpion, and resists all venoms and poisons. The seed or leaves taken in wine, is very good against the plague, and all infectious diseases, and is very good in pestilential fevers. The juice put into fresh or green wounds, doth quickly solder up the lips of them together, and is very effectual to heal all ulcers and sores in the mouth. The juice dropped into the eyes takes away the heat and inflammation of them. The distilled water of this herb, has the same properties, and may be used for the effects aforesaid.*'

HISTORY: Juice from the petals made blue ink and watercolour pigments. The colour 'cornflower blue' is named after this bright plant. A shade of azure, it replicates the hue of the cornflower, one of the few 'blue' flowers that are truly blue, most 'blue' flowers being a darker blue-purple. Its pigment structure is unlike that of any other blue flower. The French eyewash known as *Eau de Casselunettes* was made from cornflowers because of their eye-brightening properties. In the past it often grew as a weed in crop fields, hence its name of cornflower, because fields growing grains such as wheat, barley, rye or oats are generally known as 'corn fields' in Britain. Its slim stems were so tough that they could make sickles blunt. It almost became extinct across Europe as a result of pesticidal weed control in the 1970s.

Worn in Memory

In France, cornflower is the symbol of the 11 November 1918 Armistice, as like poppies, it was endemic in the cornfields of Flanders. Thus it is worn on Armistice Day.

COTTON LAVENDER
SANTOLINA CHAMAECYPARISSUS
Family Asteraceae/Compositae, Daisy, Sunflower

OTHER NAMES: Culpeper calls it Lavender cotton. Grey santolina.

DESCRIPTION: It is not a true lavender at all, but has yellow, clustered buttons of composite flowers and finely cut, grey, scented leaves, the odour of which somewhat resembles chamomile. The evergreen ornamental herb grows to about 2 feet (60 cm) tall and its flowers have an unpleasant smell. The bruised leaves can cause a severe rash on sensitive skins.

PROPERTIES AND USES: The Arabs were said to use the juice of this plant for bathing the eyes. Culpeper: '*It is under the dominion of Mercury. It resists poison, putrefaction, and heals the biting of venomous beasts. A dram of the powder of the dried leaves taken every morning fasting, stops the running of the reins in men, and whites in women. The seed beaten into powder, and taken as worm-seed, kills the worms, not only in children, but also in people of riper years; the like doth the herb itself, being steeped in milk, and the milk drank; the body bathed with the decoction of it, helps scabs and itch.*' Maud Grieve states: '*It is used as a vermifuge for children. This plant was once also esteemed for its stimulant properties, and the twigs have been used for placing amongst linen, etc., to keep away moths.*' Cotton lavender is versatile in that it can be used as an edging plant, a ground cover, an addition to a rock garden or a herb garden, spreading like a silvery carpet close to the ground. The plant repels various insect pests, especially cabbage moths.

HISTORY: The charity Plants for a Future recently reported: '*The leaves and flowering tops are antispasmodic, disinfectant, emmenagogue* [stimulating blood flow in the pelvic region], *stimulant and vermifuge. Cotton lavender is rarely used medicinally, though it is sometimes used internally as a vermifuge for children and to treat poor digestion and menstrual problems. When finely ground and applied to insect stings or bites, the plant will immediately ease the pain. Applied to surface wounds, it will hasten the healing process by encouraging the formation of scar tissue. The leaves and flowering stems are harvested in the summer and dried for later use.*'

Keeping Moths Away

The foliage can be used as a moth repellent either stuffed in sachets or hung in small bunches. The flowers can be dried as everlastings, and the fresh foliage and flowers can be used in cut flower arrangements. The dried leaves are used in pot-pourris and to distil an essential oil for perfumery.

COUCH GRASS

ELYTRIGIA REPENS
Family Poaceae, Grass

OTHER NAMES: Twitch grass, witchgrass, dog's grass, scutch, quick grass, quack grass, wheat grass, cough grass, cutch, quitchgrass, quake grass, chandler's grass, Scotch quelch, devil's grass, spear grass.

DESCRIPTION: Slender-leaved perennial grass with erect spikes similar in appearance to wheat bearing two rows of flowers. The plant has a long creeping underground stem (rhizome) system and so it has been planted in sand dunes near the coast to bind the soil together. Its names of couch and quickgrass come from the Old English *cwice*, meaning *alive*, referring to its vigorous growth.

PROPERTIES AND USES: Couch grass is a cursed by gardeners, considered an invasive weed, and is very hard to remove. Culpeper wrote: *'The dog's grass is under the dominion of Jupiter, and is the most medicinal of all the quick grasses. The roots of it act powerfully by urine; they should be dried and powdered, for the decoction by water is too strong for tender stomachs, therefore should be sparingly used when given that way to children to destroy the worms. The way of use is to bruise the roots, and having well boiled them in white wine, drink the decoction; it is opening, not purging, very safe: it is a remedy against all diseases coming of stopping, and such are half those that are incident to the body of man; and although a gardener be of another opinion, yet a physician holds half an acre of them to be worth five acres of carrots twice told over.'* Couch grass was valued by herbalists for its mucilage-rich rhizome. A tea made from the roots is used for treating urinary infections because of its antibiotic and diuretic properties. Couch grass tea will also soothe and coat an inflamed throat, hence the name cough grass.

HISTORY: Couch grass has been used in herbal medicine since classical Greek times. The Romans used it to treat kidney stones and urinary problems. The dried rhizomes of couch grass were used as incense in medieval Northern Europe where other resin-based types of incense were unavailable.

Animal Health

The common name dog grass comes from the fact that sick dogs will dig up the root and eat it. Horses and cats also eat it, possibly to rid themselves of worms. It was renowned as a vermifuge, killing worms in children. In 1694, John Pechey wrote: *'Silvius says, that Sheep and Oxen that are troubled with the stone in the wintertime are freed from it in the Spring by eating Grass.'*

COW PARSLEY

ANTHRISCUS SYLVESTRIS
Family Apiaceae/Umbelliferae, Carrot/Parsley

OTHER NAMES: Culpeper calls this *wild chervil*. Chervil is the cultivated version of this plant. Devil's parsley, devil's meat, wild beaked parsley, keck, cow mumble (Suffolk), rabbit meat (Sussex), cow-weed. It is known as Queen Anne's lace in Britain, but *Daucus carota* has that name in the USA.

DESCRIPTION: Grows up to 4 feet (1.2 m), with hollow furrowed stems and heads of small (usually) white scented flowers. It is prolific along country lanes, with a froth of white flowers in spring. Because it is easily mistaken for the poisonous hemlock and fool's parsley, it is nicknamed devils' parsley, but its leaves are edible, having a mild aniseed flavour.

PROPERTIES AND USES: It is eaten by rabbits, pigs, sheep and cattle, hence its name. It can be harvested all year round for salads, potato soups and chervil sauce as it self-seeds. Cow parsley and its cousin chervil are both made into tisanes and infusions. The tea is used to treat water retention, stomach upsets and some forms of skin eruption and is said to promote wound healing. Cow parsley is rumoured to be a natural mosquito repellent when applied directly to the skin. Until recently, a strong infusion was used for treating laminitis in horses.

HISTORY: In the Outer Hebrides, the flowering tips were harvested for the yellow-green dye used in making Harris Tweed. In Dutch it is called *'whistle herb'*, and in Britain children used to make whistles out of the dried stalks, known in places as *'kecks'*. Culpeper wrote: *'The wild Chervil bruised and applied, dissolves swellings in any part, or the marks of congealed blood by bruises or blows, in a little space.'* Cow parsley is one of the three or four plants described as *'breaking your mother's heart'*, possibly because the tiny white blossoms drop quickly. In the days when mothers had to clean carpets by hand and floors by sweeping, it was just another time-consuming chore.

Traditional Dye

Traditional Harris Tweed has flecks of colour achieved by vegetable dyes, such as yellow from cow parsley or bracken roots, orange from ragweed, green from heather or stinging nettle, red or purple-brown from lichens or roots of lady's bedstraw, purple from elderberries etc. It is no longer imbued with the traditional mordant used to fix the natural vegetable dyes that give the wool its vivid earth tones: the urine of the weavers and their families, which they collected in their crofts.

COWSLIP

PRIMULA VERIS
Family Primulaceae, Primrose

OTHER NAMES: Herb Peter, St Peter's keys, Our Lady's bunch of keys, Our Lady's keys, key of Heaven, key flower, galligaskins, paigles, palsywort, briallu mawr (Welsh for large primroses), fairy cups, palsy flower, palsywort, mayflower, drelip, cuy lippe, peggle, petty mulleins, crewel, buckles, plumrocks, password, arthritica, paralysis, cow flops, golden drops, freckled face. Peagles (Culpeper).

DESCRIPTION: A very pretty, delicately scented flower that has been over picked in the past, this hardy perennial grows to 8 inches (20 cm), with pretty clusters of small, vivid yellow flowers borne on erect stalks. A plant originally of meadows, cowslips are becoming more common, especially alongside motorways, because roadside verges are rarely sprayed with pesticides.

PROPERTIES AND USES: Herbalists used cowslips as a remedy for paralysis and for many other nervous afflictions. Today the root and flower are used internally as a relaxant or sedative and as a general tonic. Cowslips can be a helpful decongestant for colds, and are anti-inflammatory, being used to treat arthritis and gout. Culpeper noted: '*Because they strengthen the brain and nerves, and remedy the palsies, the Greeks gave them the name of paralysis. The flowers preserved or conserves, and the same quantity of a nutmeg eaten each morning, is a sufficient does for inward diseases; but for wounds, spots and sun-burning, an ointment is made of the leaves and hog's grease.*' The leaves can also be used for healing wounds. Both the flowers and leaves often used to be eaten, young cowslip leaves being eaten in salads or mixed with other herbs to stuff meat.

HISTORY: According to legend, St Peter dropped the keys to Heaven and where they landed cowslips grew. Its single flower stalk, with its head of drooping golden bells, was thought to resemble a set of keys. Cowslips have also been used for hundreds of years to treat spasms, cramps, rheumatic pain and paralysis, and it used to be called *palsywort* for this reason. It has been used since ancient times to make wine, mead, jam, tea and ointments. In the 18th century, powdered roots boiled in ale were used for treating giddiness and nervous ailments. Cowslips used to be popular in Elizabethan knot gardens. Cowslips are believed to be the favourite flower of nightingales, which were said only to frequent places where cowslips grew (often pastures where cattle had been grazing). Girls once made balls of cowslips, '*totsies*', which they threw in the air to try and divine the identity of their future husbands.

CUBEB

PIPER CUBEBA
Family Piperaceae, Pepper

OTHER NAMES: Long-tailed pepper, tailed pepper.

DESCRIPTION: A climbing perennial, extensively grown in coffee plantations, well shaded and supported by the coffee trees. The unripe fruits are gathered, dried and look similar to black pepper, but with stalks attached, the 'tails' referred to in 'tailed pepper'. They taste like a cross between allspice and black pepper.

PROPERTIES AND USES: Culpeper: '*Cubebs …of a hot taste, but not so fiery as pepper; and having each a short stalk on them like a tail: these grow on trees less than apple-trees, with leaves narrower than those of pepper; the flower is sweet, and the fruit grows clustering together. The Arabians call them quabebe, and quabebe chini; they grow plentifully in Java: they are used to stir up venery, and to warm and strengthen the stomach, being overcome with phlegm or wind; they cleanse the breast of thick tough humours, help the spleen, and are very profitable for the cold griefs of the womb. Being chewed in the mouth with mastic, they draw rheum from the head, and strengthen the brain and memory.*'

HISTORY: In John Parkinson's *Theatrum Botanicum*, we read that the king of Portugal in 1640 banned the sale of cubebs in order to promote the black pepper *(Piper nigrum)* trade, which the Portuguese dominated. Cubeb was probably brought into Europe by the Arabians as a pepper. Grieve lists it as a '*stimulant, carminative, much used as a remedy for gonorrhoea, after the first active inflammatory symptoms have subsided; also used in leucorrhoea, cystitis, urethritis, abscesses of the prostate gland, piles and chronic bronchitis.*' The Javanese growers protected their monopoly by scalding the berries to sterilize them. It was used as an incense to ward off demons.

Remedy For Infertility

In *The Book of One Thousand and One Nights* cubeb is a main ingredient in making an aphrodisiac remedy for infertility: '*He took two ounces of Chinese cubebs, one ounce of fat extract of Ionian hemp, one ounce of fresh cloves, one ounce of red cinnamon from Sarandib, ten drachms of white Malabar cardamoms, five of Indian ginger, five of white pepper, five of pimento from the isles, one ounce of the berries of Indian star-anise, and half an ounce of mountain thyme. Then he mixed cunningly, after having pounded and sieved them; he added pure honey until the whole became a thick paste; then he mingled five grains of musk and an ounce of pounded fish roe with the rest. Finally he added a little concentrated rose-water and put all in the bowl.*'

CUCKOO-PINT

ARUM MACULATUM
Family Araceae, Arum

OTHER NAMES: Culpeper calls it *Cuckow-Point* and *Spotted Wake-Robin*: '*It is also called Aaron, Janus, and Barba-Aron, Calves-Foot, Ramp, Starch-Wort, Cuckow-Pintle, Priest's-Pintle and Wake-Robin.*' Wild arum, Jack in the pulpit, devils and angels (and angels and devils), Adam and Eve, bobbins, naked boys, wake, adder's root, adder's meat, friar's cowl, parson and clerk, quaker, kings and queens, Aaron's leek, starch-root and starchwort.

DESCRIPTION: Very common, it is unmistakeable in hedgerows, with the tiny flowers borne on a poker-shaped purple inflorescence called a spadix. The spadix is partially enclosed in a pale green spathe or leaf-like hood. In autumn the lower ring of (female) flowers forms a cluster of bright orange, poisonous berries which remain after the spathe and other leaves have withered away.

PROPERTIES AND USES: All parts are toxic, but Culpeper recorded that it could be '*a most present and sure remedy for poison and the plague...The green leaves bruised, and laid upon any boil or plague-sore, do very wonderfully help to draw forth the poison...it breaks, digests, and rids away phlegm from the stomach, chest, and lungs;...provokes urine, and brings down women's courses, and purges them effectually after child-bearing, to bring away the after-birth: taken with sheep's milk, it heals the inward ulcers of the bowels...A spoonful taken at a time heals the itch; and an ounce or more, taken at a time for some days together, doth help the rupture; the leaves, either green or dry, or the juice of them, doth cleanse all manner of rotten and filthy ulcers, in whatsoever part of the body, and heals the stinking sores in the nose, called polypus... the country people about Maidstone in Kent use the herb and root, instead of soap.*' Culpeper also recommended plant preparations for eye lotions, bruises, piles, gout, scurf, freckles, spots and blemishes.

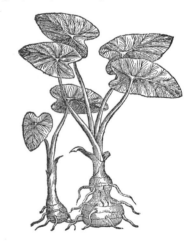

HISTORY: Carvings have been found on Egyptian walls and it was mentioned by Theophrastus and Pliny the Elder. It was believed to resuscitate bears from hibernation and to protect humans from snake bite. It has been used in 'magic' to get rid of unwelcome guests, and as a symbol of sexual intercourse in art. The starch of the root, after repeated washing, was sold as food under the name of Portland sago, or Portland arrowroot. When ground, it was used like *salop* or *saleo*, a working class drink popular before the introduction of tea or coffee. However, unless prepared correctly arum can be extremely toxic. Arum starch was used for stiffening ruffs in Elizabethan times, and Gerard says: '*The most pure and white starch is made of the roots of the Cuckoo-pint, but most hurtful for the hands of the laundresses that have the handling of it, for it chaps, blisters, and makes the hands rough and rugged and withall smarting.*' The starch was sold in Paris as '*Cyprus Powder*', a cosmetic for the skin. Presumably ladies of the time believed in the '*no pain, no gain*' principle as it must have stung and irritated. Robert Hogg, in his 1858 *Vegetable Kingdom*, reported its use in Italy to remove freckles from the face and hands.

Willy Lilly

The *pint* or *pintle* refers to the male organ, from the Middle English *pintel*, similar to Middle Low German *pint* meaning penis, and Old English *pinn*. It is pronounced to rhyme with mint, not pint. The hooded green cowl embracing an upright purple poker has such sexual symbolism that many of the 100+ common names for it are sexual in nature. *Pintle*, *pint* and *point* are all derived from the Anglo-Saxon word for penis, cuckoo from *cucu* meaning lively, and *robin* from the French for penis. The dog's type names are equally obvious in their phallic reference. *Stallions and mares, bulls and cows, lords and ladies, boys and girls, dog bobbins, dog cocks, dog's dick, dogs dibble, dog's spear, English passionflower, naked ladies* and *Willy Lilly* all allude to its male/female nature. Its '*pint*', the large phallic spadix (club) of the arum, does not rot and turn foetid, as noted in some accounts. It can raise its temperature to an amazing

57° F (14° C) above the surrounding environment, to the extent that the warmth is easily discernible to the touch. This heat volatizes a foul-smelling chemical, which attracts dung-feeding insects. Its pollen also causes the flower heads to glow at night to attract insects, giving it the name of *fairy lamp* in some areas. Using odour and light, it traps flies in its bulbous leaf bract to aid pollination. These insects are often 'owl midges', tiny, fluffy 'moth flies', family Psychodidae, of which there are 73 species. They alight on the oily hood, lose their foothold and fall into the bulb where they are trapped by a ring of downward-pointing hairs. They become dusted with pollen from male flowers, and trying to escape, transfer it to female flowers. After pollination, the ring of hairs wilts, the spathe loosens and some pollen-covered insects can escape to pollinate other arums.

CUCUMBER

CUCUMIS SATIVUS
Family Cucurbitaceae, Gourd

OTHER NAMES: *'According to the pronunciation of the vulgar, cowcumbers.'* (Culpeper).

DESCRIPTION: This familiar creeping vine roots in the ground and grows up supports, wrapping them with thin, spiralling tendrils. Large leaves form a canopy over the cylindrical green fruit, which can grow up to 20 inches (50 cm) long. Although regarded as a vegetable, it is a fruit, either grown to be eaten fresh *(slicers)* or intended for pickling *(picklers)*. Cucumbers usually contain over 90 per cent water.

PROPERTIES AND USES: Culpeper wrote: *'There is no dispute to be made, but that they are under the dominion of the Moon, though they are so much rejected for their coldness; it is by some affirmed, that if they were but one degree colder they would be poison. The best of Galenists hold them to be cold and moist but in the second degree, and then not so hot as either lettuce or purslain: they are excellent good for hot stomachs and livers; the immeasurable use of them fills the body full of raw humours, and so indeed does anything else when used to an excess. The juice of cucumbers, the face being washed with it, cleanses the skin, and is excellent good for hot rheums in the eyes; the seed is excellent to provoke urine, and cleanse the passages thereof when they are stopped; neither do I think there is a better remedy for ulcers in the bladder than cucumbers; the usual course is to use the seeds in emulsions, as they make almond milk, but a far better way by far (in my opinion) is this; when the season of the year is, take the cucumbers and bruise them well, and distil the water from them, and let such as are troubled with ulcers in their bladder drink no other drink. The face being washed with the same water, be it never so red, will be benefited by it, and the complexion very much improved. It is also excellent good for sunburning, freckles, and morphew.'*

Morphew is a skin eruption of blisters caused by scurvy. Some Englishmen in the 17th century were convinced that eating cucumbers would be fatal, although lying on a bed of cucumbers could be a cure for fever. In the later 17th century, a prejudice developed against uncooked vegetables and fruits. A number of articles in contemporary health publications state that uncooked plants brought on summer diseases, and should be forbidden to children. The cucumber acquired a reputation as: *'fit only for consumption by cows'*, which some believe is why it gained the name 'cowcumber'. Samuel Pepys wrote in his diary on 22 September 1663: *'this day Sir W. Batten tells me that Mr.*

Newhouse is dead of eating cowcumbers, of
which the other day I heard of another,
I think.'

HISTORY : Cucumber is one of the
oldest foods, having been gathered and
possibly cultivated as long ago as 9750
BCE in Southeast Asia. It is listed among
the foods of ancient Ur and the *Legend
of Gilgamesh* describes people eating
cucumbers. Cleopatra used to have her
legendarily beautiful skin rubbed with
cooked cucumber peelings. According
to Pliny the Elder, the Emperor Tiberius
ordered the cucumber on his table daily.
Roman gardeners reportedly used artificial
methods (similar to the greenhouse
system) to meet his demand. To quote
Pliny, '*It was a wonderful favourite with the
Emperor Tiberius, and, indeed he was never
without it; for he had raised beds made in
frames upon wheels, by means of which the*
cucumbers were moved and exposed to the
full heat of the sun; while, in winter, they
were withdrawn, and placed under the
protection of frames glazed with mirrorstone.
We find it stated, also, by the ancient Greek
writers, that the cucumber ought to be
propagated from seed that has been steeped
a couple of days in milk and honey, this
method having the effect of rendering them
all the sweeter to the taste.'* Reportedly, they
were also cultivated in 'cucumber houses'
glazed with oiled cloth and known as
'*specularia*'. The Romans are reported to
have used cucumbers to treat scorpion
bites, bad eyesight, and to scare away
mice. Records of cucumber cultivation
appear in France in the ninth century in
Charlemagne's gardens, England in the
14th century and in North America by
the mid-16th century. Sixty per cent of
world production of cucumbers is now
carried out in China.

Cool As a Cucumber

The slang term '*cucumber time*',
current around 1700, was also known
as '*cucumbers*', '*taylers*' (tailors),
and '*taylors' holiday*' – referring to
the season when cucumbers were
ripe, which was when tailors took
their holiday. The *Pall Mall Gazette*
explained in 1867: '*Tailors could
not be expected to earn much money
"in cucumber season". Because when
cucumbers are in, the gentry are out of
town.*' Tailors then were nicknamed
'*cucumbers*' because of this reference to
their 'cucumber time'. The Germans
have a similar phrase, '*Die Saure-
Gurken-Zeit*', literally 'pickled gherkin
time', which means that not much is
going on or you don't have much work
to do . The saying 'cool as a cucumber',
meaning imperturbable, was first
recorded in John Gay's poem *New
Song on New Similies* in 1732: '*I...cool
as a cucumber could see / The rest
of womankind.*'

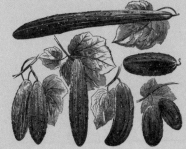

NICHOLAS CULPEPER

18 October 1616-10 January 1654

His father, the Reverend Nicholas Culpeper, lord of Ockley Manor in Surrey, died 13 days before Nicholas Culpeper was born, and the manor passed into other hands. He learnt Latin and Greek from his mother's father, the Reverend William Attersole, who introduced him to medicinal plants, astrology and medical texts by the age of ten. Aged 16, Culpeper was sent to Cambridge University to study theology and train to be a minister. More interested in medicine, Culpeper never graduated,

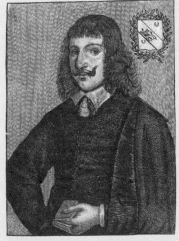

but planned to marry the heiress Judith Rivers, whom he had known since childhood. Her parents would not consent to the marriage, so the couple decided to elope to Holland until the animosity died down. However, Judith's coach was struck by lightning on her way to a rendezvous with Culpeper. She was killed and a grief-stricken Culpeper became a recluse. His mother died soon after, and his grandfather disinherited him, shamed by the affair. Culpeper now could not afford to train to become a minister or follow a medical career, and he became apprenticed to an apothecary in London, where he taught his employer Latin.

During training he collected herbs noted in Gerard's *Herbal*, and determined to help others, after suffering so much from the death of his fiancée. He took over the business in Threadneedle Street, London, on the death of his employer, and from 1635 began visiting the famed astrologer William Lilly (1602–81) who lived nearby in the Strand. Lilly told his friend to combine his new knowledge of being an apothecary, physician and astrologer into an holistic approach, and Culpeper used his Latin and Greek to pore over all the medical and astrological texts available.

In 1640 he married Alice Field, who had just inherited a considerable fortune. They had met when Culpeper successfully treated her father for gout and arthritis. Using her large dowry he was able to build a house next door to the Red Lion Inn in Spitalfields, setting himself up as an astrologer and herbalist. He quickly gained a considerable reputation among the poor people of the area, whom he charged very little or even nothing for his diagnosis and treatments. Culpeper treated anyone, sometimes seeing 40 patients a day for weeks on end. As he worked tirelessly among the poor, he realized that treatment had to be cheaper and readily available, which contributed to the formulation of his belief in 'English herbs for English bodies'. His success as a herbalist made him venomously critical of the high-charging medical men of the Royal College of Physicians. Culpeper wrote: 'They are bloodsuckers, true vampires, have learned little since Hippocrates; use blood-letting for ailments above the midriff and purging for those below. They evacuate and revulse their patients until they faint. Black Hellebore, this poisonous stuff, is a favourite laxative. It is surprising that they are so popular and that some patients recover. My own poor patients would not endure this taxing and costly treatment. The victims of physicians only survive since they are from the rich and robust stock, the plethoric, red-skinned residents of Cheapside, Westminster and St James.'

A fervent anti-Royalist, he despised the nobility and during the English Civil War (1642–51), Culpeper joined the Parliamentarian cause. In the first year of the war he volunteered to fight, but when the recruiting officer discovered his profession, he said 'We do not need you at the battle front but you can come along as a field surgeon, since most of the barbers and physicians are royal asses and we have use for someone to look after our injured.' In preparation, Culpeper collected medicinal herbs on the way to act as a field surgeon at the bloody Battle of Edgehill, which ended with no clear victor. Next, Culpeper received a commission to captain a troop of infantry, raising a company of 60 volunteers to fight at the First Battle of Newbury. On 20 September 1643, a day when 6000 men fell in battle, Culpeper was conducting battlefield surgery when a stray musket shot severely wounded him in the chest. He was conveyed back to London by carriage but never fully recovered from his injury. In cooperation with William Lilly, he now wrote 'A Prophecy of the White King', predicting the death of Charles I.

Working again among the poor in London, he continued to rail against the Society of Apothecaries and the Royal College of Physicians, the elite authoritative body for the whole medical establishment, saying 'For God's sake build not your faith upon Tradition, 'tis as rotten as a rotten Post.' He hated their 'closed shop' monopoly of drugs and medicines, keeping prices high to become wealthy, and the fact that all medical texts were only available in Latin, denying wider knowledge of them to the general public. Apothecaries were only allowed to mix medicines according to the guidelines of the College's London Pharmacopoeia, written in Latin and used by physicians to prescribe only the most expensive drugs and medicines. As he wished to make herbal medicine available to everyone, especially the poor, in 1649 Culpeper published an English translation of the *Pharmacopoeia*, calling it *A Physical Directory, or a Translation of the London Dispensary*. Of this work Culpeper wrote: '*I am writing for the Press a translation of the Physicians' medicine book from Latin into English so that all my fellow countrymen and apothecaries can understand what the Doctors write on their bills. Hitherto they made medicine a secret conspiracy, writing prescriptions in mysterious Latin to hide ignorance and to impress upon the patient. They want to keep their book a secret, not for everybody to know.*'

This sparked a major controversy and the College retaliated by attacking him for the rest of his life. In 1651 Culpeper published his *Semeiotica Uranica, or an Astrological Judgement of Diseases*. Also in 1651 he completed *A Directory for Midwives; or a Guide for women in their conception, bearing and suckling of their children, etc*. Tragedy in his family life had focused his attention on this issue. By his 14th year of marriage, he and Alice had seven children but only his daughter Mary

outlived him. In 1652 Culpeper translated from Latin Galen's Art of Physic: '*That thou mayest understand…in a general way the manifest virtues of medicines… such as are obvious to the senses, especially to the taste and smell*'. In 1653, he completed his herbal *The English Physitian, or an Astrologo-Physical Discourse of the Vulgar Herbs of this Nation*. It was followed in 1653 by *The Compleat Herball*, but by now Culpeper knew he was dying, writing to his wife of his latest books: '*…and my fame shall continue and increase thereby, though the period of my Life and Studies be at hand and I must bid all things under the Sun farewell.*' He had wasted to a skeleton from the effects of his injury, overwork, tuberculosis and possibly lung cancer from his tobacco habit. He died on 10 January 1654 at the age of just 38. Alice wrote: '*My husband left 79 books of his own making or translating in my hands.*'

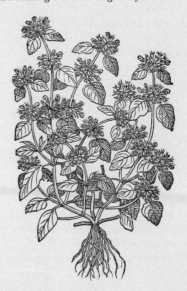

(BLACK) CURRANT

RIBES: *NIGRUM, RUBRUM* and *GLANDULOSUM*
Family Grossulariaceae, Currant/Gooseberry

OTHER NAMES: Blackcurrants were called quinsy berries or squinancy berries, as they were thought to cure quinsy (squinancy), a peritonsular abscess which is a complication of tonsillitis.

DESCRIPTION: Prolific small berries on spiked branches of shrubs which can grow to 6 feet (1.8 m) tall.

PROPERTIES AND USES: Culpeper seems to dislike blackcurrants: *'Currants…are of a moist, temperate, refreshing nature; the red and white currants are good to cool and refresh faintings of the stomach, to quench thirst, and stir up an appetite, and therefore are profitable in hot and sharp agues: it tempers the heat of the liver and blood, and the sharpness of choler, and resists putrefaction; it also taketh away the loathing of meat, and weakness of the stomach by much vomiting, and is good for those that have any looseness of the belly; Gesner says, that the Switzers [Swiss] use them for the cough, and so well they may; for, take dry currants a quarter of a pound, of brandy half a pint set the brandy on fire, then bruise the currants and put them into the brandy while it is burning, stirring them until the brandy is almost consumed, that it becomes like unto an electuary, and it is an excellent remedy to be taken hot for any violent cough, cold, or rheum. The black currants and the leaves are used in sauces by those who like the taste and scent of them, which I believe very few do of either.'* Gerard also favoured the redcurrant and whitecurrant, saying the blackcurrant had *'a stinking and somewhat loathing savour'*.

HISTORY: The juice used be boiled to an extract with sugar, called *Rob*, and used for inflammatory sore throat conditions such as quinsy. Throat lozenges are prepared from blackcurrants. The infusion of the leaves was said to be *'cleansing and diuretic'*, as was the raw juice, which was prescribed for those weak with illness. Blackcurrant jelly, tea and wine are all popular in Britain today, a fashion probably stemming from the Second World War. Most fruits rich in vitamin C, such as oranges, were not available, so the planting of blackcurrants, also rich in vitamin C, was encouraged by the British government. From 1942, nearly the entire British blackcurrant crop was made into blackcurrant cordial or syrup and distributed free to all children.

Black Corinths

The English name was given because the berries looked like the dried black Corinth grape, the Zante grape *(Vitis vinifera)*, sold in shops as currants. *Corinths* transmuted into *currants* over time.

CYCLAMEN

CYCLAMEN HEDERIFOLIUM
Family Myrsinaceae, Myrsine

OTHER NAMES: Ivy-leaved cyclamen, sowbread, stag truffle.

DESCRIPTION: The nodding pink, pale violet or white flowers, which appear before the leaves, are placed singly on fleshy stalks, 4 to 8 inches (10–20 cm) high. This herb gets its name from the Greek *cyclos*, circle, a reference either to the appearance of the reflexed lobes of the corolla, or from the spiral form of the fruit-stalk. As the fruit ripens, the flower-stalk curls spirally and buries it in the earth from its bulb-like, underground stem. The hardy plant now grows wild across Europe, probably spread by the Romans. The favourite greenhouse cyclamens which flower in winter months are varieties of a Persian species, *Cyclamen persicum*, which were introduced into European horticulture in the middle of the 18th century.

PROPERTIES AND USES: Culpeper states: '*This is a martial plant. The root of sow-bread is very forcing, and chiefly used to bring away the birth and the secundines* [afterbirth], *and to provoke the menses. The juice is commended by some against vertiginous disorders of the head, used in form of an errhine* [promoting a nasal discharge]; *it is of service also against cutaneous* [skin] *eruptions.'* The part used was the acrid tuberous rootstock, used fresh when the plant was in flower. Grieve records that '*applied externally as a liniment over the bowels* [it] *causes purging...An ointment...was made from the fresh tubers for expelling worms, and was rubbed on the umbilicus of children and on the abdomen of adults to cause emesis and upon the region over the bladder to increase urinary discharge.'*

HISTORY: Dioscorides suggested its use as a purgative, antitoxin, skin cleanser and labour-inducer. When used as a purgative, juice from the tuberous rootstock was applied externally, either over the bowels and bladder region or on the anus. Dioscorides also mentioned its use as an aphrodisiac, and old writers tell us that *sowbread*, baked and made into little flat cakes, has the reputation of being '*a good amorous medicine*', causing one to fall violently in love.

Favourite of Pigs

The species name *hederifolium* comes from *hedera* (ivy) and *folium* (leaf), because of the shape and patterning of the leaves. The older species name, *neapolitanum*, refers to Naples, where the species grew in abundance. Many English farmers called cyclamen *stag-truffle* or *sowbread* since they often observed deer and swine digging up and eating the roots.

DAFFODIL

NARCISSUS PSEUDONARCISSUS
Family Amaryllidaceae, Narcissus/Snowdrop

OTHER NAMES: Wild daffodil, Lent lily.

DESCRIPTION:
This flower has variably yellow to milky white outer petals and a golden trumpet. The subspecies Tenby daffodil, *Narcissus pseudonarcissus* subsp. *obvallaris*, looks like the wild daffodil but is half the size.

PROPERTIES AND USES:
Culpeper tells us: '*Yellow Daffodils are under the dominion of Mars, and the roots thereof are hot and dry in the third degree. The roots boiled and taken in posset drink* [a hot drink of milk curdled in wine or ale] *cause vomiting and are used with good success at the appearance of approaching agues, especially the tertian ague, which is frequently caught in the springtime. A plaster made of the roots with parched barley meal dissolves hard swellings and impostumes* [pus], *being applied thereto; the juice mingled with honey, frankincense wine, and myrrh, and dropped into the ears is good against the corrupt and running matter of the ears, the roots made hollow and boiled in oil help raw ribbed heels; the juice of the root is good for the morphew* [a scurfy eruption] *and the discolouring of the skin.*' Daffodil bulbs, farmed on Welsh mountains, are now being used to manufacture cheaply the chemical *galantamine*, which is one of the drugs used in the treatment of Alzheimer's disease.

HISTORY: In Ancient Greece they were a symbol of death. Romans introduced the daffodil into Britain, using the leaves to cure catarrh and the bulbs to make plasters. The daffodil is the national flower of Wales, always worn on St David's Day on 1 March. The word daffodil dates from 1592 and is derived from the Latin *asphodillus* and Greek *asphodelus*. Narcissus dates from 1548, and comes from the Greek *narke*, meaning numbness from the verb *narkoun*, to stupefy. Plutarch (CE 46–120) referred to the narcotic effects produced by the plant, whose bulbs contain a toxic, paralyzing alkaloid.

Lullaby of Broadway

Poultry keepers thought that the daffodil was unlucky, stopping hens from laying or eggs from hatching. A single daffodil brought into the house is also said to bring bad luck. In the 1935 song 'Lullaby of Broadway', there is the refrain '*The rumble of the subway trains / The rattle of the taxis / The daffodils that entertain / At Angelo's and Maxie's*'. In this context daffodil, or *daffydil* is an effeminate young man, with much the same meaning as *pansy* (being gay).

DAISY

BELLIS PERENNIS
Family Asteraceae/Compositae, Aster/Daisy

OTHER NAMES: Day's eye (because it opens in the sun), measure of love, poet's darling, llygad y dydd (Welsh for 'eye of the day'), lawn daisy, English daisy, common daisy, bachelor's buttons, bairnwort, billy button, boneflower, bruisewort, catposy, cockiloorie, less consound, shepherd's daisy, children's daisy, dicky daisy, hen and chickens, herb Margaret, March daisy, Margaret's herb.

DESCRIPTION:
The flower heads of this low-growing common plant are up to an inch (2.5 cm) in diameter, with white ray florets (often tipped red) and yellow disc florets. Many people think that the flower has a yellow centre with white petals, but this type of flower is known as a composite flower. Each white 'petal' is itself an individual flower, and the centre contains many tiny yellow flowers also. Differing colours and styles of flower work together, in order to attract different insects.

PROPERTIES AND USES:
In Ancient Rome, the surgeons accompanying Roman legions into battle would order their slaves to pick sacks full of daisies. Juice was extracted, bandages were soaked in this juice and would then be used to bind sword and spear cuts. It not only healed but counteracted the debility that followed injuries. Thus it always has had, in common with the ox-eye daisy, a reputation as a cure for fresh wounds, used as an ointment or poultice and applied externally. Gerard mentions it as *'Bruisewort'*, an unfailing remedy in *'all kinds of paines and aches'*, besides curing fevers, inflammation of the liver and *'alle the inwarde parts'*. Culpeper tells us: *'A decoction made of them and drank, helpeth to cure the wounds made in the hollowness of the chest. The same cureth also all ulcers and pustules in the mouth or tongue, or in the secret parts. The leaves bruised and applied to any parts that are swollen and hot, doth dissolve it, and temper the heat'*. In 1771 Dr Hill said that an infusion of the leaves was *'excellent against Hectic Fevers'*. The daisy was an ingredient of an ointment much used in the 14th century for wounds, gout and fevers. Dr Compton-Burnett, a 19th-century homeopath, stated *'It is a princely remedy for old labourers, especially gardeners.'* The plant was also beneficial for inflammatory disorders of the liver, kidney and bladder, taken internally in the form of a distilled water of the plant. Both flowers and leaves contain oil and ammoniacal salts. Homeopaths value its healing powers to treat muscular soreness not only in the limbs, but for the muscular fibres of the blood-vessels, and the plant

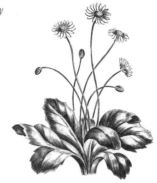

was used in baths in the treatment of paralysis. A salad of young daisy leaves is recommended in Germany as a spring medicine to stimulate metabolism.

HISTORY: Dioscorides recommended the daisy for reducing hard swellings. Pliny tells us that it was frequently used, combined with wormwood, to make into ointments for the wounded in war. The daisy in fairy tales had the power of arresting growth and children were given daisy roots and cream to keep them from growing. If you find a place where you can stand on seven daisies at once, summer has come. Making a necklace, '*a daisy chain*', is a common children's pastime.

It often represents innocence and is an emblem of Freya, the mother goddess. In the 14th century Geoffrey Chaucer mentions the daisy in the prologue to *The Legend of Good Women*: '*That well by reason men it call may, / The daisie, or else the eye of the day / The emprise* [chivalrous enterprise], *and flour of floures all*'.

She Loves Me, She Loves Me Not

Culpeper also refers to the '*greater wild daisy*', which is the much larger ox-eye daisy, *Leucanthemum vulgare*. The ox-eye daisy has similar properties in treating wounds and catarrh, but was mainly used as an antispasmodic in whooping cough and asthma, and in America the root was used to check the night sweats of consumptive people. Pliny recommended this plant to be combined with mugwort in the treatment of tumours. It is sometimes known as the moonflower or moon daisy, as at dusk it seems to glow in the half-light. It is also known as the dog daisy, marguerite, baby's pet, miss modesty and twelve disciples. In France, Germany and Holland it is associated with St John, and in Germany was known as the storm flower (*Gewitterblume*), and hung around doors to ward off lightning. Girls called Margaret were often nicknamed Daisy because the French for daisy is Marguerite. The French children's pastime of '*effeuiller la marguerite*' (plucking the daisy) is common across many countries. *The Measure of Love* is the ancient name for the daisy because it was common then, as it still is, for lovers to pull a flower to pieces to divine whether their love was reciprocated. In Britain and the United States it is known as '*She (He) Loves Me, She (He) Loves Me Not*'. The lover plucks off the petals alternately saying 'she loves me' and 'she loves me not' and the phrase spoken on picking off the last petal represents the truth.

DANDELION

TARAXACUM OFFICINALE
Family Asteraceae/Compositae Daisy/Sunflower

OTHER NAMES: Named after the French *dent de lion* (lion's teeth) either because the flowers are yellow, or because the leaves are jagged. Swine's snout, blowball, cankerwort, lion's tooth, puffball, white endive, wild endive, dant y llew (Welsh for teeth of lion), clockflower, tell-the-time, priest's crown.

DESCRIPTION:
There are more than 1000 dandelion species across Europe, with over 250 in the UK alone. There is a golden yellow flower, up to 2 inches (5 cm) across, consisting of 150 to 200 ray florets on the top of a hollow, milky stem. There is a very deep, thick, bitter root; the leaves are irregularly jagged, and the seed-head is white, globular and packed with scores of tiny parachutes ready to sail into the air.

PROPERTIES AND USES: Culpeper tells us: '*It is under the dominion of Jupiter. It is of an opening and cleansing quality, and therefore very effectual for the obstructions of the liver, gall and spleen, and the diseases that arise from them, as the jaundice, and hypochondriac; it opens the passages of the urine both in young and old; powerfully cleanses impostumes* [removes pus] *and inward ulcers in the urinary passages, and by its drying and temperate quality doth afterwards heal them; for which purpose the decoction of the roots or leaves in white wine, or the leaves chopped as pot-herbs, with a few Alexanders, and boiled in their broth, are very effectual. And whoever is drawing towards a consumption, or an evil disposition of the whole body, called cachexia* [wasting or weight loss], *by the use hereof for some time together, shall find a wonderful help. It helps also to procure rest and sleep to bodies distempered by the heat of ague-fits, or otherwise. The distilled water is effectual to drink in pestilential fevers, and to wash the sores.*' The plant's properties are used for constipation, eczema, acne, liver problems, poor digestion, and is a natural diuretic and detoxifier. In recent studies, it was shown to have a positive effect on weight management, and its phytosterols prevent the body from accumulating cholesterols. Dandelion root makes a reasonable coffee substitute, leaves were cultivated for salads until the 20th century, and some of us remember the classic drink of dandelion and burdock.

HISTORY: Dandelions were first mentioned in China in the Tang *Materia Medica* of the seventh century. It was recommended to restore health by the

Arabian physician, Avicenna, in the 11th century, and in the 13th century dandelions were used by the 'Physicians of Myddfai' in Wales to treat jaundice, in a remedy that also contained cornflower *(Centaurea cyanus)*, garden parsley *(Petroselinum crispum)* and old ale. According to the Doctrine of Signatures, dandelions had been *'signed'* in yellow to cure diseases with a yellow hue, such as yellow jaundice. The plant is sacred to St Bridget and the milky white sap that comes from the stems is said to nourish lambs and calves. It is also supposed to rid a person of warts. The slang name indicating that dandelions will make one urinate in bed is common in many languages, e.g. in Spanish *'piscialetto'*, in France *'pissenlit'* and Culpeper's piss-a-beds.

Dandelion Clock

The fluffy dandelion seedhead is like a barometer. In fine weather the ball extends fully, but when rain approaches, it shuts like an umbrella. If the weather is inclined to be showery it keeps shut all the time, only opening when the threat of rain is past. The globe of seeds is also used as a *'Dandelion clock'* or *'Tell Time'*. In folklore, the number of breaths it took to blow off all the seeds was the hour number. Alternatively, blow three times on the seed head. The number of seeds left reveals the hour. To determine how long you have left to live, blow once on the seed head. How long you have left to live is determined by the number of seeds that are left on the head. The dandelion is also called the 'rustic oracle' – its flowers open about 5 a.m. and shut at 8 p.m., serving the shepherd for a clock. In the daisy tradition of *'she loves me, she loves me not'*, instead of picking the petals off a daisy, blow the seeds off a dandelion globe. If you can blow all the seeds off with one blow, then you are loved with a passionate intensity. If some seeds remain, then your lover has reservations about the relationship. If a lot of seeds still remain on the globe, you are not loved at all, or only very little. If separated from the object of your love, carefully pluck one of the feathery heads, wish a tender thought, turn towards the place where your loved one lives, and blow. The seedball will convey your message faithfully. If you wish to know if your beloved is thinking of you, blow again. If there is left upon the stalk a single seed, it is a proof you are not forgotten. Similarly, the dandelion oracle can be consulted as to whether a future lover lives east, west, north or south, and whether he/she is coming or not.

DEADLY NIGHTSHADE

ATROPA BELLADONNA
Family Solanaceae, Nightshade

OTHER NAMES: Belladonna, banewort, black cherry, devil's cherries, naughty man's cherries, devil's herb, great morel, dwales and dwayberry.

DESCRIPTION: *'The flower is bell-shaped; it hath a permanent empalement of one leaf, cut into five parts; it hath five stamina rising from the base of the petal; in the centre is situated an oval germen, which becomes a globular berry, having two cells sitting on the empalement, and filled with kidney-shaped seed. It is of a cold nature; in some it causeth sleep; in others madness, and, shortly after, death. This plant should not be suffered to grow in any places where children have been killed by eating the berries'* – Culpeper.

PROPERTIES AND USES: All parts of the plant contain alkaloid poisons, and even small doses can send the taker into a coma. Compounds in the plant are narcotic and sedative, and effects include mental confusion, cramps, delirium, hallucinations and unconsciousness.

HISTORY: The scientific name refers to one of the Greek Fates, Atropos, who held the shears which cut the thread of human life. Poisoning by belladonna has the symptom of a complete loss of voice, along with continuous movements of the fingers and hands and bending of the trunk. It is supposedly the plant which poisoned Mark Antony's troops during the Parthian Wars. Culpeper relates that Macbeth poisoned an army of Harold

Harefoot's invading Danes, using a liquor infused with deadly nightshade. It was given to the Danes during a truce, so they did not suspect poison. When they fell into a deep sleep, the Scots fell upon them and murdered them easily.

Bright Pupils

In Italian, belladonna means 'fair lady', and the active ingredients atropine and hyoscyamine in its juice dilate the pupils, for which reason they are used in eye examinations. It was especially popular as a female beauty enhancer in 16th century Venice and throughout history, as enlarged pupils are thought to be attractive.

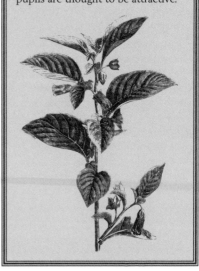

DILL

ANETHUM GRAVEOLENS
Family Umbelliferae/Apiaceae, Carrot

OTHER NAMES: Dillweed, dilly, aneton, garden dill, llys y gwewyr (herb of anguish, Welsh).

DESCRIPTION: It has small umbels with numerous yellow flowers, grows 2–3 feet (60–90 cm) in height, with graceful, highly aromatic, dark green feathery leaves.

PROPERTIES AND USES: Culpeper writes: '... *it strengthens the brain. The dill being boiled and drank, is good to ease swellings and pains; it also stayeth the belly and stomach from casting. The decoction therefore helpeth women that are troubled with the pains and windiness of the mother, if they sit therein...The Seed is...used in Medicines that serve to expel Wind and the pains proceeding therefrom. The Seed being toasted or fried and used in Oils or Plasters, dissolves the Impostumes* [pustular sores] *in the Fundament* [posterior], *and dries up all moist Ulcers (especially in the secret parts.) The Oil made of Dill is effectual to warm, to resolve Humours and Impostumes, to ease pains and to procure rest. The Decoction of Dill be it Herb or Seed (only if you boil the Seed you must bruise it) in white Wine, being drunk is a gallant expeller of Wind and provoker of the Terms* [periods].' It is a carminative, easing dyspepsia, flatulence, bloating and unsettled stomachs. Dill water (gripe water) is an effective remedy for colic in babies and is mildly antibacterial. Its leaves (dill weed), flower heads and seeds are used as a seasoning, the fresh, feather-like leaves for eggs, fish, dressings, sauces and salads. Flower heads are used for pickling. Cucumbers pickled in dill vinegar are known as dill pickles in the USA. Scandinavians use it in gravadlax, marinating fresh salmon with salt, sugar, pepper and finely chopped dill leaves. Dill is also used in sauerkraut and coleslaw.

HISTORY: In the Bible, dill was used to pay taxes and the Greeks regarded dill as a sign of wealth. Dill's strong aroma caused ancient peoples, such as the Scythians, to use it to embalm their dead. Twigs of dill were found in the tomb of Pharaoh Amenhotep. In the Middle Ages, if someone believed they had been bewitched, they would drink a mixture containing dill leaves to seek protection from the curse. Dill was used in monasteries to chase off the *Bublteufel* (incubus or devil of temptation), and was also used to help suppress fertility.

Sacred Herbs

Dill is one of the 'nine sacred herbs' of pagan festivals which was later consecrated to Mary. The flowering herbs found in Mary's grave are dill, yarrow, mugwort, arnica, calendula, valerian, tansy, lovage and sage.

PEDANIUS DIOSCORIDES

*c.*40–90 CE

This Greek physician, surgeon, pharmacologist and botanist was born in Anazarbus (later Caesarea) in Anatolia, Cilicia, Asia Minor. It was part of the Roman empire and is now Turkey. As a surgeon in the Roman army, Dioscorides travelled across the known world of North Africa and Europe, and he deliberately sought out new medicinal plants and minerals to tend to the troops. Between 50 and 70 CE, he wrote a five-volume encyclopaedia about herbal medicine and related medicinal substances, *De Materia Medica* (Regarding Medical Materials in five volumes). The work focused not only upon the preparation and properties of drugs, but upon their testing, and it was the most important pharmacological work in Europe and the Middle East for 1600 years. This precursor to all modern pharmacopeias was circulated in Latin, Greek and Arabic. Some of the most important Greek manuscripts survive in Mount Athos monasteries. The most famous manuscript is the superb '*Vienna Dioscorides*' produced in Constantinople around 512–13, and now in the Austrian National Library. This oldest and most valuable work in the history of botany and pharmacology was illustrated by a Byzantine artist for presentation to Juliana Anicia, the daughter of the Roman Emperor Anicius Olybrius.

De Materia Medica is the premier historical source of information about the medicines used by the Greeks, Romans, and other cultures of antiquity. The work presents about 600 plants in all, but some of the botanical identifications remain uncertain. The Chinese separately had developed their own materia medica, with one dating from 168 BCE being rediscovered sealed in a tomb. In the Islamic world, other materia medica expanded lists of other useful plants to over 1300 species. In Europe, Avicenna's *The Canon of Medicine* (1025) is another early pharmacopeia which lists 800 drugs, plants and minerals. The origins of clinical pharmacology are said to date back to Avicenna's works, Peter of Spain's *Commentary on Isaac*, and John of St Amand's *Commentary on the Antedotary of Nicholas*. In particular, Avicenna introduced clinical trials, randomized controlled trials and efficacy tests. During the Middle Ages and into the modern era, the body of knowledge termed materia medica was slowly transformed by the methods and expanding knowledge of medicinal chemistry into the modern scientific discipline of pharmacology. Around 1600, there was a flowering of scientific thought, and Dioscorides's message that investigation and experimentation were crucial to pharmacology began to emerge and modern research into medicines began. While Culpeper used his extensive knowledge of Dioscorides's work, he does not slavishly accept everything, judging each plant by his personal knowledge of it and in the light of later works.

DITTANDER

LEPIDIUM LATIFOLIUM
Family Brassicaceae, Mustard/Cabbage

OTHER NAMES: Pepperwort, pepper-weed, garden ginger, poor-man's pepper, dittany, peppergrass, broadleaved pepperweed, tall whitetop.

DESCRIPTION: A perennial growing around 4 feet (1.2 m) high, with long and broad bluish-green leaves and small white flowers which are held in large terminal heads. It is often found growing in salt marshes. Culpeper always tried to tell people where they could obtain herbs for nothing, e.g. here he writes: *'It grows naturally in many places of this Land, as at Clare in Essex, near also unto Exeter in Devonshire, upon Rochester common in Kent; in Lancashire and divers other places; but is usually kept in Gardens.'*

PROPERTIES AND USES: Culpeper says: *'The herb is under the direction of Mars. Pliny and Paulus Aeginetus say that Pepper-Wort is very effectual for the Sciatica, or any other Gout or pain in the Joints, or any other inveterate grief; the Leaves hereof to be bruised and mixed with old Hogs grease and applied to the place; and to continue thereon four hours in Men, and two hours in women, the place being afterwards bathed with Wine and Oil mixed together, and then wrapped with Wool or Skins after they have sweat a little. It also amends the Deformities or discolouring of the Skin, and helps to take away Marks, Scars, and Scabs, or the foul marks of burning with fire or iron. The Juice hereof is in some places used to be given in Ale to drink to women with child, to procure them a speedy delivery in Travail.'* Other herbalists also recommend it for gout, joint pains, scars, skin discoloration and child delivery.

HISTORY: Culpeper tells us: *'The Root is slender running much under ground, and shooting up again in many places; and both Leaves and Root, are very hot and sharp of taste like Pepper, for which cause it took the name* [pepperwort].' All parts of the plant, including the root, are hot and spicy to eat and the young leaves taste of creamy horseradish sauce. Dittander's flavour is hot and peppery, recalling mustard, watercress and nasturtium, and it was used as a hot condiment before the introduction of horseradish. The German name for dittander, *Pfefferkraut*, also indicates its use as a flavouring before pepper became widely available.

Leper Hospitals

Often we can learn about the use of a herb from its Latin name. *Lepidium latifolium* was cultivated for use in treating leprous sores, and can sometimes be found growing near old hospital sites. *Lepidium* is a genus of plants which includes about 175 species found worldwide, including cress and pepperweed.

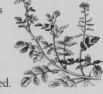

135

DITTANY OF CRETE

ORIGANUM DICTAMNUS
Family Labiatae, Mint

OTHER NAMES: Dictanum of Candie, Cretan oregano, Crete dittany, dittany of Candie, hop marjoram, Spanish hops, hop plant, eronda, diktamo.

DESCRIPTION: It grows up to 6 inches (15 cm) tall with a 16 inch (41 cm) spread, and has tiny pink flowers on tubular grey-green bracts which mature to purple. The grey-green leaves are aromatic and covered in white down.

PROPERTIES AND USES: Culpeper described dittany as a treatment for poisoned wounds, to draw out splinters and broken bones, and to drive away *'venomous beasts'*. Gerard wrote: *'It prevaileth much against all wounds, and especially those made with invenomed weapons, arrows...it draweth forth also splinters of wood, bones, or such like.'* The herb has been utilized to heal wounds, soothe pain and ease childbirth. The root has been used in a salve to treat sciatica, and as a remedy against gastric or stomach ailments and rheumatism. As a tea its aromatic healing properties can be used as an anticonvulsive and a menstrual tonic. It is said to strengthen the heart muscles

Healing for Wild Goats

In ancient times dittany of Crete was famous for of expelling weapons embedded in soldiers. Wild goats were reputed to seek out the plant after being struck by arrows; the goats were thought to eat the plant, and the arrows would fall out immediately. Shepherds saw this and would then ingest and later make compresses of the leaves to heal open wounds. The legend may predate the story in Virgil's *Aeneid* (*c.*29–19 BCE), the epic of the Trojan Wars. The hero Aeneas was severely wounded by a deeply embedded arrow that could not be extricated. His mother, the goddess Aphrodite (the Roman Venus), travelled to Mount Ida on the island of Crete and retrieved some dittany of Crete, which was applied to the wound, causing the arrow to drop out and the wound to cure immediately. Aphrodite's sister, the goddess Artemis, also has connections with dittany of Crete, and her statues in temples were often crowned with a wreath of dittany to honour her.

There are rivers, mountains, gorges and bays on Crete all named after an earlier Minoan goddess, Diktynna, who is also associated with the herb.

Highly Prized

Aphrodite, the Greek goddess of love, is also linked to dittany of Crete as she used it to treat her wounded son Aeneas during the Trojan Wars. Possibly because of this link with Aphrodite/Venus, dittany of Crete has reputed aphrodisiac qualities, and Cretans called it *eronda*, which means love. Young men, called *'erondades'*, were often given the task of harvesting dittany from steep cliffs as a proof of devotion. They worked like rock climbers in teams with ropes and long sticks. The Venetians during their occupation of Crete tried to transport the plant back to Italy but it would not thrive there, so Crete remained the only source of the herb. At one time dittany could command a price as high as gold and high demand threatened its eradication. It is gathered while in bloom, and exported for use in pharmaceuticals, perfumery and to flavour drinks such as absinthe, with the bulk of exports going to Italy as one of the ingredients in vermouth.

and arteries. Adding cinnamon and honey it soothes coughs. The leaves have been used for flavouring salads and vermouth. It has a pleasant aromatic flavour, especially when mixed with parsley, thyme, garlic, salt and pepper. It was often combined with more herbs such as rue and parsley to make a pepper sauce for fish or omelettes. Its chartreuse and pink flowers are still used in Crete to make tea.

HISTORY: The Minoans in Crete used it for curing ailments and beautifying their skin and hair. Hippocrates recommended it for stomach and digestive system diseases, rheumatism, arthritis, and used it to regulate menses and to tone and heal. Dittany is mentioned in Charlemagne's list of herbs. In Saxon kitchens it was an ingredient of a sauce to be used with fish. In ancient times it was believed that a snake would allow itself to be burned to death, rather than cross the path of dittany of Crete. Juice of dittany was commonly drunk in wine to treat snakebite, and the compressed leaves used as a poultice on wounds and bruises. A dittany compress was also believed to help expel foreign substances from the body. Dittany was believed to induce abortions in early pregnancy, to ease the pain of childbirth, and to reduce the severity of menstrual cramps.

Gift From Zeus

Origanum is a blend of the Greek words for joy and mountains. The word *dictamnus* is also a blending of two words. The first part refers to Dikti, the mountain where Zeus was born and *thamnos* means shrub. The rare endemic plant which is known as *diktamo* grows in the birthplace of Zeus – the Diktaeon Andron cave on Mount Dikti on the Greek island of Crete. Zeus, ruler of the Olympian gods, was born in the cave and in thanks for his upbringing on Crete gave the pink coloured and healing aromatic plant to the Greek island.

DOCTRINE OF SIGNATURES

This idea stems from the theory that God has marked everything that he created with a sign. This 'signature' was his indication of the reason why the living thing was created. The doctrine had been followed by apothecaries and herbalists for centuries, and there are allusions to this sort of idea in the writings of the Roman physician Galen (131–200 CE). However, it did not become part of mainstream medical thinking until the writings of Jakob Böhme (Jacob Boehme, 1575–1624). He was a master shoemaker in Görlitz, Germany, who when aged 25 had a mystical vision in which he saw the relationship between God and man. Amongst his voluminous Christian writings was *De Signatura Rerum; or The Signature of All Things* (1621). The Swiss physician Paracelsus (Theophrastus Bombastus von Hohenheim, 1493–1541), an important advocate of the Doctrine of Signatures, stated that '*Nature marks each growth… according to its curative benefit.*' Greatly influenced by the works of Paracelsus, Böhme believed that God must have revealed himself in the things that he created on Earth, since this was the only way that that man could have any knowledge of his true being. In the book, Böhme asserted '*the greatest understanding lies in the signature, wherein man…may*

learn to know the essence of all essences; for by the external form of all creatures… the hidden spirit is known; for nature has given to everything its language according to its essence and form.' The book stated a spiritual philosophy, but was quickly adopted for its medical applications. Paracelsus is considered by modern scholars to be the father of modern chemistry, and he did much in his lifetime to popularize the Doctrine of Signatures in its medical application. As an example, Paracelsus observed that Christmas rose (*Helleborus niger*) bloomed in winter, and concluded that it had rejuvenative powers. He introduced the plant into the pharmacopoeia of the time and recommended it for people over 50 years old. It was later found that this plant did have a beneficial effect on arteriosclerosis.

Windy Solution

The ultimate assertion of the usefulness of the Doctrine was probably that proposed by Thomas Hill in 1577. As lentils caused flatulence, he advised that they should be sowed in exposed gardens to reduce wind damage to other plants.

The Doctrine states that, by observation, one can determine from the colour of the flowers or roots, the shape of the leaves and roots, the place of growing, or other 'signatures', what the plant's purpose was in God's plan. Thus the liverwort, *Hepatica acutiloba*, has a three-lobed leaf that supposedly bears a resemblance to the liver, and the herbalist would not only name it, but prescribe the plant for liver ailments. The shape, colour, smell and markings of plants were thought to indicate their usefulness in medicine. *Pulmonaria* has heart-shaped leaves spotted with silver, resembling a diseased lung, so was prescribed for consumption, and came to be called lungwort, or lung-plant. The fine hairs of quince were an indicator that it could cure baldness, and red roses cured nosebleeds, as plants with a red signature were used for blood disorders. The petals of the iris were commonly used as a poultice for bruising because of the signature of colour, the petals resembling in hue the bruise they were to alleviate. Plants with yellow flowers or roots, such as goldenrod were believed to cure conditions of jaundice by the signature of colour.

John Gerard states in his herbal when speaking of St John's Wort, '*The leaves, flowers and seeds stamped, and put into a glass with oile of olive, and set in the hot sunne for certaine weeks togather and then strained from those herbes, and the like quantity of new put in, and sunned in like manner, doth make an oile of the colour of blood, which is a most precious*

Chinese Medicine

The Chinese extend the Doctrine whereby the colour and taste of a food is considered to be a reflection of its medicinal importance. It is believed that yellow and sweet foods relate to the spleen; red and bitter foods relate to the heart; green and sour foods relate to the liver; and black and salty foods relate to the lungs. Herbs were also categorized as hot, dry, cold or damp – and this is still an important aspect of herbal healing in different parts of the world.

remedy for deep wounds...' Here, the doctrine demands that the preparation be made before the signature evidences itself, an early type of preventative medicine. Eyebright, a plant whose flower looks like bright blue eyes, was used to treat eye diseases. The use of eyebright for this purpose was still common in the 1800s. The Doctrine was taken up universally by medieval alchemists, apothecaries and herbalists across Europe, but similar beliefs were held by Native Americans, Middle Eastern and Asian cultures. Folk healers in Christian and Muslim countries claimed that God, or Allah, deliberately made plants to resemble the parts of the body they could cure, a concept easy to accept by the common people. Today the idea of 'like cures like' is at the heart of modern homeopathy.

EARLY PURPLE ORCHID

ORCHIS MASCULA
Family Orchidaceae, Orchid

OTHER NAMES: *'It has almost as many several names attributed to the several sorts of it, as would almost fill a sheet of paper; as dog-stones, goat-stones, fool-stones, fox-stones, satiricon, cullians, together with many others too tedious to rehearse.'* – Culpeper. Long purples, great orchis, cuckoos, granfer griggles, salep, saloop, hare's bollocks, dog-stones, adder's meat, bloody butchers, goosey ganders, kecklegs, standerwort, standergrass, Gethsemane (see Plant Names in Folklore on pages 266–267).

DESCRIPTION:
Culpeper includes several species of the *Orchis* genus of the orchid family, including the military and pyramidical orchids. A single flower stem rises from the tuberous root, bearing flowers that as a rule are a rich purple colour, mottled with lighter and darker shades. Every tint, from purple to pure white can be found. Each flower has a long spur which turns upwards, and the leaves are lance-shaped on the plant which can grow to 12 inches (30 cm) high. The orchid family is the largest and most diverse of the flowering-plant kingdom, with more than 25,000 species observed so far. Each year, as many as 300 new species are added to the list and some scientists estimate that more than 5000 orchids remain undiscovered. A further 100,000 hybrids have been cultivated by dedicated horticulturalists.

PROPERTIES: *'They are hot and moist in operation, under the dominion of Dame Venus, and provoke lust exceedingly, which, they say, the dried and withered roots do restrain. They are held to kill worms in children; as also, being bruised and applied to the place, to heal the king's evil.'* Culpeper recommended it for 'king's evil' i.e. scrofula, referring to a variety of skin diseases, in particular a form of tuberculosis affecting the lymph nodes of the neck. It is said to be astringent, demulcent and an expectorant. It has been used as a diet of nutritive value for children and convalescents, being boiled with water, flavoured and prepared in the same way as arrowroot. Starch from the tubers is called *'sahlep'*, *'salop'*, *'salep'* or *'saloop'*, being rich in mucilage, and forming a soothing and demulcent jelly that is used in the treatment of irritations of the gastrointestinal canal. Thus it was used by infants and invalids suffering from chronic diarrhoea and bilious fevers.

Before coffee supplanted it, it was sold at stalls in the streets of London. The best *English salep* came from Oxfordshire, but the tubers were chiefly imported from the east. In Turkey, an ice cream made from salep (flour produced from the tubers of dried wild orchids) is so popular that the trade is threatening the plants' future, as a thousand orchids are required to make every kilo of it. The dessert is called *salepi dondurma* (fox-testicle ice cream).

HISTORY: According to the Greek physician Dioscorides, married couples used *Orchis mascula* to determine the sex of their unborn child. When the man ate the larger tuber, they would have a boy; if the woman ate the smaller tuber, they would have a girl. In his *Theatrum Botanicum*, John Parkinson wrote: *'If a man ate a large orchid tuber, he would begat many children.'* Parkinson in 1640 noted that orchids were among the drugs dispensed in London to cure conditions as diverse as fever, swellings and sores. Orchids were also thought to possess powerful aphrodisiac properties. One Greek philosopher wrote that the ground root of a species, named after the fertility god Priapus, allowed a man to perform 70 consecutive acts of sexual intercourse. As a result the particular orchid was so assiduously gathered that it almost became extinct. Vanilla is a rare example of an orchid used for food, with the seeds and pulp found in vanilla orchid pods being used to make vanilla extract, most of which is produced in Madagascar. The island churned out three million tons of vanilla extract in 2005, much of it destined for Coca-Cola. The US drinks maker is the world's biggest consumer of vanilla extract.

The Dog's Bollocks

Culpeper believed that orchids were *'hot and moist in operation; under the dominion of Venus, and provoke lust exceedingly'*. Theophrastus, the ancient Greek 'father of botany' first named the plant 'orchis', meaning 'testicle'. Due to the appearance of the paired subterranean tuberoids, its root is called *Adam and Eve root*. We associate hares with lust, and another name for the orchis is hare's bollocks. Another is *Dog-stones*, stones meaning testicles. Thus this most common of British orchids is by definition the *'dog's bollocks'*.

From *Love's Martyr,* 1601

There's Standergrass, Hare's bollocks, or
*   great Orchis,*
Provoking Venus, and procuring sport,
It helps the weakened body that's amiss,
And falls away in a consumptuous sort,
It heals the Hectic fever by report:
But the dried shrivelled root being
*   withered,*
Hinders the virtue we have uttered.
If Man of the great springing roots doth eat,

Being in matrimonial copulation,
Male children of his wife he shall beget,
This special virtue hath the operation,
If Women make the withered roots their
*   meat,*
Faire lovely Daughters, affable, and wise,
From their fresh springing loins there
*   shall arise.*

Robert Chester

EGYPTIAN MEDICAL HERBS

From the Ebers Papyrus of *c.*1534 BCE, from the reign of Amenhotep I

Acacia *(Acacia nilotica)* A vermifuge, eases diarrhoea and internal bleeding, also used to treat skin diseases.

Aloe vera For worms, relieves headaches, soothes chest pains, burns, ulcers and for skin disease and allergies.

Balsam apple *(Malus sylvestris)* or apple of Jerusalem. A laxative, skin allergies, soothes headaches, gums and teeth, for asthma, liver stimulant, weak digestion.

Basil *(Ocimum basilicum)* Excellent for heart.

Bayberry *(Myrica cerifera)* Diarrhoea, soothes ulcers, shrinks haemorrhoids, repels flies.

Camphor tree Reduces fevers, gum pains, soothes epilepsy.

Caraway *(Carum carvi)* Soothes flatulence, digestive, breath freshener.

Cardamom *(Elettaria cardamomum)* Spice in foods, a digestive, soothes flatulence.

Cubeb pepper *(Piper cubeba)* Urinary tract infections, larynx and throat infections, gum ulcers and infections, soothes headaches.

Deadly nightshade *(Atropa belladonna)* Pain reliever.

Dill *(Anethum graveolens)* Soothes flatulence, relieves dyspepsia, laxative and diuretic properties.

Fenugreek *(Trigonella foenum-graecum)* Respiratory disorders, cleanses the stomach, calms the liver, soothes pancreas, reduces swelling.

Garlic *(Allium sativum)* Gives vitality, soothes flatulence and aids digestion, mild laxative, shrinks haemorrhoids, rids body of 'spirits'.

Henna *(Lawsonia inermis)* Astringent, stops diarrhoea, closes open wounds.

Juniper tree *(Juniperus phoenecia)* A digestive, soothes chest pains and stomach cramps.

Liquorice *(Glycyrrhiza glabra)* Mild laxative, expels phlegm, soothes liver, pancreas and chest and respiratory problems.

Meadow saffron *(Citrullus colocynthis)* Soothes rheumatism, reduces swelling.

Mint *(Mentha x piperita)* Soothes flatulence, aids digestion, stops vomiting, breath freshener.

Myrrh *(Commiphora myrrha)* Stops diarrhoea, relieves headaches, soothes gums, toothaches and backaches.

Onion *(Allium cepa)* Diuretic, induces perspiration, prevents colds, soothes sciatica, relieves pains and other cardiovascular problems.

Parsley *(Petroselinum crispum)* Diuretic.

Poppy *(Papaver somniferum)* Relieves insomnia, relieves headaches, anaesthetic, soothes respiratory problems, deadens pain.

Sandalwood *(Santalum albus)* Aids digestion, stops diarrhoea, soothes headaches and gout.

Sesame *(Sesamum indicum)* Soothes asthma.

Tamarind *(Tamarindus indica)* Laxative.

Thyme *(Thymus* species) Pain reliever.

Turmeric *(Curcuma longa)* Closes open wounds, also used to dye skin and cloth.

EYEBRIGHT

EUPHRASIA OFFICINALIS
Family Orobanchaceae, Broomrape

OTHER NAMES: Red eyebright.

DESCRIPTION: An elegant little plant, 2 to 8 inches (5–20 cm) high with deeply cut leaves and numerous small white or purplish flowers. *Euphrasia* is a genus of around 450 species of herbaceous flowering plants which are semi-parasitic on grasses.

PROPERTIES AND USES:
Culpeper writes: '*It is under the sign of the Lion, and Sol claims dominion over it. The juice or distilled water of eye-bright, taken inwardly in white wine or broth, or dropped into the eyes, for divers days together, helps all infirmities of the eyes that cause dimness of sight. Some make conserve of the flowers to the same effect. Being used any of the ways, it also helps a weak brain, or memory. This tunned up with strong beer, that it may work together, and drank; or the powder of the herb mixed with sugar, a little mace, and fennel-seed, and drank, or eaten in broth; or the said powder made into an electuary with sugar, and taken, has the same powerful effect to help and restore the sight decayed through age; and Arnoldus de Ville Nova says, it has restored sight to them that have been blind a long time before.*'
Herbalists use eyebright as a poultice with or without concurrent administration of a tea for the redness, swelling and visual disturbances caused by blepharitis and conjunctivitis. The herb is also used for eyestrain and to relieve inflammation caused by colds, coughs, sinus infections, sore throats and hay fever.

HISTORY: Historically, eyebright's use for eye problems was due to the Doctrine of Signatures – the purple and yellow blotches resembled a bruised eye, so it was called eyebright and bestowed with ophthalmic properties. In Milton's *Paradise Lost* the Archangel Michael employs the herb to give Adam clear sight: '*...to nobler sights, Michael from Adam's eyes the film removed, Then purged with euphrasine and rue, His visual orbs, for he had much to see...*' There is considerable evidence that compounds in the herb are anti-inflammatory and antibacterial.

Improving the Memory

Eyebright has a history of use as a general tonic and to improve memory, being usually drunk as a tea or infused in alcohol. Gervase Markham in *Countrie Farm* in 1616 suggested '*Drink every morning a small draught of eyebright wine*'. Gerard wrote: '*Three parts of the powder of eye-bright, and one part of maces mixed therewith, takes away all hurts from the eyes, comforts the memory and clears the sight, if half a spoonful be taken every morning fasting with a cup of white wine...*'

FENNEL

FOENICULUM VULGARE
Family Apiaceae/Umbelliferae, Carrot

OTHER NAMES: Common fennel (Culpeper), sweet fennel, ffenigl (Welsh).

DESCRIPTION: A perennial standing 4 to 5 feet (1.2 to 1.5 m) high, with bright, yellow flowers in large, flat terminal umbels and feathery ornamental leaves. Note that this is not Florence fennel (*Foeniculum vulgare* var. *azoricum*), which has edible celery-like stalks, an edible bulb, and is only 2 feet (60 cm) high.

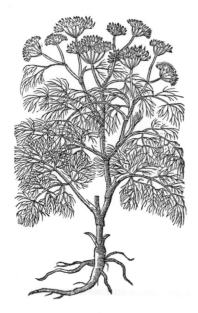

PROPERTIES AND USES: Stalks, leaves and seeds are edible. Culpeper relates: '*One good old fashion is not yet left off, viz. to boil fennel with fish; for it consumes that phlegmatic humour which fish most plentifully afford and annoy the body with, though few that use it know wherefore they do it; I suppose the reason of its benefit this way is, because it is an herb of Mercury, and under Virgo, and therefore bears antipathy to Pisces...The Leaves or Seed boiled in Barley Water and drunk is good for Nurses to increase their Milk and make it more wholesome for the Child: The Leaves, or rather the Seed boiled in Water stays the Hiccough, and takes away that loathing which oftentimes happens to the Stomachs of Sick, and Feverish Persons, and allays the heat thereof. The Seed boiled in Wine and drunk, is good for those that are bitten by Serpents, or have eaten Poison full Herbs or Mushrooms...The Seed is of good use in Medicines to help shortness of breath, and Wheezing by stopping of the Lungs. It helps also to bring down the Courses and to cleanse the parts after delivery... Both Leaves, Seeds, and Roots hereof are much used in Drinks or Broths, to make people more spare and lean that are too fat.*' Culpeper recorded its reputation as a diet aid, and in the 17th century William Coles wrote that fennel was much used '*for those that are grown fat, to abate their unwieldiness and cause them to grow more gaunt and lank.*' Drinking a cup of fennel seed tea before eating a heavy meal can take the edge off your appetite. As a diuretic fennel seeds are detoxifying and have been recommended to reduce cellulite. Sarah Garland wrote '*the seeds were eaten in quantities with fish and with hard fruit because of their digestive qualities.*

In the 11th century a large household is recorded as having consumed 8.5 pounds (3.9 kg) of fennel seed in a month.' Fresh leaves can be used as flavouring in soups and sauces, and fennel seeds make an excellent tea. Fennel teas are useful for chronic coughs and act as an expectorant to help clear mucus from the lungs, syrup prepared from fennel juice was formerly given for chronic coughs. The seeds are a digestive aid and are known to help with babies' colic, and adults find they assist with problems of abdominal cramps, flatulence, indigestion and bloating. Fennel not only improves digestion, but also can reduce bad breath and possibly body odour. The fresh stems of fennel can be eaten like celery, and the seeds add an anise flavour to fish and other dishes. If you expect to eat a vegetable that you have trouble digesting, like cabbage, try adding fennel seeds to your recipe. Oil of fennel relieves muscular or rheumatic pains and is warming and soothing in massage oil blends. Fennel is one of the plants that repels fleas, and powdered fennel was used in stables and kennels.

HISTORY: Fennel was supposed to have bestowed immortality upon Prometheus. It has been used to treat digestive ailments since the time of the Egyptians. In the third century BCE Hippocrates recommended its use for infant colic. The Romans and the Greeks cultivated it and Pliny gave 22 uses for it, especially as an eye herb.

Marathon

The Greek name for fennel was marathon, derived from '*maraino*', to grow thin, reflecting the widely held belief that drinking fennel tea would have a slimming effect. In Ancient Greece, the famous battle against the Persians in 490 BCE was fought on a field of fennel.

Pliny also related that snakes casting off their skins ate fennel to restore their eyesight. Dioscorides recommended it as an appetite-suppressant and for nursing mothers to increase milk production. In some countries it is regarded as an aphrodisiac. In the Middle Ages, fennel was used together with St Johns wort and other herbs as a preventative against witchcraft and other evil influences, being hung over doors on Midsummer's Eve to ward off evil spirits. It was also used to increase breast milk. Recent studies support its traditional use as a digestive aid. It has been shown to relieve intestinal spasms and cramping in the smooth muscle lining of the digestive tract, helping to relieve discomfort. An expert panel in Germany, that evaluates the safety and effectiveness of herbs, endorses fennel for the treatment of digestive upsets, including indigestion, wind pains, irritable bowel syndrome and infant colic. Some studies have shown the effectiveness of fennel to be comparable to well-known proprietary treatments such as Mylanta, Gaviscon and Maalox.

FENNEL - HOG'S FENNEL

PEUCEDANUM OFFICINALE
Family Apiaceae/Umbelliferae, Carrot

OTHER NAMES: Culpeper says it is *'called also Sow-Fennel, Hoar-Strange, Hoar-Strong, Sulphur-Wort and Brimstone Wort.'* Milk parsley, marsh parsley, sulphur weed, marsh smallage.

DESCRIPTION: Culpeper tells his readers that it *'grows plentifully in the salt low marshes near Faversham in Kent'*. Now rare, it still grows here and at the 'backwaters' at Walton-on-Naze in Essex. Related to dill, it resembles fennel, and grows to 3–5 feet (90–152 cm), with large umbels of yellow flowers. *'Peucedanum'* indicates that its leaves resemble those of the pine tree.

PROPERTIES AND USES:
Culpeper recorded: *'The Juice of Sow-Fennel (say Dioscorides and Galen) used with Vinegar and Rosewater, or the Juice with a little Euphorbium put to the Nose, helps those that are troubled with the Lethargy, Frenzy, turning or Giddiness of the Head, Falling-Sickness, long and inveterate Headache, the Palsy, Sciatica, and Cramp, and generally all the Diseases of the Sinews, used with Oil and Vinegar. The Juice dissolved in Wine, or put into an Egg, is good for the Cough, or shortness of Breath and for those that are troubled with the Wind in the Body; It purges the Belly gently, helps the hardness of the Spleen, gives ease to Women that have sore travail in Childbirth, and eases the pains of the Reins and Bladder, and also of the Womb. A little of the Juice*
dissolved in Wine and dropped into the Ears, eases much of the pains in them; and put into an hollow Tooth, eases the pain thereof. The Root is less effectual in all the aforesaid Diseases: yet the Powder of the Root cleanses foul Ulcers being put into them; and takes out Splinters of broken Bones or other things in the Flesh and heals them up perfectly, as also it dries up old and inveterate running Sores, and is of admirable Virtue in all green Wounds.'

HISTORY: This plant is now naturalized in North America, where in addition to the name of *sulphurwort*, it is called *chucklusa*. The juice is used for epilepsy and as a vinegar substitute in Russia. Its active ingredients act a diuretic and as an emmenagogue, stimulating blood flow in the uterus and pelvic area.

Smell of Sulphur

The thick root has a strong odour of sulphur, hence the popular names of the plant, *sulphurwort, sulphur weed* and *brimstonewort*. When wounded in the spring, the plant yields a considerable quantity of a yellowish-green juice, which dries into a gummy resin and retains the strong sulphuric scent of the root.

FEVERFEW

TANACETUM PARTHENIUM
Family Asteraceae/Compositae, Daisy/Sunflower

OTHER NAMES: Culpeper calls it common feverfew. Featherfew, flirtwort, bachelor's buttons, featherfoil, febrifuge plant, pyrethrum parthenium, altamisa, chamomile grande, featherfoil, midsummer daisy, nosebleed, wild chamomile, wild quinine. The Welsh name, wermod wen, means white wormwood. Culpeper also describes corn feverfew and sea feverfew.

DESCRIPTION: A hardy perennial growing to 15 inches (38 cm) with clusters of small daisy-like flowers and bright green, bitter, serrated leaves. Its bright white flower is similar to chamomile, and the plant is popular in flower gardens.

PROPERTIES AND USES: Culpeper recommends it for headaches, and states: '*Venus commands this herb, and has commended it to succour her sisters* [women], *to be a general strengthener of their wombs, and to remedy such infirmities as a careless midwife has there caused.*' Up to four leaves eaten daily sandwiched in bread (the bitter leaves can otherwise hurt the mouth) has a preventative effect on migraine. Alternatively, a few drops can be taken of a tincture made from the leaves and flowers. Feverfew inhibits platelets aggregating in the bloodstream, thus preventing blockage of small capillaries. This action has a mild tranquillizing effect and is especially good for headaches caused by tension or fatigue. (Do not mix with any warfarin treatment, as feverfew also thins the blood). Taken hot, feverfew will bring down fevers and act as a decongestant for coughs and catarrh. It has an antihistamine action, offering allergy relief to hay fever and asthma sufferers.

A household disinfectant can be made from the leaves. It is a fly and flea repellent, and must be kept away from plants which need to be pollinated by bees, as bees also dislike its pungent aroma.

HISTORY: Feverfew was known as *parthenium* because it was used to save the life of someone who had fallen from the Parthenon, the Doric temple of Athena on the Acropolis in Athens. Dioscorides recommended it for many complaints, such as arthritis, phlegm (one of the 'four humours', lack of emotion) and melancholy (another of the four humours), and also for '*St. Anthony's Fire* [erysipelas], *to all hot inflammations and hot swellings*'. Feverfew has been used in the treatment of headaches since the first century. It has also been used for inflammation, arthritis, menstrual discomforts, fever and other aches and pains. Double-blind medical studies in England proved that feverfew tea helps migraine sufferers, possibly by controlling levels of serotonin.

FIG-TREE

FICUS CARICA
Family Moraceae, Fig/Mulberry

OTHER NAMES: Edible fig, tree of life and knowledge.

DESCRIPTION: *'The Fig-tree seldom grows to be a tree of any great bigness in our parts, being clothed with large leaves bigger than vine-leaves, full of nigh veins, and divided for the most part into five blunt-pointed segments, yielding a thin milky juice when broken. It bears no viable flowers.'* – Culpeper.

PROPERTIES AND USES: Culpeper describes it thus: *'They prosper very well in our English gardens, yet are fitter for medicine than for any other profit that is gotten by the fruit of them. The tree is under the dominion of Jupiter. The milk that issues out from the leaves or branches where they are broken off, being dropped upon warts, takes them away. The decoction of the leaves is excellent good to wash foreheads with. It clears the face also of morphew* [a scurfy eruption], *and the body of white scurf, scabs, and running sores. If it be dropped into old fretting ulcers, it cleanses out the moisture, and brings up the flesh; because you cannot have the leaves green all the year, you may make an ointment of them whilst you can. A decoction of the leaves being drunk inwardly, or rather a syrup made of them, dissolves congealed blood caused by bruises or falls, and helps the bloody flux. The ashes of the wood made into an ointment with hog's grease, helps kibes* [ulcerated chilblains, especially on the heel] *and chilblains. The juice being put into a hollow tooth, eases pain; as also deafness and pain and noises in the ears, being dropped into them. An ointment made of the juice and hogs' grease, is as excellent a remedy for the biting of mad dogs, or other venomous beasts, as most are; a syrup made of the leaves, or green fruits, is excellent for coughs, hoarseness, or shortness of breath, and all diseases of the breast and lungs: it is very good for the dropsy and falling-sickness.'*

Figs can be eaten fresh or dried, and are used for their mild laxative action, being used in the preparation of laxative confections and syrups. Possibly the laxative property resides in the saccharine juice of the fresh fruit and in the indigestible seeds and skin of the dried fruit. Syrup of figs, a mild laxative, is suitable for children. Figs are demulcent as well as nutritive. Demulcent decoctions are prepared for the treatment of catarrhal affections of the nose and throat. Roasted and split into two portions, the soft pulpy interior of figs can be applied as emollient poultices to gumboils, dental abscesses and other circumscribed maturing tumours. In the Book of Isaiah in the Old Testament they were used by Hezekiah as a remedy for boils. The milky juice of the freshly-broken stalk of a fig has been used to remove warts on the body.

HISTORY: In Genesis, Adam and Eve used fig leaves to cover '*their nakedness*' after eating the fruit from the *Tree of Knowledge of Good and Evil*. Figs were one of the principal articles of sustenance in Greece, especially among the Spartans. Warriors and athletes fed almost entirely on figs, considering that they increased their strength and swiftness. Figs were such an important staple food in Ancient Greece that there was a law forbidding the exportation of the best fruit from their trees. The term *sycophant*, meaning a servile, self-seeking flatterer, literally translates as '*one who shows the fig*'. The term dates back to the Ancient Greek fig trade and originally referred to one who informed on fig smugglers. In Latin mythology the shrub was dedicated to Bacchus and employed in religious ceremonies. The wolf that suckled Romulus and Remus rested under a fig tree, which was therefore held sacred by the Romans, and Ovid states that as part of the celebrations of the first day of the year by Romans, figs were offered as presents. Both Greek and Roman mythology associate the fig with Dionysus (the Roman

---

Early Cultivation

The edible fig was one of the first plants to be cultivated by humans. Nine subfossil figs dating to about 9400–9200 BCE were found in an early Neolithic village 10 miles (16 km) north of Jericho in the Jordan Valley. This find predates the domestication of wheat, barley and legumes, and may be the first known instance of agriculture. It is proposed that they may have been planted and cultivated intentionally, 1000 years before the next crops to be domesticated, wheat and rye.

Bacchus), god of wine and drunkenness, and with Priapus, a satyr who symbolized sexual desire. In Italy, Pliny details 29 kinds of known figs. According to Buddhist legend, the founder of the religion achieved enlightenment in 528 BCE while sitting under a *bo*, a kind of fig tree. In Victorian times, nude statues had fig leaves added to spare the blushes of any modest viewers.

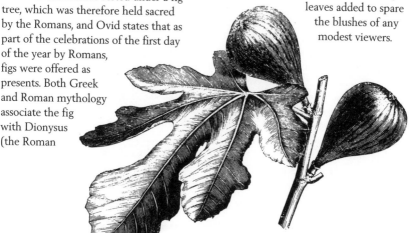

FINES HERBES, HERBES DE PROVENCE AND FIVE SPICE MIX

Fines herbes is a combination of herbs that forms a mainstay of Mediterranean cuisine. The ingredients are usually fresh parsley, chives, tarragon and chervil. These 'fine herbs' are not the pungent and resinous herbs that appear in a shop-bought bouquet garni – which, unlike *fines herbes*, release their flavour in long cooking. Marjoram, cress, cicely or lemon balm may be added to *fines herbes*, of which marjoram may be dried, but the essence of taste and flavour is to use fresh 'fine herbs'. You can simply finely chop a tablespoon each of fresh oregano, savory, thyme, marjoram and rosemary, put them into a bowl and mix together. Make into a bouquet garni for French Provençal dishes, or simply use the mix to complement any salads, vegetables, meat dishes, eggs, cheese, soups, stews, sauces and even hot desserts. *Fines herbes* are most commonly sprinkled on top of food after it has been cooked. An alternative *fines herbes* recipe using fresh herbs is to mix a tablespoon each of finely chopped or minced chives, chervil, parsley and tarragon. If using dried herbs in cooking, use a teaspoon each of chives, chervil, parsley and tarragon.

Fresh vegetables, fish, game meats, soups and stews can be flavoured with the seasoning blend known as *Herbes de Provence*. If using fresh herbs use one stem of each herb and tie them together into a bundle. If using dried herbs, place one teaspoon of each herb in the middle of a double layer of cheese cloth and tie the ends together with a piece of string. Place the bundle of herbs into the cooking liquid of the dish that is being prepared, and remove and discard the bundle prior to serving. A recipe using fresh herbs could be made up of basil, lavender flowers, fennel, rosemary, savory and thyme. For a recipe using dried herbs, try crumbled bay leaf, celery seeds, lavender flowers, marjoram, parsley, tarragon and thyme.

The Chinese tried to invent a 'wonder powder' balancing the yin and yang of food, encompassing all five flavours – sweet, sour, bitter, pungent and salty. Five Spice Mix is a traditional Chinese recipe, using a mix of powders to flavour poultry and meat dishes in Chinese-style cooking. It can also be added to soy sauce or teriyaki sauce and used as a marinade for meat, fish or poultry. Grind a teaspoon of each of the following ingredients into a fine powder using a pestle and mortar: black pepper, cinnamon, cloves, (sweet) fennel seeds and star anise or one star anise pod. There are many, many variations of this recipe.

FLAX

LINUM USITATISSIMUM
Family Linaceae, Flax

OTHER NAMES: Linseed, linen plant. Welsh llin amaeth (farmed linseed).

DESCRIPTION: A hardy annual which grows up to 4 feet (1.2 m) high with a spread of 12–24 inches (30–60 cm). Its sky-blue flowers make an unforgettable waving sea of sky blue in a field of planted flax.

PROPERTIES AND USES: Culpeper observes: '*Of the bark of the stalks of this plant, which is tough, and made up of a great many slender filaments, is made linen cloth…The seed, which is usually called linseed, is emollient, digesting, and ripening; of great use against inflammations, tumours, and impostumes* [pus-filled sores], *and is frequently put into fomentations and cataplasms, for those purposes. Cold-drawn linseed oil is of great service in all diseases of the breast and lungs, as pleurisies and pneumonia, coughs, asthma and consumption. It likewise helps the colic and stone, both taken at the mouth, and given in clysters* [enemas using a syringe].' Poultices treat boils and the plant is used to cure constipation. Flaxseed, or linseed, oil helps maintain a healthy heart and circulation, and the plant is used in cancer treatments. The oil is used in paint as an emulsifier, and the plant fibres make linen, used for clothing, fishing nets, ropes, sacks, candle wicks etc.

HISTORY: In Georgia, dyed flax fibres dating to 30,000 BCE have been found. Flax was one of the first crops to be cultivated, from 5000 BCE, being used to produce seed and textile fibre. It is used to make linen, linseed and rope, and the Egyptians wrapped mummies in linen cloth. Pictures on walls at Thebes show flax plants. Greeks used it to make sails for boats – cotton was not grown in Europe until the Moors introduced it into Spain in the ninth century. In the New Testament, it wrapped the body of Christ in the tomb, and it was the plant to which the plague of hail was so disastrous in the Book of Exodus. The Latin name for flax means 'most useful'. Flax flowers were believed in the Middle Ages to be a protection against sorcery. The Bohemians thought that seven-year-old children who danced among the flowers would grow up to be beautiful. Then, as now, flaxseed was used for the laxative effect of the mucilage the seeds give out when soaked in water. Sixty per cent of the world's flax production now comes from Canada and China.

Healthy Flax Seed

Flax seed (making linseed oil) is rich in Omega-3 alpha-linolenic acid, helping prevent heart disease, diabetes, arthritis, inflammation and immune system problems.

FLORAL CLOCK

Insects visit flowers to collect nectar and thereby help in pollination, which is essential for the survival of plants. Some believe that there is also some kind of 'time agreement' between plants and their insect visitors, which is precise to the hour. Only during this 'agreed period' do insects visit the flowers, and the flowers in their turn produce the nectar and pollen. Thus neither the visit of the insects, nor the pollen is wasted, and this 'clock' is independent of the weather. The great Swedish botanist Carl Linnaeus (1707–78) observed over a number of years that the flowers of many plants opened and closed periodically and that these times varied from species to species. Based on this finding, he was said to have planted a *'floral clock'* in his garden. Carefully chosen plants were arranged in segments around a circle, in the order of their daily blooming time. Linnaeus called it a *Horologium Florae*, in his *Philosophia Botanica* (1751). Linnaeus did not understand the mechanism of the response of plants to different day lengths *(photoperiodism)*. This periodic opening and closing of flowers is brought about by the interaction of an endogenous rhythm and the day length (light/dark signal). It appears that the plant is capable of measuring the time after which the light has reappeared. However, even today scientists appear to not know which receptors are used, and all we know about blooming time measurement is that the pigment *phytochrome* is involved. As well as the *circadian rhythm*, temperature and humidity are probable stimuli, as well as light intensity.

Linnaues's garden at Uppsala was situated at 60 degrees north, so many of the plants he selected for his flower clock were long-day species, adapted to short nights and daily photoperiods of 12 hours or more. However, his plants also included species of the intermediate type, which produce flowers regardless of the day length. These day-neutral types, such as dandelion, are not useful time keepers, since their times of opening vary with the season. During the first half of the 19th century keepers of botanic gardens attempted to construct flower clocks, but with little success as many of the plants listed by Linnaeus do not flower at the same month/times in different countries. Not only do the times of opening and closing of some of flowers vary with the month but also with the weather, as in rainy or cold weather blooms may remain closed or their opening may be later. The plant's aspect (whether it is on the north or south side of a hill, or on a valley floor, or shaded by trees, or near the warmer climates of coastlines) will also affect flowering. In *Philosophia Botanica*, Linnaeus described three groups of flowers:

Meteorici – flowers which change their opening and closing times according to the weather conditions.
Tropici – flowers which change their times for opening and closing according to the length of the day.
Aequinoctales – flowers which have fixed times of the day or night for opening and closing. Because of this characteristic, only aequinoctales are suitable for use in a flower clock.

LINNAEUS'S SUGGESTED PLANTS FOR A FLORAL CLOCK

Botanical name	Common name	Opening time	Closing time
Tragopogon pratensis	Goat's beard	3 a.m.	-
Leontodon hispidum	Rough hawkbit	by 4 a.m.	-
Helminthotheca echioides	Bristly ox-tongue	4–5 a.m.	-
Cichorium intybus	Chicory	4–5 a.m.	-
Crepis tectorum	Hawk's beard	4–5 a.m.	-
Reichardia tingitana	False sowthistle	by 6 a.m.	10 a.m.
Sonchus oleraceus	Sow thistle	5 a.m.	12 p.m.
Taraxacum officinale	Dandelion	5 a.m.	8–9 a.m.
Crepis alpina	Hawk's beard	5 a.m.	11 a.m.
Tragopogon hybridus	Goat's beard	5 a.m.	11 a.m.
Rhagadiolus edulis	Endive daisy	5 a.m.	10 a.m.
Lapsana chondrilloides	Nipplewort	5 a.m.	-
Convolvulus tricolor	Morning glory	5 a.m.	-
Hypochaeris maculata	Spotted cat's ear	6 a.m.	4–5 p.m.
Hieracium umbellatum	Hawkweed	6 a.m.	5 p.m.
Hieracium murorum	Hawkweed	6 a.m.	2 p.m.
Crepis rubra	Red hawksbeard	6 a.m.	1–2 p.m.
Sonchus arvensis	Field milk-thistle	6 a.m.	-
Sonchus palustris	Marsh sow-thistle	by 7 a.m.	2 p.m.
Leontodon autumnale	Hawkweed	7 a.m.	3 p.m.
Hieracium sabaudum	Hawkweed	7 a.m.	1–2 p.m.
Cicerbita alpina	Blue sow-thistle	7 a.m.	12 p.m.
Lactuca sativa	Garden lettuce	7 a.m.	10 a.m
Calendula pluvialis	Marigold	7 a.m.	3–4 p.m.
Nymphaea alba	White waterlily	7 a.m.	5 p.m.
Anthericum ramosum	St Bernard's lily	7 a.m.	3–4 p.m.
Hypochaeris achyrophorus	Aster	7–8 a.m.	2 p.m.
Hedypnois rhagadioloides	Scaly hawkbit	7–8 a.m.	2 p.m.
Trichodiadema babrata	Desert rose	7–8 a.m.	2 p.m.
Hieracium pilosella	Mouse-ear hawkweed	8 a.m.	-
Anagallis arvensis	Scarlet pimpernel	8 a.m.	
Petrorhagia prolifera	Proliferous pink	8 a.m.	1 p.m.
Hypochaeris glabra	Smooth cat's-ear	9 a.m.	1 p.m.
Malva caroliniana	Red-flowered mallow	9–10 a.m.	1 p.m.
Spergularia rubra	Sand spurrey	9–10 a.m.	2–3 p.m.
Mesembryanthemum crystallinum	Ice-plant	9–10 a.m.	3–4 p.m.
Cryophytum nodiflorum	Ice-plant	10–11 a.m	3 p.m.
Calendula officinalis	Pot marigold	-	3 p.m.
Hieracium aurantiacum	Hawkweed	-	3–4 p.m.
Alyssum alyssoides	Pale madwort	-	4 p.m.
Papaver nudicaule	Iceland poppy	-	7 p.m.
Hemerocallis lilioasphodelus	Day-lily	-	7–8 p.m.

FOXGLOVE

DIGITALIS PURPUREA
Family Plantaginaceae, Plantain

OTHER NAMES: Purple foxglove, fairy gloves, fairy fingers, fairy petticoats, fairy weed, fairy thimbles, witches' thimbles, witches' gloves, witches' bells, virgin's glove, Our Lady's glove, gloves of Our Lady, the great herb, fox bells, dead men's bells, floppy-dock, floptop folk's glovers, dog's finger, cow-flop.

DESCRIPTION: It grows up to 5–6 feet (1.5–1.8 m), and is a hardy, pretty biennial with purple bell-shaped flowers.

PROPERTIES AND USES: Culpeper writes: *'The plant is under the dominion of Venus, being of a gentle cleansing quality, and withal very friendly to nature. The herb is familiarly and frequently used by the Italians to heal any fresh or green wound, the leaves being but bruised and bound thereon; and the juice thereof is also used in old sores, to cleanse, dry, and heal them. The decoction hereof made up with some sugar or honey, is available to cleanse and purge the body both upwards and downwards, sometimes of tough phlegm and clammy humours, and to open obstructions of the liver and spleen. It has been found by experience to be available for the king's-evil, the herb bruised and applied, or an ointment made with the juice thereof, and so used; and a decoction of two handfuls thereof with four ounces of polypody in ale, has been found by late experience to cure divers of the falling sickness, that have been troubled with it above twenty years. I am confident that an ointment thereof is one of the best remedies for a scabby head.'* Infusions were made from the leaves to treat sore throats and catarrh, and a compress of leaves was made for bruises and swellings.

HISTORY: In 1785, the physician William Withering learned of the herbalist remedy for dropsy (oedema), using foxglove leaves, but it was unpredictable and could be fatal. He found that the plant affected the heart, stimulating the kidneys to cleanse the body of the fluids which caused dropsy. He experimented to find the correct dosages, leading to the purification of the active ingredients digitoxin and digoxin, which are used in heart stimulants today. In 1799, physician John Ferriar showed that digitalis slows the pulse, and increases the force of heart contractions and the amount of blood pumped per heartbeat.

Dead Man's Thimbles

The mottlings of the foxglove's blossoms were said to be marks where elves had placed their fingers, and they were also a warning sign of the harmful juices secreted by the plant, giving it the popular name of *'dead man's thimbles'*.

FUMITORY

FUMARIA OFFICINALIS
Family Fumariaceae, Fumitory/Fumewort/Bleeding Heart

OTHER NAMES: Earth smoke, smoke of the earth, fumus, vapour, beggary, fumus terrae, fumiterry, drug fumitory, wax dolls.

DESCRIPTION: It is a small and slender plant, with weak, straggling, or climbing stems 4 to 12 inches (10–30 cm) long, and clusters or spikes of small flowers of a pinkish hue, topped with purple, or more rarely, white. The leaves taste bitter and saline.

PROPERTIES AND USES: *'The juice or syrup…is very effectual for the liver and spleen, opening the obstructions thereof, and clarifying the blood from saltish, choleric, and adust humours, which cause leprosy, scabs, tetters* [a form of herpes, ringworm or eczema]*, and itches, and such like breakings out of the skin; and, after the purgings, strengthens all the inward parts. It is also good against the yellow jaundice, eradicating it by urine, which it procures in abundance…The distilled water also, with a little water and honey of roses, helps all the sores of the mouth or throat, being gargled often therewith. The juice dropped into the eyes, clears the sight, and takes away redness and other defects in them, although it procures some pain for the present, and causes tears. Dioscorides says, it hinders any fresh springing of hairs on the eyelids (after they are pulled away) if the eyelids be anointed with the juice hereof with gum arable dissolved therein. The juice of the Fumitory and docks mingled with vinegar, and the places gently washed or wet therewith, cures all sorts of scabs, pimples, blotches, wheals, and pushes which rise on the face or hands, or any other parts of the body.'* – Culpeper. It is used in eruptive skin diseases such as eczema. Fumitory is claimed as an aperient, depurative, cholagogue (stimulating the flow of bile), skin cleanser, diuretic, laxative, sedative, stomach pacifier, sudorific (sweat inducer), liver detoxifier, blood purifier and tonic.

HISTORY: The dried leaves were smoked in the manner of tobacco for disorders of the head. Dr Cullen recommended a leaf infusion to clear the skin and get rid of freckles. The plant was burned, so that its smoke might expel evil spirits, in the famous geometrical botanical gardens of St Gall in Switzerland.

Smokescreen

The common name *'earth smoke'* may come from the appearance of fumitory's whitish, blue-green flowers when viewed from afar. However, Pliny said that using the juice of the plant for eye infections brings on such a flow of tears, that the sight becomes dim as when affected by smoke. There is also a legend that the plant was produced, not from seed, but from vapours arising out of the earth.

GALL-OAK

QUERCUS LUSITANICA
Family Fagaceae, Beech

OTHER NAMES: *Quercus infectoria*, olivier, oak gall, nut-galls, Lusitanian oak, dyer's oak.

DESCRIPTION: A small, crooked, shrubby oak 4–6 feet (1.2–1.8 m) high native to Morocco, Portugal and Spain, and also Asia. The gall nuts that are used commercially for dyes are produced by the action of wasps. Culpeper says: *'This tree flowers and bears acorns, as also round woody substances, which are called galls, and the timber is very hard. There are other kinds, much shorter, bearing leaves more or less cut or jagged on the edges, and producing a great quantity of galls, and no acorns: some bear large galls, others small; some knobbed or bunched, and others smooth: they are of different colours white,*

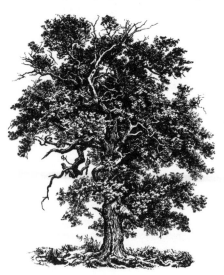

red, yellow, and green…chiefly grow in hot countries, Italy, Spain, &c.' The galls are the result of a puncture made in the bark by a wasp (*Diplolepis gallae tinctoriae* or *Cynips quercusfolii*) to deposit its egg. A small tumour soon appears, forming a dense mass about the egg. The egg hatches into the larval wasp while still inside these galls, and it eats its way out through a small opening. The excrescences vary from the size of a large pea to that of a chestnut, are nearly round and hard. Those in which the egg has not yet turned into a larva are most compact and heavy, and dark blue or bluish-green. When the larva has developed, the external colour lightens. Those of large size and greyish appearance are more or less consumed internally by the grub, and consequently of less commercial value.

PROPERTIES AND USES: Culpeper relates: *'The small gall is Saturnine, of a sour harsh nature, dry in the third degree, and cold in the second. It is effectual in drawing together and fastening loose and faint parts, as the overgrowing of the flesh: it expels and dries up rheums* [watery mucus expelled from the eyes, nose and mouth during sleep] *and other fluxes, especially those that fall upon the gums, almonds of the throat, and other places of the mouth. The other whiter gall also binds and dries, but not so much as the former, having a less quantity of that sour harshness in it: it is good against the dysentery and bloody flux. The decoction of them in water, is of a* mean astriction [binding or confining], *but more powerful in harsh red wine. Being sat over, it remedies the falling of the mother, or the galls being boiled and bruised, and applied to the fundament when fallen, or to any swelling or inflammation will prove a certain cure. The pods of burned galls being quenched in wine and vinegar are good to staunch bleeding in any place. They will dye hair black, and are one of the chief ingredients for making ink: it is also used by dyers for colouring black. The oak apple is much of the nature of galls, though inferior in quality, but may be substituted for them with success to help rheums, fluxes, and other such like painful distempers.'*

The common oak gall wasp *(Cynips quercusfolii)*, induces characteristic 1-inch (2.5-cm) spherical galls on the underside of oak leaves in other varieties of oak across the world. These turn reddish in the autumn and are commonly known as *'oak apples'*. Dr William Cook, in his 1869 The *Physiomedical Dispensatory*, wrote: *'Oak galls…are one of the strongest natural astringent herbs available and also are antiseptic. Useful in leucorrhoea and other vaginal discharges and in profuse menstruation. Also useful in chronic diarrhoea, dysentery, bleeding haemorrhoids, gleets* [bodily discharges, for instance from the urethra of gonorrhoea sufferers], *varicose veins and long standing gonorrhoea. They are also used as a gargle and mouthwash to treat sore throat, stomatitis* [inflammation of any parts of the mouth], *pharyngitis, laryngitis and tonsillitis. The blood-clotting agents active in Oak Bark are also helpful to cease nosebleeds…'*

HISTORY: Oak galls preserved during the eruption of Mount Vesuvius in 79 CE have been found, and they probably

---

Indelible Ink

Oak galls have been used externally to blacken hair since ancient times. Containing tannic acid, they were ground and mixed with iron sulphate, gum arabic and liquid (e.g. rainwater, beer or wine) to form an indelible black ink. The use of iron gall ink eventually became popular from the fifth century CE, owing to the fact that it does not easily rub off or erase. Iron gall ink turns light brown over time, as we see on old parchments. Dr William Cook noted *'Their decoction or tincture forms bluish-black precipitates with salts of iron, and is a basis in all black writing inks.'*

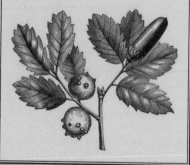

---

intended for use in medicines. Pliny the Elder (23–79 CE) recorded an experiment in which he noted the reaction of iron sulphate on a sheet of papyrus that had been soaked in tannic acid: *'The fraud may also be detected by using a leaf of papyrus, which has been steeped in an infusion of nut-galls; for it becomes black immediately upon the genuine verdigris being applied.'* Native North Americans used poultices of ground gall nuts on sores, cuts and burns.

GARLIC

ALLIUM SATIVUM
Family Alliaceae (formerly Liliaceae), Lily

OTHER NAMES: Poor man's treacle, rustic treacle, stinkweed, stinking rose, clove garlic, nectar of the gods, camphor of the poor.

DESCRIPTION: All parts of the plant are edible, and Culpeper tells us that *'It is a Native of the East, but for its use is cultivated every where in gardens.'* The differences between garlic and onions is in the bulbs and leaves. Garlic produces heads that a divided into sections (cloves), but onions produce a single multilayer globe. Garlic leaves are flat and almost grass-like, while onions tend to be hollow and erect. Culpeper also mentions *'Broadleaved Wild Garlic'*, *Allium ampeloprasum*, which is the ancient broadleaf wild leek, the ancestor of all leeks and *elephant garlic*. He recommends this plant for opening the lungs, relieving asthma, relieving wind, as a diuretic and for illnesses of the kidney and dropsy, especially anasarca (swelling of the skin).

PROPERTIES AND USES: Culpeper noted: *'Mars owns this herb. This was anciently accounted the poor man's treacle, it being a remedy for all diseases and hurts (except those which itself breeds.) It provokes urine, and women's courses, helps the biting of mad dogs and other venomous creatures, kills worms in children, cuts and voids tough phlegm, purges the head, helps the lethargy, is a good preservative against, and a remedy for any plague, sore, or foul ulcers; takes away spots and blemishes in the skin, eases pains in the ears, ripens and breaks*

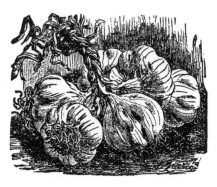

impostumes, or other swellings; and for all those diseases the onions are as effected. But the Garlic has some more peculiar virtues besides the former, viz. it has a special quality to discuss inconveniences, coming by corrupt agues or mineral vapours, or by drinking corrupt and stinking waters; as also by taking wolf-bane, hen-bane, hemlock, or other poisonous and dangerous herbs. It is also held good in hydropic [relating to dropsy] diseases, the jaundice, falling-sickness, cramps, convulsions, the piles or haemorrhoids, or other cold diseases. Many authors quote many other diseases this is good for; but conceal its vices. Its heat is very vehement; and all vehement hot things send up but ill-savoured vapours to the brain. In choleric men it will add fuel to the fire; in men oppressed by melancholy, it will attenuate the humour, and send up strong fancies, and as many strange visions to the head; therefore let it be taken inwardly with great moderation; outwardly you may make more bold with it.' Along with the related onion, garlic helps to lower hypertension, serum triglyceride and cholesterol levels. Both garlic and onions help thin the blood by discouraging platelets from sticking together. Garlic contains allicin, one of the most impressive broad-spectrum antimicrobial substances found in nature, and over 30 other medicinal compounds have been identified in the plant. Garlic oil or the juice of garlic adds a significant protective quality to cells which help to reduce fatty deposits. Garlic increases the potency of other medical preparations; helps nonsteroidal anti-inflammatory drugs provide greater pain relief; and boosts the infection-fighting capacity of many antibiotics.

HISTORY: It has been a cultivated plant for over 6000 years, originating in central Asia. Garlic was placed by the Greeks on piles of stones at crossroads as a supper for Hecate, their goddess of magic, witchcraft, the night, moon, ghosts and necromancy. According to Pliny, garlic and onion were invoked as deities by the Egyptians at the taking of oaths. It was used as a currency and clay models of bulbs were placed in Tutankhamen's tomb. During the building of the Pyramids, the workers were given garlic daily to imbue them with vitality and strength. The word derives from Old English *garleac*, '*spear leek*'. For all of recorded history it has been considered an aphrodisiac. It was therefore forbidden to monks, who believed it to be a stimulant

> ## Garlic and Vampires
> Culpeper wrote: '*The offensiveness of the breath of him that hath eaten garlic will lead you by the nose to the knowledge hereof, and (instead of a description) direct you to the place where it groweth in gardens, which kinds are the best, and most physical.*' The penetrating odour is so diffusive that if a bulb is applied to the soles of the feet, the breath will smell of it. In the USA in the 1920s it was known disparagingly in slang as *Italian perfume, halitosis* and *Bronx vanilla*. It is also said to protect against vampires – presumably you simply breathe upon them.

which aroused passions. Widows, adolescents and those who had taken up a vow or were fasting could not eat garlic because of this stimulant quality. During years of plague in Europe, many people ate garlic daily in an attempt to protect themselves. Louis Pasteur verified its antiseptic properties in 1858. Garlic is a strong antibacterial, antifungal, antiviral and antiparasitic herb and throughout history has been used for such purposes. Its properties as a '*superfood*' have been verified in countless studies. During the two World Wars, when the supply of sulphur drugs ran out, the British relied on garlic's antiseptic qualities for effectively treating wounds.

GOLDENROD

SOLIDAGO VIRGAUREA
Family Asteraceae, Aster/Daisy

OTHER NAMES: Aaron's rod, cast the spear, farewell summer refer to *Solidago virgaurea*, but Culpeper names three types of goldenrod. Common goldenrod was named as *Solidago fragrans* (fragrant), a synonym for *Solidago serotina* or *Solidago odora* (sweet goldenrod). Narrow-leaved goldenrod was named as *Solidago angustifolia*, which appears to now be named *Solidago sempervivens* (seaside, beach or evergreen goldenrod). The small *Solidago cambrica*, Welsh goldenrod, may be a variety of *S. virgaurea* and is extremely rare and seems confined to the mountainous valleys of Snowdonia National Park. Goldenrod is native to Europe, and there are many different species of goldenrod that possess the same medicinal properties. Frequently, many species, such as *Solidago canadenis*, *Solidago gigantea*, *Solidago serotina*, *Solidago odora*, *Solidago nemoralis*, *Solidago radiata* and *Solidago spathulata*, along with many others are used interchangeably with *Solidago virgaurea*.

DESCRIPTION: The hardy perennial *Solidago virgaurea*, with its spikes of golden yellow daisy-like flowers and bright green pointed leaves, may indeed be Culpeper's 'Common Golden Rod' as it also grows about 2 feet (60 cm) high.

PROPERTIES AND USES:
According to Culpeper apropos the common goldenrod, '*Venus rules this herb. It is a balsamic vulnerary herb, long famous against inward hurts and bruises, for which it is most effectual in a distilled water, and in which shape it is an excellent and safe diuretic; few things exceed it in the gravel, stone in the reins and kidneys, strangury, and where there are small stones so situated, as to cause heat and soreness, which are too often followed with bloody or purulent urine; then its balsamic healing virtues co-operate with its diuretic quality, and the parts at the same time are cleansed and healed. It is a sovereign wound-herb, inferior to none, both for inward and outward use. It is good to stay the immoderate flux of women's courses, the bloody flux, ruptures, ulcers in the mouth or throat, and in lotions to wash the privy parts in venereal cases. No preparation is better than a tea of the herb for this service: and the young leaves, green or dry, have the most virtue.*' He says that the narrow-leaved goldenrod is a native perennial of Ireland, seldom found in Britain, and grows in rocky hills: '*It resembles the preceding in virtues as in form. Venus claims the herb, and applied outwardly it is good for green wounds, old ulcers and*

sores. *As a lotion it is effectual in curing ulcers in the mouth and throat, and privy parts of man or woman. The decoction helps to fasten the teeth that are loose.'* The Welsh goldenrod is 6 or 7 inches (15–18 cm) high, *'a pretty perennial, a native of the Welsh mountains, and a favourite food for the goats…It possesses the same virtues as the first kind, though in an inferior degree. The leaves and tops are the parts used. It is accounted one of our best vulnerary plants, much used in apozems [infusions], and wound-drinks; and outwardly in cataplasms and fomentations. It is somewhat astringent, and useful in spitting of blood, and is of great service against the stone.'*

Solidago odora was sold as a medicinal herb for problems with: mucus, kidney/bladder cleansing and stones, diarrhoea, colds and digestion. A tea was made from the leaves and flowers for sore throat, snake bite, fever, kidney and bladder problems, period pains, fevers, nausea, cramps, colic, colds, measles, cough and asthma. A poultice was used for boils, burns, headache, toothache, wounds and sores. Poultices also staunched bleeding from wounds. Goldenrod is now used as an anti-inflammatory treatment for cystitis, urethritis and arthritis. Goldenrod has also been used to help prevent kidney stones. Traditionally, goldenrod has been used as a diuretic and also as 'irrigation therapy', taken along with fluids to increase urine flow in the treatment of diseases of the lower urinary tract. Leaves and flowers were used to make a yellow dye for textiles. A companion plant, it attracts lacewings which feed on aphids and whitefly. As it flowers in late summer, it heralds the change of the seasons, thus is called *'farewell summer'*.

Goldenrod Rubber

Thomas Edison experimented with goldenrod to produce rubber, which it contains naturally. He created a fertilization and cultivation process to maximize the rubber content in each plant, and experiments produced a 14-foot-tall (4.3-m) plant yielding up to 12 per cent latex in 1929. The rubber was resilient and long lasting, and the tyres on the Model T car given to him by his friend Henry Ford were made from goldenrod rubber. Edison died before he could bring his project into production and goldenrod rubber never became commercially successful, however, examples of the compound can still be found in his laboratory, elastic and rot-free after more than 80 years.

HISTORY: Originally imported from the Middle East, it was cultivated and naturalized all over Europe and in common use from the 16th century. *Solidago* means to 'make whole' and its ointment healed wounds. It was expensive until found growing wild in London.

HAWTHORN

CRATAEGUS MONOGYNA
Family Rosaceae, Rose

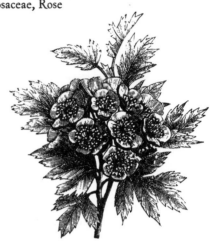

OTHER NAMES: Common hawthorn may, may blossom, mayflower, whitethorn, bread and cheese tree, hagthorn, red haw, ladies' meat, quick, tree of chastity. In some countries the berries are known as pixie pears, cuckoo's beads and chucky cheese.

DESCRIPTION: Hawthorn is a thorny deciduous shrub or tree that grows up to 45 feet (14 m) high, and is often used as livestock hedging because of its dense thorns. There are more than 200 species of hawthorn growing around the world. The white blossoms make a splendid show in spring. *Crataegus* is derived from the Greek '*kratos*' (strength), referring to the hardness and toughness of the wood. The wood of the hawthorn allegedly makes one of the hottest fires known to man and is considered to be better than oak for burning in ovens. Charcoal made from hawthorn was said to melt pig-iron without the aid of a blast furnace.

PROPERTIES AND USES: Culpeper says: '*It is a tree of Mars. The seeds in the berries beaten to powder being drunk in wine, are held singularly good against the stone, and are good for the dropsy. The distilled water of the flowers stays the lask* [diarrhoea]; *and the seeds, cleeted* [unfastened] *from the down, then bruised and boiled in wine, will give instant relief to the tormenting pains of the body. If cloths and sponges are wet in the distilled water, and applied to any place wherein thorns, splinters, &c, are lodged, it will certainly draw them forth.*' Hawthorn berries have been used as a heart tonic for at least two millennia, and hawthorn is used in treating angina, irregular heartbeat, and Reynaud's disease. Hawthorn's medical properties are cardiac, diuretic, astringent, and tonic. Scientific study has validated that it dilates coronary arteries, improves oxygenation and energy metabolism in the heart, and decreases lactic acid, the waste product of exertion that causes heart muscle pain. Hawthorn has the ability to normalize blood pressure, lowering high blood pressure and restoring low blood pressure to normal levels. Hawthorn is also used for insomnia, as a digestive aid and to cure sore throats. The active constituents in hawthorn are noted for their antioxidant and astringent properties. Hawthorn's diuretic properties make it useful for treating dropsy and kidney trouble. Hawthorn wood was used for making long-lasting printing blocks.

The young leaves and berries of the hawthorn used to be known as 'bread and cheese', the young leaves having a nutty taste, and leaves and flowers were used to make herbal tea, jam, wine and liqueurs.

HISTORY: The tree was regarded as sacred, probably from a tradition that it furnished the Crown of Thorns. Joseph of Aramathea was said to have planted his hawthorn staff in the soil at Glastonbury, creating the Glastonbury Thorn. Along with ash and oak, it was one of the *'three sacred trees'* of the Celts. The original Glastonbury Thorn was supposed to flower annually on Christmas Day, but was chopped down by Cromwellians during the English Civil War. A replacement was vandalized in 2010. It is a form of the tree, growing locally, which flowers twice a year, *Crataegus monogyna* 'Biflora'. Hawthorn has been a symbol of fertility and was said to offer protection from lightning. It is still thought unlucky to bring hawthorn flowers into the house. Hawthorn flowers were thought to bear the smell of the Plague of London. The flowers are mostly fertilized by carrion insects, attracted by the suggestion of decay in the perfume, called *'the stench of death'*. Flowers give off trimethylene as they deteriorate, the same chemical odour that is given off when corpses decay. In past times, May blossom signified new life and the word *nuts* in the traditional song *'Here we go gathering nuts in May'* is a corruption of the words *'knots'*, the pieces of hawthorn (May) wood gathered for ceremonial use. The Maypole was originally constructed from hawthorn, so that it would last for years. Across Europe, branches were cut from the hawthorn on May or Beltane Eve and were used to decorate the doors of houses and the blossoms made into garlands for the Maypole on May Day. Garlands hung over the doorway prevented evil spirits from entering the home. Hawthorn was referred to as the *'faerie bush'* and it was considered bad luck to cut it for fear of offending the fairies which inhabited it. A schoolboy trick that this author remembers only too well involved removing the red skin from a haw and dropping the downy seed covering down the back of someone's shirt. The resultant *'itchie'* irritated the skin of the unfortunate victim.

Hawthorn Lore

Though the hawthorn tree now flowers around the middle of the month of May, it flowered much nearer the beginning of the month before the introduction of the Gregorian calendar in 1752. Thus the old proverb *'ne'er cast a clout before May is out'* means 'never get rid of clothing before the May blossoms'. A Scots proverb: *'Mony haws, Mony snaws'* means that many haws on the May indicate a harsh, snowy winter. This popular nursery rhyme alludes to the hawthorn tree:

'The fair maid who, the first of May,
Goes to the fields at break of day
And washes in dew from the hawthorn tree
Will ever after handsome be.'

HAZELNUT

CORYLUS AVELLANA
Family Betulaceae, Birch

OTHER NAMES: Culpeper calls it hasel-nut, common hazel, cob nut.

DESCRIPTION: The hazel tree typically grows 10–25 feet (3–8 m) tall, but can reach 45 feet (14 m), and bears the familiar catkins and nuts.

PROPERTIES AND USES:

Culpeper gives a rather odd account: *'They are under the dominion of Mercury. The parted kernels made into an electuary, or the milk drawn from the kernels with mead or honeyed water, is very good to help an old cough; and being parched, and a little pepper put to them and drank, digests the distillations of rheum from the head. The dried husks and shells, to the weight of two drams, taken in red wine, stays lasks and women's courses, and so doth the red skin that covers the kernels, which is more effectual to stay women's courses. And if this be true, as it is, then why should the vulgar so familiarly affirm, that eating nuts causes shortness of breath, than which nothing is falser? For, how can that which strengthens the lungs, cause shortness of breath? I confess, the opinion is far older than I am; I knew tradition was a friend to error before, but never that he was the father of slander. Or are men's tongues so given to slander one another, that they must slander Nuts too, to keep their tongues in use? If any part of the Hazel Nut be stopping, it is the husks and shells, and no one is so mad as to eat them unless physically; and the red skin which covers the kernel, you may easily pull off. And so thus have I made an apology for Nuts, which cannot speak for themselves.'*

The name hazelnut generally applies to the nuts of any of the species of the genus

Turkish Delights

There are many cultivars of the hazel, some being grown for specific qualities of the nut including large nut size and early and late fruiting cultivars, whereas other are grown as pollinators. Turkey accounts for 75 per cent of the world's annual hazelnut production of around 850,000 tonnes. Hazelnuts have been grown along the Black Sea coast in northern Turkey since at least 300 BCE, and hazelnut farming has been the chief form of livelihood in the region, with hazelnut orchards extending up to 20 miles (32 km) inland from the coast.

Nut Crack Night

Holy Cross Day, 14 September, was formerly a school holiday so that children could go 'nutting'. On Halloween, '*Nut Crack Night*', lovers would roast hazelnuts over fires. If they burned steadily, their romance would flourish, but if they flew apart there would be trouble ahead. In another tradition, hazelnuts were given the names of potential husbands and thrown into the fire by girls. The loudest crack and the brightest flame indicated their true love. In eastern England, hazel boughs were collected on Palm Sunday and placed in vases on windowsills to protect against lightning. People would cut a hazel stick before sunrise on May Day and draw a circle round themselves with it to protect against fairies, serpents and evil. Adder bites were treated by laying cross-shaped pieces of hazel wood against the wound, and St Patrick was said to have used a hazel wand to drive the serpents out of Ireland. In '*The Discoverie of Witchcraft*' (1534), a hazel wand was recorded as being used as a charm against witches and thieves. In 19th-century Devon, brides used to be met outside church by an old woman holding a basket of hazelnuts to encourage fertility. It was believed that a 'good nut year' would mean many babies. In legend and folklore, the hazel, hawthorn and apple are associated with being at the border between the real and the magical world of elves, fairies and the like.

Corylus. An exception is *Corylus maxima*, which gives us the longer, less spherical, *filbert* nut. Its oil is used as a carrier oil in aromatherapy, with a slightly astringent action that is good for all skin types. For medicinal use, the hazelnut or cobnut, the kernel of the seed, is used raw or roasted, or ground into a paste. Hazelnuts are rich in protein and unsaturated fat, and contain significant amounts of thiamine and vitamin B6. They are extensively used in confectionery.

HISTORY: At Roman weddings hazel torches were burned on the wedding night to bring happiness to the couple. Hazelnuts were also often ground up with flour to make bread. Milk from the nuts can be used to treat chronic cough, and mixed with pepper for runny noses and eyes. The wood was traditionally grown as fast-growing coppice, the poles cut being used for wattle-and-daub buildings and agricultural fencing. It is very common in older hedgerows that were the traditional field and lane boundaries. Hazel is a favourite wood for walking sticks, shepherds' crooks and poles for gardening purposes. The wood bends easily so is ideal for weaving fences, and its stems were bent into a U-shape to hold down thatch on roofs. Young hazel shoots are used to make baskets and containers. Hazel is traditionally the favoured forked rod used for dowsing or divining. Hazelnut butter is presently being promoted as a more nutritious spread than its peanut butter counterpart.

HEARTSEASE

VIOLA TRICOLOR
Family Violaceae, Violet/Pansy

OTHER NAMES: Culpeper says *'It is called in Sussex pansies'*. Viola, wild pansy, little faces, love-in-idleness, trilliw (Welsh for three hues), herb of trinity, three faces in a hood, full me to you, biddy's eyes, pancies, lady's delight, cupid's delight, johnny jump-up (USA), tittle my fancy, love-in-vain, kiss behind the garden door, herb constancy, jump up and kiss love, love-lies-bleeding, live-in-idleness, loving idol, love idol, cull me, cuddle me, call-me-to-you, jackjump-up-and-kiss-me, meet-me-in-the-entry, kiss-her-in-the-buttery, kit-run-in-the-fields, pink-o'-the-eye, kit-run-about, godfathers and godmothers, stepmother, herb trinitatis, pink-eyed-John, bouncing Bet, flower o'luce, bird's eye, bullweed, bonewort (Anglo-Saxon).

DESCRIPTION: The modern garden pansy *(Viola wittrockiana)* is a plant of complex hybrid origin involving at least three species, *Viola tricolor* (the small purple, white and yellow 'wild pansy' or 'heartsease'), *Viola altaica* and *Viola lutea* (mountain pansy).

PROPERTIES AND USES: Culpeper: *'This is a Saturnine plant, of a cold, slimy and viscous nature. A strong decoction of the herb and flowers is an excellent cure for the venereal disorder, being an approved anti-venereal; it is also good for the convulsions in children, falling sickness, inflammation of the lungs and breast, pleurisy, scabs, itch &c. It will make excellent syrup for the aforesaid purposes.'* The flowers have also been used to make yellow, green and blue-green dyes. Viola tricolor can be used both internally and as a compress or ointment in the treatment of eczema, psoriasis and acne and it is a suitable remedy for clearing cradlecap in babies. The flowers contain a high concentration of rutin, which helps prevent bruising and heals broken capillaries.

HISTORY: Gerard states: *'It is good as the later physicians write for such as are sick of ague, especially children and infants, whose convulsions and fits of the falling sickness it is thought to cure. It is commended against inflammation of the lungs and chest, and against scabs and itchings of the whole body and healeth ulcers.'*

Good for the Heart

The flowers were considered good in diseases of the heart, from which may have arisen its name of *heartsease*. It was called *herba trinitatis*, because it has in each flower three colours. *Stepmother* refers to the differently shaped petals, supposed to represent a stepmother, her own daughters and her stepchildren.

(BLACK) HELLEBORE

HELLEBORUS NIGER
Family Ranunculaceae, Buttercup

OTHER NAMES: Culpeper also calls it: *'Setter-wort, Setter-grass, Bear's-foot, Christmas-herb, and Christmas-flowers.'* Christe herbe, Christmas rose, Melampode.

DESCRIPTION: A perennial, low-growing plant with dark, shining, smooth leaves and flower-stalks rising directly from the root. Its large white blossoms appear in the depth of winter, earning it the name of *Christmas rose.* John Gerard writes of the black hellebore: *'It floureth about Christmas, if the winter be mild and warm…called Christ herbe.'*

PROPERTIES AND USES: *'It is an herb of Saturn, and therefore no marvel if it has some sullen conditions with it, and would be far safer, being purified by the art of the alchemist than given raw. If any have taken any harm by taking it, the common cure is to take goat's milk. If you cannot get goat's milk, you must make a shift with such as you can get. The roots are very effectual against all melancholy diseases, especially such as are of long standing, as quartan [the fourth stage of] agues and madness; it helps the falling sickness, the leprosy, both the yellow and black jaundice, the gout, sciatica, and convulsions; and this was found out by experience, that the root of that which grows wild in our country, works not so churlishly as those do which are brought from beyond sea, as being maintained by a more temperate air. The root used as a pessary, provokes the terms exceedingly; also being beaten into powder, and strewed upon foul ulcers, it consumes the dead flesh,* and instantly heals them; nay, it will help gangrenes in the beginning.' – Culpeper. Its rhizome possesses drastic purgative, emmenagogue (stimulating blood flow) and anthelmintic (expelling parasitic worms) properties, but is violently narcotic. It was formerly used in dropsy and amenorrhoea, nervous disorders and hysteria. Applied locally, the fresh root is violently irritant. The generic name of this plant is derived from the Greek *elein* (to injure) and *bora* (food), and indicates its toxic nature. The specific name *niger* refers to the dark-coloured rootstock.

HISTORY: According to Pliny, black hellebore was used as a purgative in mania by Melampus, a soothsayer and physician, 1400 years before Christ, hence the name *Melampodium.* Parkinson in 1641 wrote: *'a piece of the root being drawne through a hole made in the eare of a beast troubled with cough or having taken any poisonous thing cureth it, if it be taken out the next day at the same houre.'*

From *Anatomy of Melancholy,* 1621

*'Borage and hellebore fill two scenes,
Sovereign plants to purge the veins
Of melancholy, and cheer the heart
Of those black fumes which make it
smart.'*

Robert Burton

HEMLOCK

CONIUM MACULATUM
Family Apiaceae, Carrot/Parsley

OTHER NAMES: Poison hemlock, devil's porridge (Ireland), poison parsley, spotted hemlock.

DESCRIPTION: With a usual height of 2–5 feet (60 cm to 1.5 m), (although it can grow to 10 feet/3 m) it looks like many other members of the parsley family, but there are bold red/purple blotches on the stem, finely divided leaves and typical umbels of tiny white flowers. It smells of mice, or to Culpeper *'a very strong, heady, and disagreeable smell'*.

PROPERTIES AND USES: Culpeper: *'Hemlock is exceeding cold and very dangerous, and consequently must not be taken inwardly: It may safely be applied to Inflammations, Tumours, and Swelling in any part of the Body (save the Privy parts) as also to St. Anthony's Fire Wheals, Pushes, and creeping Ulcers that rise of hot sharp Humours, by cooling and repelling the heat. The leaves bruises, and laid to the brow or forehead, are good for those whose eyes are red or swelled, and for cleansing them of web or film growing thereon…If any shall through mistake eat the Herb Hemlock instead of Parsley, or the Root instead of a Parsnip (both which it is very like) it will cause a kind of Frenzy, or Perturbation of the senses, as if they were stupefied or drunk. The Remedy is as Pliny says, to drink of the best and strongest pure Wine, before it strike to the Heart, or Gentian put into Wine or a draught of good vinegar, wherewith Tragus doth affirm that he cured a Woman that had eaten the Root.'* Coniine, which is found in hemlock, is a neurotoxin which disrupts the workings of the central nervous system and is toxic to humans and all classes of livestock. Ingestion in any quantity can result in respiratory collapse and death. It was often mistaken for cow parsley by children making whistles from its hollow stems, and led to accidental poisoning.

HISTORY: Linnaeus, in 1737, restored the classical Greek name *Conium*, being derived from the Greek word *konas*, meaning to whirl about, because the plant, when eaten, causes vertigo and potentially death. The Latin specific name *maculatum* (spotted) refers to the stem markings. In tradition, the purple streaks on the stem represent the brand put on Cain's brow after he had murdered Abel. Hemlock was used in Anglo-Saxon medicine, and the name hemlock seems to be derived from the Anglo-Saxon *hem* (border, shore) and *leác* (leek or plant). In Ancient Greece, hemlock was used to poison condemned prisoners. After being condemned to death for impiety in 399 BCE, the philosopher Socrates was given a potent infusion of the hemlock plant. Plato described Socrates's death in the *Phaedo*: 'The man...laid his hands on him and after a while examined his feet and legs, then pinched his foot hard and asked if he felt it. He said "No"; then after that, his thighs; and passing upwards in this way he showed us that he was growing cold and rigid. And then again he touched him and said that when it reached his heart, he would be gone. The chill had now reached the region about the groin, and uncovering his face, which had been covered, he said – and these were his last words – "Crito, we owe a cock to Asclepius. Pay it and do not neglect it." "That," said Crito, "shall be done; but see if you have anything else to say." To this question he made no reply, but after a little while he moved; the attendant uncovered him; his eyes were fixed. And Crito when he saw it, closed his mouth and eyes.' William Coles in his 1656 *Art of Simpling* recorded: 'If Asses chance to feed much upon Hemlock, they will fall so fast asleep that they will seem to be dead, in so much that some thinking them to be dead indeed have flayed off their skins, yet after the Hemlock had done operating they have stirred and wakened out of their sleep, to the grief and amazement of the owners.'

Ingredients of the Witches Brew

To be most effective, hemlock root had to be dug out at night. In the witches' cauldron described in Shakespeare's *Macbeth* (1605), we see the first witch place a live toad in the mixture. The three witches then chant:

'*Double, double toil and trouble;*
Fire, burn; and, cauldron, bubble.'

The second witch added:
'*Fillet of a fenny snake*
In the cauldron boil and bake:
Eye of newt, and toe of frog,
Wool of bat, and tongue of dog,
Adder's fork, and blind-worm's sting,
Lizard's leg, and owlet's wing.'

The third witch then added:
'*Scale of dragon, tooth of wolf,*
Witches' mummy; maw and gulf
Of the ravined salt-sea shark,
Root of the hemlock, digged i'the dark;

Liver of blaspheming Jew;
Gall of goat, and slips of yew
Slivered in the moon's eclipse;
Nose of Turk, and Tartar's lips,
Finger of birth-strangled babe
Ditch-delivered by a drab,
Make the gruel thick and slab:
Add thereto a tiger's chaudron,
For th'ingredients of our cauldron.'

The witches repeat their toil and trouble refrain, and the second witch adds baboon's blood.

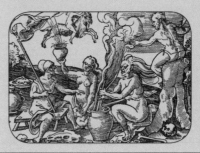

HEMP

CANNABIS SATIVA
Family Cannabaceae (formerly Urticaceae), Nettle

OTHER NAMES: Cannabis, marijuana, pot, ganja, hash, weed etc.

DESCRIPTION: This tall, roughish annual usually grows from 3 to 10 feet (90 cm to 3 m) high. The distinctive leaves are coarsely and sharply serrate, attenuate at both ends, dark-green above, pale and downy beneath.

PROPERTIES AND USES: *'It is a plant of Saturn, and good for something else, you see, than to make halters only. The seed of Hemp consumes wind, and by too much use thereof disperses it so much that it dries up the natural seed for procreation; yet, being boiled in milk and taken, helps such as have a hot dry cough… The Dutch make an Emulsion out of the Seed, and give it with good success to those that have the Jaundice, especially in the beginning of the Disease if there be no Ague accompanying it, for it opens Obstructions of the Gall, and causes digestion of Choler. The Emulsion or Decoction of the Seed stays Lasks* [halts diarrhoea] *and continual Fluxes, eases the Cholic, and allays the troublesome Humours in the Bowels, and stays bleeding at the mouth, nose or any other place; it will destroy the worms either in man or beast…'* – Culpeper. Hemp oil is one of the few dietary sources of gamma-linolenic acid (GLA), promoting healthy hormones and being beneficial for PMS symptoms. The green colour in hemp seed oil is a result of the high level of chlorophyll which is naturally present in the seeds. Hemp seed is a highly nutritious food, and contains antioxidants, protein, carotene, phytosterols, phospholipids, as well as a number of minerals including calcium, magnesium, sulphur, potassium, iron, zinc and phosphorus. It is a source of complete protein and contains all 20 known amino acids, including the nine essential amino acids. It also contains vitamins A, B1, B2, B3, B6, C, D and E. It was used throughout history for making cloth and ropes. Female hemp plants were processed for domestic purposes, and provide hemp used for cordage.

HISTORY: The famous Muslim sect who attacked both Islamic Seljuq rulers and the Crusaders from 820–1231 derived their name *Hashashin* from the drug, and from that our word *assassin* is derived. Although illegal across the developed world because of the dried leaves' intoxicating properties, *Cannabis sativa* subsp. *indica* has considerable medicinal value. Among its various uses, it

Duck Wormer

In November 2010, a French farmer was given a one-month suspended jail sentence and fined 500 Euros (£428) for feeding his ducks marijuana to rid them of worms. Police arrested Michel Rouyer after they discovered 12 cannabis plants and about 11 pounds (5 kg) of the drug during a visit to his home after a theft. Mr Rouyer said there was '*no* *better worming substance*' for ducks and that his flock was in excellent health. A police spokesman (never having read Culpeper) said it was the first time they had heard such a claim. M. Rouyer, who lives in the village of La Gripperie-Saint-Symphorien on France's Atlantic coast, did also admit to smoking some of the cannabis.

is an antibiotic for gram-positive bacteria, relieves nausea induced by chemotherapy, has been used to treat glaucoma and eases arthritic pains. Modern varieties, known as 'skunk', are far more powerful and dangerous than the original plant. The 16th-century English poet Thomas Tusser noted: '*Where plots full of nettles be noisome to eye / Sow thereupon hempseed, and nettle will die.*' Cannabis was reintroduced into British medicine in 1842 by Dr W O'Shaughnessy, an army surgeon who had served in India. In Victorian times it was widely used for a variety of ailments, including muscle spasms, menstrual cramps, rheumatism, and the convulsions of tetanus, rabies and epilepsy; it was also used to promote uterine contractions in childbirth, and as a sedative to induce sleep. It is said to have been used by Queen Victoria against period pains.

With the growing demand currently for ecologically sound biomass crops to use as biofuels, an environmental disaster has occurred where rainforest has been replaced with palm oil trees. Other crops such as sugar cane, rapeseed, soya, cornstalks and kenaf also carry attendant problems. The drug abuse of just one variety of hemp, *Cannabis sativa*, has undermined its potential as a solution to worldwide problems. Hemp is the fastest-growing crop on Earth, producing two or three crops a year in hot countries. It will grow almost anywhere so there is no need to clear forests for its cultivation, has hardly any natural predators and requires no chemicals to grow it. Its percentage of essential fatty acids is higher than that of any other plant in the world. Hemp contains both omega-6 and omega-3 essential fatty acids in a proportion of 3:1. This proportion is the recommended balance of omega-6 to omega-3 acids, making it a simple way to complete one's diet. Essential fatty acids are necessary for our health, and are responsible for the good condition of our skin, hair, eyes, etc. transferring oxygen to the every cell in our body. Hemp seeds are comparable to sunflower seeds, and may be used for food and milk, tea, and for baking, like sesame seeds.

HENBANE

HYOSCYAMUS NIGER
Family Solanaceae, Nightshade

OTHER NAMES: Black henbane, hog bean, stinking nightshade, henbell, foetid nightshade, devil's eye, Jupiter's bean, devil's tobacco, poison tobacco, witches' herb.

DESCRIPTION: Covered with sticky hairs, its grey-green, sharply toothed leaves surround bell-shaped creamy yellow or pale purple flowers, marked with deep purple veins. The stem can rise to 4 feet (1.2 m), and the whole plant, according to some, looks and smells like death.

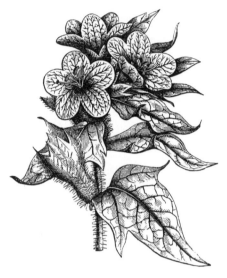

PROPERTIES AND USES: John Gerard describes it: *'The leaves, the seeds and the juice, when taken internally cause an unquiet sleep, like unto the sleep of drunkenness, which continues long and is deadly to the patient. To wash the feet in a decoction of Henbane, as also the often smelling of the flowers causes sleep.'* Culpeper writes: *'I wonder how astrologers could take on them to make this an herb of Jupiter: and yet Mizaldus, a man of penetrating brain, was of that opinion as well as the rest: the herb is indeed under the dominion of Saturn and I prove it by this argument: All the herbs which delight most to grow in saturnine places are saturnine herbs. Both Henbane delights most to grow in saturnine places, and whole cart loads of it may be found near the places where they empty the common Jakes, and scarce a ditch to be found without it growing by it. Ergo, it is a herb of Saturn. The leaves of Henbane do cool all hot inflammations in the eyes…It also assuages the pain of the gout, the sciatica, and other pains in the joints which arise from a hot cause. And applied with vinegar to the forehead and temples, helps the headache and want of sleep in hot fevers…The oil of the seed is helpful for deafness, noise and worms in the ears, being dropped therein; the juice of the herb or root doth the same. The decoction of the herb or seed, or both, kills lice in man or beast. The fume of the dried herb stalks and seeds, burned, quickly heals swellings, chilblains or kibes [ulcerated chilblains] in the hands or feet, by holding them in the fume thereof. The remedy to help those that have taken Henbane is to drink goat's milk, honeyed water, or pine kernels, with sweet wine; or, in the absence of these, Fennel seed, Nettle seed, the seed of Cresses, Mustard or*

Radish; as also Onions or Garlic taken in wine, do all help to free them from danger and restore them to their due temper again. Take notice, that this herb must never be taken inwardly; outwardly, an oil, ointment, or plaster of it is most admirable for the gout…to stop the toothache, applied to the aching side…' Henbane was a key component of the 'soporific sponge' used to achieve anaesthesia for surgery. Opium, henbane, hemlock, mulberry juice, mandrake, ivy and lettuce were soaked into a sponge,which was placed over the patient's nose before and during surgery to render him insensible.

HISTORY: The oldest surviving record of henbane, dating to 4000 BCE is an inscription on a Sumerian clay tablet, and henbane is also mentioned in the Egpytian *Ebers Papyrus* of 1500 BCE. The Egyptians knew it as '*Sakran*' (the drunken), referring to the plant's intoxicating properties, but perhaps also with an allusion to the practice of fortifying alcoholic beverages with its seeds. Dioscorides used it to procure sleep and allay pains. The powerful hallucinogen was used as a painkiller, to treat ulcers and as a remedy for whooping cough. In 1648 Simon Paulli wrote in *Flora Danica*: *'Among other herbs which are poisonous and harmful, Henbane is not the least, so that the common man, not without fear should spit at that herb when he hears its name spoken, not to mention when he sees it growing in great quantity where his children are running at play.'* The seedheads look like a piece of jawbone complete with a row of teeth, so it was used in dentistry from ancient times. Gerard describes sharp practice involving it: *'Drawers of teeth, who run about the country and*

Celebrity Poisoner

In 1910, an American homeopath living in London, 'Dr' Crippen, allegedly used scopolamine, an alkaloid extracted from henbane, to poison his wife. In August 2008, celebrity chef Antony Worrall Thompson was interviewed by *Healthy and Organic Living* magazine, which calls itself *'the only magazine dedicated to providing information and advice for modern women who want to discover how to lead a healthy and organic lifestyle'.* Asked whether he used any wild foods in his dishes, he replied *'The weed henbane is great in salads.'* In the following month's publication Worrall Thompson said that he meant to say 'fat hen', not henbane.

---

pretend they cause worms to come forth from the teeth by burning the seed (of henbane) in a chafing dish of coals, the party holding his mouth over the fume thereof, do have some crafty companions who convey small lute strings into the water, persuading the patient that these little creepers came out of his mouth, or other parts which it was intended to ease.'

HERBAL AUTHORITIES

Dioscorides and Culpeper have separate entries in this book, but the following men also contributed greatly to our understanding of herbs and medicine:

Nicolás Bautista Monardes (1493-1588)

The genus *Monarda* (bergamot, bee balm etc.) was named for this Spanish botanist and physician. In *Diálogo llamado pharmacodilosis* (1536), Monardes examined humanism, and suggested studying classical authors, mainly Dioscorides. In *De Secanda Vena in pleuriti Inter Grecos et Arabes Concordia* (1539), he outlined and emphasized the importance of Greek and Arab medicinal practice. In 1540 he wrote a treatise upon roses and citrus fruits: *De Rosa et partibus eius*. His magnum opus was *Historia medicinal de las cosas que se traen de nuestras Indias Occidentales*, published in three parts under varying titles in 1565, 1569 and completed in 1574. It was translated into Latin by Charles l'Écluse, and then into English by John Frampton as *Joyfull News out of the New Found World*. Because of this publication, Monardes made tobacco a household remedy throughout western Europe for headaches, arthritis, various wounds, and stomach cramps. Nowhere does Monardes write that tobacco might be smoked by white men for pleasure, but he recommended it as a cure for toothaches – and also for bad breath, which says a great deal about the state of 16th-century oral hygiene.

John Gerard (1545-1612)

He is mentioned in the entry upon the Barbers Company Physic Garden. Gerard studied medicine and travelled widely as a ship's surgeon. From 1577 onward, he supervised the gardens of Elizabeth I's chief advisor William Cecil, Lord Burghley, in London. In 1596, he published a list of rare plants cultivated in his garden at Holborn, which gives us an insight into the practices of his time. In 1597 his famous *Great Herball, or Generall Historie of Plantes* was published. By 1608 he was Master of the Barber Surgeon's Company. In 1633 an enlarged and amended version of his *Herball* was printed for which he he extensively used the *Materia Medica* of Dioscorides, the writing of the Italian Matthiolus and the works of the German botanists Leonhart Fuchs and Conrad Gessner.

John Parkinson (1567-1650)

A wonderful herbalist and botanist, he was Apothecary to James I and a founding member of the Worshipful Society of Apothecaries in 1617. Parkinson later became Royal Botanist to Charles I. In 1629 he produced *Paradisi in Sole Paradisus Terrestris (Park-in-Sun's Terrestrial Paradise)*, which described the most efficient and effective cultivation of plants. It was followed in 1640 by the comprehensive and wonderfully illustrated *Theatrum Botanicum (The Theatre of Plants)*. Parkinson kept his own botanical garden at Long Acre in Covent Garden, and disseminated information between European plantsmen, botanists and herbalists.

HOLLY

ILEX AQUIFOLIUM
Family Aquifoliaceae, Holly

OTHER NAMES: Common holly, bat's wings, holy tree, Christ's thorn, Christmas holly. Culpeper also calls it hulver (holly) bush and holm.

DESCRIPTION: Holly can grow to 40 feet (12 m) high, and has glossy prickly leaves and bright red berries. *Ilex* is a genus of around 600 flowering plants, the only living genus in its family.

PROPERTIES AND USES: Culpeper: '*The tree is Saturnine. The berries expel wind, and therefore are held to be profitable in the cholic. The berries have a strong faculty with them; for if you eat a dozen of them in the morning fasting when they are ripe and not dried, they purge the body of gross and clammy phlegm: but if you dry the berries, and beat them into powder, they bind the body, and stop fluxes, bloody-fluxes, and the terms in women. The bark of the tree, and also the leaves, are excellently good, being used in fomentations for broken bones, and such members as are out of joint. Pliny says, the branches of the tree defend houses from lightning, and men from witchcraft.*' The leaves have been used in homeopathy for fevers, rheumatism and bronchitis.

HISTORY: Pliny describes the holly under the name of *Aquifolius*, needle leaf. The botanical name *Ilex* was the original Latin name for the holm oak (*Quercus ilex*), which has similar foliage to common holly. In legend, holly first sprang up under the footsteps of Christ, and its thorny leaves and scarlet berries, like drops of blood, have been thought symbolical of his sufferings, for which reason the tree is called '*Christ's thorn*' across much of Europe. Holly is a traditional Christmas decoration, often used in wreaths. These decorations are said to be derived from a Roman custom of sending holly boughs, accompanied by other gifts, to friends during the festival of the Saturnalia, a custom that the early Christians adopted. The wood is hard and whitish, often being used for white chess pieces, with ebony for the black. Other uses include turnery, walking sticks and decorative inlay woodwork such as Tunbridge ware. Looms in the 1800s used holly for cloth spinning rods, as the dense wood was less likely than other woods to snag threads.

Bird Food

Holly berries are moderately poisonous to humans, but are an extremely important food item for numerous species of birds. In the autumn and early winter the berries are hard and unpalatable, but after being frozen or frosted several times, they soften, and become milder in taste. Holly hedges and trees also provide secure shelter for birds.

HONEYSUCKLE

LONICERA PERICLYMENUM
Family Caprifoliaceae, Honeysuckle

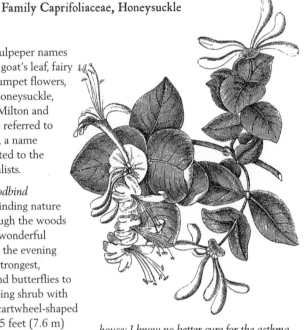

OTHER NAMES: Culpeper names it woodbine. Woodbind, goat's leaf, fairy trumpets, honeybind, trumpet flowers, sweet suckle, common honeysuckle, European honeysuckle. Milton and Chaucer amongst others referred to honeysuckle as *eglantine*, a name more commonly attributed to the *sweet briar* rose by herbalists.

DESCRIPTION: *Woodbind* describes the twisting, binding nature of the honeysuckle through the woods and hedgerows. It has a wonderful fragrance, particularly in the evening when the scent is at its strongest, attracting bees, moths and butterflies to its sweet nectar. A climbing shrub with pink, white and yellow cartwheel-shaped flowers, it can grow to 25 feet (7.6 m) high if supported. The flowers give way to red berries which are toxic if eaten.

PROPERTIES AND USES: Culpeper says: '*Honeysuckles are cleansing, consuming and digesting, and therefore no way fit for inflammations. Take a leaf and chew it in your mouth and you will quickly find it likelier to cause a sore mouth and throat than cure it. If it be not good for this, what is it good for? It is good for something, for God and nature made nothing in vain. It is a herb of Mercury, and appropriated to the lungs; the celestial Crab claims dominion over it, neither is it a foe to the Lion; if the lungs be afflicted by Jupiter, this is your cure. It is fitting a conserve made of the flowers should be kept in every gentlewoman's house; I know no better cure for the asthma than this besides it takes away the evil of the spleen: provokes urine, procures speedy delivery of women in travail, relieves cramps, convulsions, and palsies, and whatsoever griefs come of cold or obstructed perspiration; if you make use of it as an ointment, it will clear the skin of morphew, freckles, and sunburnings, or whatever else discolours it, and then the maids will love it. Authors say, the flowers are of more effect than the leaves, and that is true: but they say the seeds are the least effectual of all. But there is a vital spirit in every seed to beget its like; there is a greater heat in the seed than any other part of the plant; and heat is the mother of action.*' According to Maud Grieve, '*a dozen or more of the*

100 species of Lonicera or Honeysuckle are used medicinally'. Today, there are at least 180 species of honeysuckle recorded. Honeysuckle is astringent, depurative, expectorant, laxative, diuretic and has been used in the treatment of respiratory illnesses and catarrh. The flowers have been used in external applications for skin infections. The leaves and flowers of the honeysuckle are rich in salicylic acid, so may be used to relieve headaches, colds, flu, fever, aches, pains, arthritis and rheumatism. The leaves have anti-inflammatory properties and contain antibiotics active against staphylococci and coli bacilli. The flowers can be used for making teas, vinegars, jams and jellies. They can also be used for decorating cakes and desserts and for making country wine. One old remedy recommends curing asthma and freckles with honeysuckle wine. At least one writer tells us that inhaling the fragrant flowers, along with visualizing the way you want your body to look, can help you to lose weight.

HISTORY:

Honeysuckle can be found in the Chinese pharmacopoeia *Tang Ben Cao*, with remedies dating to the 3rd century BCE, first published in 659 CE. The Chinese used the honeysuckle *Lonicera japonica* as a cleanser and for removing poisons from the body. Pliny recommended that honeysuckle should be mixed with wine to cure spleen disorders. The flowers have been highly valued for medicinal purposes by many cultures worldwide, and their use was recommended by Dioscorides and

Sweet Nectar

Children still suck nectar from the narrow end of the flower's thin tube, hence the name honeysuckle. Its leaves are a favourite food of goats, hence the Latin name *caprifolium* (goats' leaf), and the French *chèvre-feuille*, German *Geisblatt* and Italian *capri-foglio*.

Gerard. Gerard says that honeysuckle is '*neither cold nor binding, but hot and attenuating or making thin…the ripe seed gathered and dried in the shadow and drunk for four days together, doth waste and consume away the hardness of the spleen and removeth wearisomeness, helpeth the shortness and difficulty of breathing, cureth the hicket* [hiccough], *etc. A syrup made of the flowers is good to be drunk against diseases of the lungs and spleen.*'

In Scotland, it was believed that if honeysuckle grows around the entrance to the home it would prevent a witch from entering. Bringing the flowers into the house was said to bring money with them. Honeysuckle is a symbol of fidelity and affection, and those who wear honeysuckle flowers are said to be able to dream of their true love. In Victorian times young girls were banned from bringing honeysuckle into the home, because it was believed to cause dreams that were far too risqué for their sensibilities. Its clinging habit in the '*language of flowers*' symbolizes that two people are united in love and devotion.

HOP

HUMULUS LUPULUS
Family Cannabaceae, Hemp/Hop

OTHER NAMES: Humulus, lupulus, hop vine.

DESCRIPTION: A twining climber with bristly stems and coarsely toothed leaves. Tiny green male flowers are produced in branched clusters and larger female flowers appear in 'hops', beneath soft, pale green, aromatic bracts. The dried female flower clusters (hops) and hops grain are normally used. Although referred to as the hop 'vine', it is technically a *bine*. Vines use tendrils, suckers and other appendages for attaching themselves, but bines have stout stems with stiff hairs to aid in climbing.

PROPERTIES AND USES: Culpeper notes: '*It is under the dominion of Mars. This, in physical operations, is to open obstructions of the liver and spleen, to cleanse the blood, to loosen the belly, to cleanse the reins from gravel, and provoke urine. The decoction of the tops of Hops, as well of the tame as the wild, works the same effects. In cleansing the blood they help to cure the French diseases, and all manner of scabs, itch, and other breakings-out of the body; as also all tetters, ringworms, and spreading sores, the morphew and all discolouring of the skin. The decoction of the flowers and hops, do help to expel poison that any one hath drank. Half a dram of the seed in powder taken in drink, kills worms in the body, brings down women's courses, and expels urine. A syrup made of the juice and sugar, cures the yellow jaundice, eases the head-ache that comes of heat, and tempers the heat of the liver and stomach, and is profitably given in long and hot agues that rise in choler and blood. Both the wild and the manured are of one property, and alike effectual in all the aforesaid diseases. By all these testimonies beer appears to be better than ale. Mars owns the plant, and then Dr. Reason will tell you how it performs these actions.*' It is a potent sedative and has hormonal as well as antibacterial effects, and is a bitter tonic herb that is diuretic, relieves pain and relaxes spasms. Hops are taken internally for nervous tension, insomnia, anxiety, irritability, nervous digestion (including irritable bowel syndrome) and premature ejaculation. Hops are used externally for skin infections, eczema, herpes and leg ulcers. Hops help to promote sleep and interestingly are said to decrease the desire for alcohol. The young shoots can be eaten raw or cooked like asparagus. The main commercial application of hops is in the flavouring in beer.

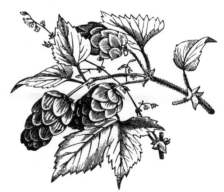

Hair Raising

The antiseptic and antidandruff properties of hops are of use in many of today's shampoos and it has recently been included in the group of products which are marketed to enhance hair growth. There are a number of antibaldness shampoos available featuring hops, often combined with nettles, burdock, pot marigold and rosemary. Hops can also be incorporated into bath gels because they stimulate the skin's metabolism.

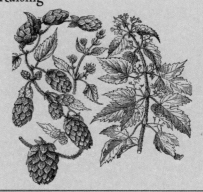

HISTORY: The English name hop comes from the Anglo-Saxon *hoppan* (to climb). Hops were cultivated continuously from the eighth century in Bohemian gardens in Bavaria and other parts of Europe. However, the first documented use of hops in beer as a 'bittering agent' is from the 11th century. The liquor prepared from fermented malt formed the favourite drink of Saxons and Danes, called *ale* (from the Scandinavian *öl* – the Viking's drink). Ale was brewed either from malt alone, or from malt mixed with honey and flavoured with heath tops, ground ivy, and various other aromatic herbs, such as marjoram, horehound, buckbean, wormwood, yarrow, woodsage or germander and broom. Long after the introduction of hops, the liquor flavoured in the old manner retained the name of ale, while the word of German and Dutch origin, *Bier* or *Beer*, was given only to alcohol made with the newly introduced bitter catkins. Henry VIII forbade brewers from putting hops and sulphur into ale, Parliament having been petitioned against the hop as *'a wicked weed that would spoil the taste of the drink and endanger the people'*. In England hops were not used extensively for making ale until around 1600. Hops became popular in brewing for their many benefits, including balancing the sweetness of the malt with bitterness, contributing a variety of desirable flavours, and having an antibiotic effect that favours the activity of brewer's yeast over less desirable microorganisms. Traditional herb combinations for ales were abandoned when it was noticed that ales made with hops were less prone to spoilage, and gradually hop-bittered alcohol began to be called beer. Hops were at first thought to engender melancholy, but the diarist John Evelyn wrote in 1670: *'Hops transmuted our wholesome ale into beer, which doubtless much alters its constitution. This one ingredient, by some suspected not unworthily, preserves the drink indeed, but repays the pleasure in tormenting diseases and a shorter life.'*

HORSERADISH

ARMORACIA RUSTICANA (SYN. *COCHLEARIA ARMORACIA*)
Family Brassiceae/Cruciferae, Cabbage

OTHER NAMES: Red cole, mountain radish, great raifort, German mustard.

DESCRIPTION: It grows up to 4 feet (1.2 m) tall with a large leaf spread and tiny white flowers, and is mainly cultivated for its large white, tapered root, which can be 2 feet (60 cm) long. It is difficult to eradicate the plant when established.

PROPERTIES AND USES:
Culpeper: *'The juice of Horse-raddish given to drink, is held to be very effectual for the scurvy. It kills the worms in children, being drank, and also laid upon the belly. The root bruised and laid to the place grieved with the sciatica, joint-ache, or the hard swellings of the liver and spleen, doth wonderfully help them all. The distilled water of the herb and root is more familiar to be taken with a little sugar for all the purposes aforesaid.'*
In 1656 William Coles commented: *'Of all things given to children for worms, horseradish is not the least, for it soon killeth and expelleth them.'* Known primarily as a food condiment, horseradish is used as a herb to lessen joint inflammation and treat whooping cough and infected sinuses. It is also used as a diuretic, a circulatory stimulant, and an antibacterial agent. Horseradish root has antiseptic and stimulant properties, and aids in digesting rich and oily foods. Young, fresh leaves have a mild, pleasant flavour and are excellent in salads and sandwiches.

HISTORY: *Armoracia* is the original Latin name for the related wild radish. John Gerard (*The Herball, or Generall Historie of Plantes,* 1597) wrote that *'the Horse Radish stamped with a little vinegar put thereto, is commonly used among the Germans for sauce to eat fish with and such like meats as we do mustard.'* Horseradish means a *'coarse'* radish, as a description to distinguish it from the edible radish; the prefix *'horse'* is often thus used, e.g. horse-mint, horse chestnut.

Saucy Horseradish

Fresh root is grated alone, or with apple, as a condiment for fish, or with vinegar and cream to accompany roast beef, cold chicken or hard-boiled eggs. Horseradish sauces may be gently warmed, but cooking destroys the volatile oils, which are responsible for the pungency. The author's favourite condiment, Tewkesbury mustard, is mentioned by Falstaff in Shakespeare's *Henry IV Part 2* – *'his wit's as thick as Tewkesbury mustard'* – and contains grated horseradish root. Its 'kick' comes from a glycoside called sinigrin that releases horseradish's acrid sulphur-bearing oil through enzymatic action.

(BLACK) HOREHOUND

BALLOTA NIGRA
Family Lamiaceae, Mint/Deadnettle

OTHER NAMES: Culpeper calls it hen-bit, but that is a different plant, *Lamium amplexicaule*. Black hoarhound, madwort, stinking horehound, black stinking horehound, foetid horehound, black archangel.

DESCRIPTION: It has bushy heart-shaped hairy leaves which have a grey mottle, and can be recognized by its whorls of hairy white, lavender or reddish-purple flowers. It can grow up to 3 feet (90 cm) in height. The scent is aromatic from a distance, but becomes more offensive as one nears it. When bruised, the plants smell of stale perspiration.

PROPERTIES AND USES: It settles nausea and vomiting which derive from the nervous system rather than the stomach. For instance, in motion sickness the nausea is triggered through the inner ear and the central nervous system. It was used particularly for morning sickness in pregnancy and also acts as a mild sedative. Black horehound had a reputation as a normalizer of menstrual function, and also as a mild expectorant. The leaves were used topically relieve insect sting, allergenic itch or sunburn.

HISTORY: *Ballota* comes from the Greek *ballo*, to reject, indicating that livestock would not eat it. *Nigra*, black, refers to the darkened leaves when the plant has flowered. *Madwort* derives from the practice whereby the leaves were mixed with a pinch or two of salt, prepared as a dressing and applied directly to any wound caused by the bite of a mad dog. The resultant effect was to calm any otherwise uncontrollable spasms. Dioscorides and Gerard believed that it could cure the bite of a rabid dog. In William Meyrick's *Herbal* (1790) we read that an infusion of its leaves are good for '*hypochondrical and hysterical complaints*'. It was used as an antiemetic, for mild depression, and taken for nervous dyspepsia, arthritis, gout, menstrual disorders and bronchial complaints. It is claimed that the plant acts as an antispasmodic, expectorant, stimulant and vermifuge (to expel intestinal worms).

Lucifer's Herb

Black horehound's second most common name is *black archangel, Lucifer*, while *Ballota vulgare* is called *white archangel, Michael*, who cast Lucifer from heaven. Black horehound, Lucifer's herb, is thus the herb of sorcery and occultism, whereas white horehound was believed to have the ability to repel spells cast against a household.

(WHITE) HOREHOUND

MARRUBIUM VULGARE
Family Lamiaceae/Labiatae, Mint

OTHER NAMES: White archangel, white horehound, common hoarhound, marrubio, bull's blood, eye of the star, hoarhound, seed of Horus, soldiers' tea, llwyd y cwn (dogs' hoar, Welsh), houndbane, huran, grand-bonhomme, *herbe vierge* (widow's herb, French), devil's eye.

DESCRIPTION: It grows 18 inches (46 cm) high with a 12-inch (30-cm) spread, looking a little like a white, or 'dead', nettle with clusters of small cream or purple-coloured flowers. Its wrinkled aromatic leaves smell of musty thyme. The stems and leaves are covered with downy hairs, giving a silvery-grey effect, and horehound is also spelt *hoarhound* from the Anglo-Saxon *har*, meaning grey. We still use the old word hoary when referring to a white frost. All parts of the plant are poisonous, which explains some of its alternative names. Excess dosage can cause dysphagia (difficulty in swallowing), dry mouth, pupil dilation, tachycardia (speeding up of the heart), restlessness, hallucinations, delirium and coma.

PROPERTIES AND USES: Culpeper noted: '*It is an herb of Mercury. A decoction of the dried herb, with the seed, or the juice of the green herb taken with honey, is a remedy for those that are short-winded, have a cough, or are fallen into a consumption, either through long sickness, or thin distillations of rheum upon the lungs. It helps to expectorate tough phlegm from the chest, being taken from the roots of Iris or Orris. It is given to women to bring down their courses, to expel the after-birth, and to them that have taken poison, or are stung or bitten by venomous serpents. The leaves used with honey, purge foul ulcers, stay running or creeping sores, and the growing of the flesh over the nails. It also helps pains of the sides. The juice thereof with wine and honey, helps to clear the eyesight, and snuffed up into the nostrils purges away the yellow jaundice, and with a little oil of roses dropped into the ears, eases the pains of them. Galen says, it opens obstructions both of the liver and spleen, and purges the breast and lungs of phlegm: and used outwardly it both cleanses and digests. A decoction of Horehound (says Matthiolus) is available for those that have hard livers, and for such as have itches and running tetters [skin diseases]. The powder hereof taken, or the decoction, kills worms. The green leaves bruised, and boiled in old hog's grease into an ointment, heals the biting of dogs, abates the swellings and pains that come by any pricking of thorns, or such like means;*

and used with vinegar, cleanses and heals tetters. There is a syrup made of Horehound to be had at the apothecaries, very good for old coughs, to rid the tough phlegm; as also to void cold rheums from the lungs of old folks, and for those that are asthmatic or short-winded.' Leaves and stems can be boiled and used in cough drops and syrups. White horehound is still used as in cough mixtures as an expectorant, and for bronchitis and whooping cough. Infusing the leaves gives an insecticide, excellent against caterpillars, which can be used as a fly-killer when mixed with milk. The plant makes a bitter tonic that stimulates digestion, easing bloating and wind. Horehound also contains a potent pain reliever and nervous system stimulant.

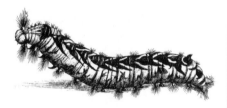

HISTORY: The Egyptians and Romans grew white horehound to treat coughs and colds, and Egyptian priests called it the *'seed of Horus'*, *'bulls blood'* and *'the eye of the star'*. It was a principal ingredient in a Roman antidote for vegetable poisons. Its name may come from the Hebrew *marrob* (a bitter juice), and it was one of the bitter herbs which the Jews were ordered to take for the Feast of Passover. Gerard recommended it, in addition to its uses in coughs and colds, for *'those that have drunk poyson or have been bitten of serpents,'* and it was also administered for *'mad dogge's biting... Syrup made of the greene fresh leaves and*

sugar is a most singular remedie against the cough and wheezing of the lungs...and doth wonderfully and above credit ease such as have been long sicke of any consumption of the lungs, as hath beene often proved by the learned physitions of our London College.' For centuries white horehound has been traditionally used as a reliable liver and digestive remedy, as well as being used to help reduce fevers and treat the symptoms of malaria. Recently the plant has been found to have a normalizing effect on an irregular heartbeat.

Horehound Ale

Before the first documented use of hops in beer as a bittering agent in the 11th century, brewers used a wide variety of bitter herbs and flowers, including horehound. The German name for horehound means *'mountain hops'*. Horehound ale/beer was brewed until the 20th century in the east of England, and a non-alcoholic variety is sold today.

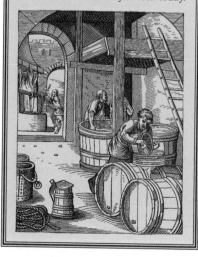

HORSETAIL

EQUISETUM ARVENSE
Family Equisetaceae, Horsetail

OTHER NAMES: Field horsetail, common horsetail, giant horsetail, shave-grass, bottle-brush, paddock-pipes, Dutch rushes, pewterwort, scouring rush, corncob plant, snake grass, puzzle grass.

DESCRIPTION: An herbaceous perennial with a hairy, tuberous rhizome. The stems are erect and grow to 2 feet (60 cm) tall, without leaves or hairs; they have black-toothed sheaths with whorls of spreading, green branches.

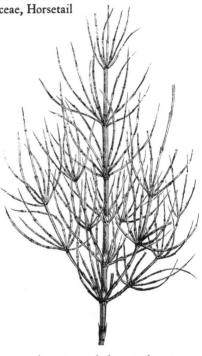

PROPERTIES AND USES: Culpeper: *'This herb belongs to Saturn. It is very powerful to stop bleeding either inward or outward, the juice of the decoction being drunk, or the juice, decoction, or distilled water applied outwardly. It also stays lasks or fluxes in man or woman, and heals the inward ulcers, and the excoriation of the entrails, bladder, &c. It solders together the tops of green wounds, and cures all ruptures in children. The decoction, taken in wine, provokes urine, and helps the stone and strangury; and the distilled water drank two or three times a day, and a small quantity at a time, also eases the entrails or guts, and is effectual in a cough that comes by distillation from the head. The juice or distilled water, used as a warm fomentation is of service in inflammations, pustules or red wheals, and other breakings-out in the skin, and eases the swelling heat and inflammation of the fundament, or privy parts, in men or women.'* Besides being useful in kidney and bladder trouble, horsetail can be used for haemorrhage, cystic ulceration and ulcers in the urinary passages. An external decoction will stop the bleeding of wounds and quickly heal them, and will also reduce the swelling of eyelids. Several of the species have been used medicinally, and the older herbalists considered them useful for healing wounds, and recommended them as a diuretic, for consumption and for dysentery. The ashes of the plant were considered very valuable in treating acidity of the stomach, dyspepsia, etc. The young shoots of the larger species of horsetail were formerly said to be eaten in Europe, dressed like asparagus, or fried with flour and butter. It is recorded that the poorer classes among the Romans occasionally ate them as a vegetable, but they are neither palatable nor very nutritious. They are used in Korean cuisine today. Linnaeus stated that the reindeer, which refuses ordinary hay, will eat a species of horsetail, and that it is cut as fodder in the north of Sweden for cows, with a view to increasing their milk, but that horses will not touch it. Another species, he states, forms excellent food for horses in some parts of Sweden, but cows are apt to lose their teeth by feeding on it and to be afflicted with diarrhoea.

HISTORY: A quantity of silica is deposited in the stems, especially in the epidermis or outer skin. In one species, *E. hyemale*, the epidermis contains so many abrasive silicates that bunches of the stem were commonly sold for polishing metal and used to be imported from Holland for the purpose, hence the popular name of *Dutch rushes*. It is also called by old writers *shavegrass*, and was formerly used by white-smiths and cabinet-makers. Gerard tells us that it was used for scouring pewter and wooden kitchen utensils, and so was named *pewterwort*, and that fletchers and comb-makers also rubbed and polished their work with it. In later days, the dairymaids of the northern counties of England used it for scouring their milk-pails. This accounts also for its common name of *scouring-rush*, as it was employed for scouring (cleaning) metal items such as cooking pots or drinking mugs, particularly those made of tin. In German, the corresponding name is *Zinnkraut* (tin-herb).

Living Fossil

This class of plants, the Equisetaceae, has no direct affinity with any other group of plants, being nearest allied to the ferns. The class Equisetopsida includes only a single genus, *Equisetum*, the name derived from the Latin words *equus* (a horse) and *seta* (a bristle), a reference to the peculiar bristly appearance of the jointed stems of the plants. Equisetum is known as a 'living fossil'. Over 200 millions years ago, huge plants of this order dominated the vegetation during the Carboniferous Period, with the well-known tree-size fossils of the genus *Calamites* being the stems of gigantic Equisetaceae. *Calamites* are found in coal deposits, and some Equisetopsida were as tall as 100 feet (30 m). This family of vascular plants reproduces by spores rather than seeds. The plant has a very high diploid number – 216 (108 pairs of chromosomes) – which is roughly five times greater than the human diploid number of 46. The Australian bulldog ant has the lowest diploid number possible, 1. The higher the number, the more likely it is that the organism has lost the ability to evolve, so humans may evolve into different forms, but the horsetails are in an evolutionary cul-de-sac and are unlikely to evolve further. The adder's tongue fern has the highest diploid number, 1200, of any organism, and the highest mammal count of 102 is found in a South American desert rodent, the viscacha rat.

HOUSELEEK

SEMPERVIVUM TECTORUM
Family Crassulaceae, Orpine

OTHER NAMES: Sengreen (Culpeper), liveforever, llysiau pentai (plants of the housetops, Welsh), hens and chicks, sengreen, ayron, ayegreen, bullock's eye, Thor's beard, Jupiter's beard, thunderbeard, Jupiter's eye, thunder flower.

DESCRIPTION:
A familiar hardy evergreen succulent, which grows in gardens and often appears on walls and roofs. There is a succulent multiple rosette of leaves with occasional pink, star-shaped flowers, growing around 9 inches (23 cm) high. It is called *hens and chicks* as it often propagates by lateral rosettes splitting from the mother plant.

PROPERTIES AND USES: Culpeper writes: *'The ordinary houseleek is good for all inward and outward heats, either in the eyes or other parts of the body. A posset made of the juice is singularly good in all hot agues, for it cools and tempers the blood and spirits and quenches the thirst. It is also good to stay all defluxions or sharp and salt rheums in the eyes, the juice being dropped into them. If the juice be dropped into the ears, it eases pain. It stops immoderate flooding of the menstrual, and helps the humours of the bowels. It cools and restrains all hot inflammations St. Anthony's fire* [erysipelas], *scaldings and burnings, the shingles, fretting ulcers, cankers, tetters,*

ringworms and the like; and is a certain ease to those who are affected by the gout.' After describing the use of the leaves in the cure of warts and corns, Culpeper relates: '...*it eases also the headache, and the distempered heat of the brain in frenzies, or through want of sleep, being applied to the temples and forehead. The leaves bruised and laid upon the crown or seam of the head, stays bleeding at the nose very quickly. The distilled water of the herb is profitable for all the purposes aforesaid. The leaves being gently rubbed on any place stung with nettles or bees, doth quickly take away the pain, and discharge the blisters proceeding therefrom.'* Gerard tells us the: *'Juice of Houseleek, Garden Nightshade and the buds of Poplar, boiled in hog's grease, make the most singular Populeon* [ointment] *that ever was used in Chirurgerie* [surgery].' The leaves were snapped in half to release the gel-like sap, to apply to insect bites, stings, burns and minor wounds in a similar manner to aloe vera. An infusion of the leaves treated bronchitis. Traditionally, to remove a corn or wart, cut a leaf in half and apply it to the corn for a few hours, and then soak the foot or hand in water before scraping off the corn or wart. The Natural History Museum's *Country Cures* website relates how a Cumbrian boy had a bandaged hand caused by ringworm from cattle. A gipsy cured it by recommending '*You have the cure on your wall. Take the leek, boil it and then dab the boy's hand with the water.*' She also recommended it for warts. A 1991 account from East Sussex reads: '*My father-in-law was brought up in Norfolk. When he was suffering from impetigo* [bacterial skin infection] *a visiting gypsy woman recommended breaking off a piece of houseleek and rubbing the sores with it. The houseleek was growing on the cottage roof. My father-in-law (who is still alive) says the cure did work.*'

HISTORY: Galen recommended houseleek for erysipelas and shingles, and Dioscorides as a remedy for weak and inflamed eyes. Pliny wrote that it never failed to produce sleep. In the 14th century it was used as an ingredient of a preparation for neuralgia called *hemygreyne*, i.e. *megrim*, and an ointment used at that time for scalds and burns. The names *ayegreen* and *sengreen* mean evergreen. The generic name *Sempervivum*

is from the Latin *semper* (always) and *vivare* (to live), as the plant thrives under almost all conditions. *Tectorium* bears witness to its usual place of growth – a roof. It was deliberately grown on roofs and can be seen on thatched roofs in Brittany today, especially along the apex. When fixed, it spreads fast by means of its offsets, and can easily be made to cover the whole roof of a building, whether of tiles, thatch or wood, by sticking the offsets on with a little earth. (Houseleek is now being used as a roof covering for new 'green' buildings. It seems to help preserve thatched roofs.) Culpeper noted: '*Jupiter claims dominion over this herb, from which it is fabulously reported, that it preserves whatever it grows upon from fire and lightning*', and Charlemagne ordered it to be planted upon the roof of every house in his empire. As in Brittany, Welsh countryfolk believed it protected their homes from storms, kept evil spells away, and ensured their prosperity.

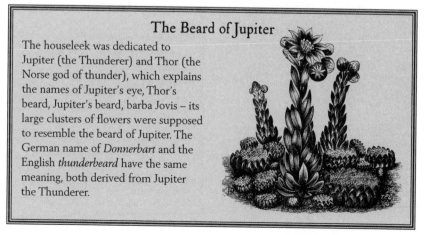

The Beard of Jupiter

The houseleek was dedicated to Jupiter (the Thunderer) and Thor (the Norse god of thunder), which explains the names of Jupiter's eye, Thor's beard, Jupiter's beard, barba Jovis – its large clusters of flowers were supposed to resemble the beard of Jupiter. The German name of *Donnerbart* and the English *thunderbeard* have the same meaning, both derived from Jupiter the Thunderer.

HYSSOP

HYSSOPUS OFFICINALIS
Family Lamiaceae/Labiatae, Mint

OTHER NAMES: Blue hyssop (there is also a pink hyssop variety, *Hyssop officinalis roseus*). Isop (Welsh).

DESCRIPTION: Hardy evergreen bush with a height of 30 inches (76 cm) and a spread of 36 inches (91 cm), with dense spikes of dark blue flowers, and lance-like leaves tasting of mint and sage.

PROPERTIES AND USES: *'The herb is Jupiter's, and the sign Cancer. It strengthens all the parts of the body under Cancer and Jupiter; which what they may be, is found amply described in my astrological judgment of diseases. Dioscorides says, that Hyssop boiled with rue and honey, and drank, helps those that are troubled with coughs, shortness of breath, wheezing and rheumatic distillation upon the lungs.'* – Nicholas Culpeper. Hyssop helps fight infection, particularly in the respiratory tract and thus helps with colds, catarrh and chest infections. Hyssop has been one of the main expectorant and decongestant herbs commonly used to treat respiratory conditions such as influenza, colds and bronchitis. It also increases circulation, causing sweating and lowering fevers. Hyssop has a regulating effect on the blood pressure, tending to lower it if it is high, and raise it if is low. The leaves, stems and flowers have a highly aromatic odour and when distilled produce an essential oil used by perfumers, its value being greater than oil of lavender. It is also employed for the manufacture of liqueurs, being an important constituent in Chartreuse. Honey obtained from hyssop is much favoured. The leaves are used as a medicinal tea for colds and flu. Hyssop essential oil relieves stress, and can help clear bruises. Flowers can be used in salads, and the leaves, chopped thinly, add a mint flavour to salads or stews.

HISTORY: The *Hyssopos* of Dioscorides was named from *azob* (*aesob*, the Hebrew name meaning holy herb), because it was used for cleaning sacred places. Historically used as a cleansing herb, it is mentioned in the Old Testament as a symbol of purity, and is one of the 'bitter herbs' to be taken over Passover. Hippocrates (*c.*460–*c.*377 BCE) prescribed hyssop for chest complaints. Because of its aroma it was formerly employed as a strewing herb. It said to be a sprig of hyssop that was used to offer up the sponge soaked in vinegar and sour wine for Jesus when he was on the Cross.

Butterfly Deterrent

Hyssop makes an excellent low hedging plant, and is used as a companion plant to deter the cabbage white butterfly from brassicas. It also seems to stimulate grape production, and is thought to repel slugs from lettuce.

IRIS - FLAG IRIS

IRIS GERMANICA
Family Iridaceae, Iris

OTHER NAMES: Blue flag, blue flower de luce, German iris, German flag.

DESCRIPTION: The sword-like leaves are bluish-green, narrow and flat, and the flower-sterns are 2 to 3 feet (60 to 90 cm) high. The flowers are large and deep blue, or purplish-blue in colour, but closely related species range from pale blue to white. The flowers have an agreeable scent, reminiscent of orange blossoms.

PROPERTIES AND USES: Culpeper often refers to the plant in his works, saying that *'it strengthens the stomach exceedingly, Orris, or Flower-de-luce…takes away the pains thereof coming of cold… the smell of it strengthens the brain…They are hot and dry…relieves faint hearts, takes away windiness in degree, resists poison, helps shortness of the breath, provokes the menses. Root being green and bruised…it helps ulcers in the head, and blackness and blueness of a stroke…amends the ill colour of the face.'* The root has been used as an expectorant and a remedy for colds and coughs. It is also said to relieve nausea and flatulence and improve circulation. The dried root is the valuable *'orris'* root, scented of violet and used in perfumes, cosmetic powders, toothpastes and breath fresheners. Pieces of the dried root were also given to infants to chew. Three species of iris furnish the orris root of commerce, the *Iris germanica*, or blue flag; the *Iris pallida*, or pale flag, and the *Iris albicans (florentina)*, or white flag.

HISTORY: Theophrastus, Dioscorides and Pliny wrote of *orris root*, and Charlemagne ordered its planting. The plant was named after the rainbow goddess Iris, from the variety of colours in the flowers of the genus. Dedicated to Juno, it seems to be the origin of the sceptre. Orris root powder was sometimes known as *'love drawing powder'*.

A Perfume for a Sweet Bag

'Take half a pound of Cypress Roots, a pound of Orris, 3 quarter of a pound of Calamus, 3 Orange stick with Cloves, 2 ounces of Benjamin, 3 quarters of a pound of Rhodium, a pound of Coriander seed, and an ounce of Storax and 4 pecks of Damask Rose leaves, a peck of dried sweet Marjoram, a pretty stick of Juniper shaved very thin, some lemon pele dried and a stick of Brazil; let all these be powdered very grossly for ye first year and immediately put into your bags; the next year pound and work it and it will be very good again.'

Mary Doggett, *Mary Doggett: Her Book of Receipts*, 1682.

IRIS - YELLOW FLAG

IRIS PSEUDACORUS
Family Iridaceae, Iris

OTHER NAMES: Culpeper also names it the *flower de luce, myrtle flag,* and *myrtle grass*. Iris aquatica, yellow iris, water flag, Jacob's sword, dragon flower, flaggon, daggers, levers.

DESCRIPTION: Culpeper says: '*It usually grows in watery ditches, ponds, lakes, and moor sides, which are always overflowed with water.*' Its name means 'false acorus', referring to the similarity of its leaves to those of a plant that favours the same habitat, *Acorus calamus* (sweet flag), which also has a prominently veined mid-rib and sword-like leaf shape. It is a herbaceous perennial plant growing to 3–5 feet (90 cm to 1.5 m) tall, with long erect leaves and bright yellow flowers with the typical iris form. It tolerates poor soils and total immersion and is very invasive. Along with stinking iris, it is native to Britain.

PROPERTIES AND USES: In Culpeper: '*It is under the dominion of the Moon. The root of this Water-flag is very astringent, cooling, and drying; and thereby helps all lasks* [diarrhoea] *and fluxes, whether of blood or humours, as bleeding at the mouth, nose, or other parts, bloody flux, and the immoderate flux of women's courses. The distilled water of the whole herb, flowers and roots, is a sovereign good remedy for watering eyes, both to be dropped into them, and to have cloths or sponges wetted therein, and applied to the forehead. It also helps the spots and blemishes that happen in and about the eyes, or in any other parts. The said water fomented on swellings and hot inflammations of women's breasts, upon cancers also, and those spreading ulcers called Noli me tangere, do much good. It helps also foul ulcers in the privities* [private parts] *of man or woman; but an ointment made of the flowers is better for those external applications.*'

'*Noli me tangere*' (touch me not) was the name then applied to several varieties of ulcerous skin diseases, but is now restricted to *Lupus exedens*, an ulcerative affliction of the nose.

HISTORY: The rhizome has historically been used as a herbal remedy, most often as an emetic. Yellow iris is now used as a form of water treatment since it has the ability to take up heavy metals through its roots.

Fleur-de-lys

Clovis (*c.*466–511 CE), the Merovingian king of the Franks, first wore the flower as a heraldic device in the sixth century, and Louis VII adopted it as the fleur-de-lys emblem of France.

IRIS - STINKING GLADWIN

IRIS FOETIDISSIMA
Family Iridaceae, Iris

OTHER NAMES: Stinking iris, gladdon, gladwyn, roast beef plant, adder's meat, spurge plant.

DESCRIPTION: It has mauve flowers, and is one of only two native British irises. The long strap-like leaves form dense evergreen clumps, often on chalky soils. Culpeper relates that *'the root is like that of the Flower-de-luce, but reddish on the outside, and whitish within, very sharp and hot in the taste, of as evil a scent as the leaves.'* In the autumn and winter, it puts on a spectacular display when its almost disproportionately large seed pods burst open to reveal brilliant orange, or sometimes red, seeds.

PROPERTIES AND USES: Culpeper notes: *'It is used by many country people to purge corrupt phlegm and choler, which they do by drinking the decoction of the roots... The powder thereof drank in wine, helps those that are troubled with the cramps and convulsions, or with the gout and sciatica, and gives ease to those that have griping pains in their body and belly, and helps those that have the strangury...The root boiled in wine and drank, doth effectually procure women's courses, and used as a pessary, works the same effect, but causes abortion in women with child...The root is very effectual in all wounds, especially of the head; as also to draw forth any splinters,*

thorns, or broken bones, or any other thing sticking in the flesh, without causing pains, being used with a little verdigris and honey, and the great Centaury root. The same boiled in vinegar, and laid upon an eruption or swelling, doth very effectually dissolve and consume them; yea, even the swellings of the throat called the king's evil; the juice of the leaves or roots heals the itch, and all running or spreading scabs, sores, blemishes, or scars in the skin, wheresoever they be.'

HISTORY: Theophrastus recommended it as a purgative in the fourth century BCE. In his English translation of the Flemish botanist Rembert Dodoens's *A New Herbal*, Henry Lyte, calling it '*Stinking Gladin*', said that the leaves were '*of a loathsome smell or stinke, almost like unto the stinking worm, called in Latin Cimex*'. Despite this, the plant was highly valued as a medicinal herb, especially for making poultices for drawing out splinters and even arrow heads.

Burning Rubber

The leaves, when they are crushed, do not necessarily smell of roast beef despite the common name, but more like burning rubber. *Gladwyn* is an old name for a sword, referring to the shape of the leaves.

ION THE GARDENER

Mayster (Master) Ion Gardener wrote the first practical English text, *The Feate of Gardening c.*1440. It was a set of instructions in verse on the cultivation, grafting, and the culture of herbs. All of the herbs listed were Old World, commonly grown all over Europe for hundreds of years, and the plants could make a perfect replica 15th-century garden. Here is his list of plants:

Gardener	Modern	Classification
Adderstongue	Adder's tongue	*Ophioglossum vulgatum* or *Arum maculatum*
Afodyl	Daffodil	*Narcissus pseudo-narcissus*
Apyl	Apple	*Pyrus malus*
Asche Tree	Ash Tree	*Fraxinus excelsior*
Avens	Herb bennet	*Geum urbanum*
Betony	Bishop's wort	*Stachys betonica*
Bigold or Bygu	Corn marigold	*Chrysanthemum segetum*
Borage	Borage	*Borago officinalis*
Bryswort	Bruisewort	*Bellis perennis* (daisy), or *saponaria officinalis* (soapwort)
Bugu	Bugle	*Ajuga reptans*
Calamynte	Basil thyme	*Calamintha officinalis*
Camemyl	Chamomile	*Anthemis noblis*
Carsyndills	Cresses	*Lepidium sativum*
Centory	Cornflower	*Centaurea cyaneus*
Centory	Great centaury	*Centaurea nigra*
Centory	Little centaury	*Erythraea centaurium*
Clarey	Clary sage	*Salvia horminodes* or *sclarea*
Comfrey	Comfrey	*Symphytum officinale*
Coryawnder	Coriander	*Coriandrum sativum*
Cowslippe	Cowslip	*Primula veris*
Egrimoyne	Agrimony	*Agrimonia eupatoria*
Elysawder	Alexanders	*Smyrnium olustratum*
Feldwort	Felwort	*Gentiana amarella*
Feltwort	Common mullein	*Verbascum thapsus*
Floscampi	Ragged Robin	*Lychnis flos-cuculi* or *Lychnis diurna*
Foxglove	Foxglove	*Digitalis purpurea*
Fynel	Fennel	*Foeniculum vulgare*
Garleke	Garlic	*Allium sativum* or *Allium ursinum*
Gladyn	Stinking gladwin	*Iris foetidissima* or *Iris pseudacorus*
Gromel	Gromwell	*Lithospermum officinale*
Growdyswyly	Groundsel	*Senecio vulgaris*
Hasel tree	Hazel tree	*Corylus avellana*
Haw thorn	Hawthorn	*Cratoegus oxycantha*
Henbane	Henbane	*Hyoscamus niger*
Herb Ion	St John's wort	*Hypericum perforatum*
Herbe Robert	Herb Robert	*Geranium robertianum*
Herbe Walter	Sweet woodruff	*Galium odoratum*
Hertystonge	Hartstongue	*Scolopendrium vulgare*
Holyhocke	Hollyhock, single	*Alcea rosea*

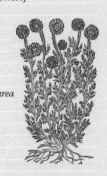

Honysoke	Honeysuckle	*Lonicera periclymenum*
Horehound	Horehound	*Marrubium vulgare*
Langbefe	Viper's bugloss	*Echium vulgaris* or *Heleminthia echioides*
Lavyndull	Lavender	*Lavendula vera*
Letows	Lettuce	*Lactuca sativa*
Primrose	Primrose	*Primula vulgaris*
Leke	Leek	*Allium porrum*
Lyly	Lily	*Lilium candidum* and others
Lyverwort	Liverwort	*Anemone hepatica* or *Marchantia polymorpha*
Merege	Celery?	*Apium graviolens?*
Moderwort	Motherwort	*Artemisia vulgare* or *Lysimachia numullaria*
Mouseer	Mouse ear	*Hieracium pilosella* or *Cerastium triviale*
Myntys	Mint	*Mentha* varieties
Nept, Neppe	Catmint	*Nepeta cataria*
Oculus Christi	Wild clary sage	*Salvia verbanaca*
Orage	Orach	*Atriplex hortensis*
Orpy, Orpies	Orpine, Stonecrop	*Sedum telephium*
Owyns, Oynet	Onion	*Allium cepa*
Parrow	Yarrow?	*Achillea millefolium?*
Pellyter	Pellitory of the wall	*Parietaria officinalis*
Percely, Perseley	Parsley	*Petroselinum sativus*
Pere	Pear	*Pyrus communis*
Peruynke	Periwinkle	*Vinca major* or *minor*
Primrole	Primrose	*Primula vulgaris*
Polypody	Common polypody	*Polypodium vulgare*
Pympenold	Pimpernel	*Anagalis arvensis* or *Poterium sanguisorba*
Redenaye	Red rye grass	*Lolium perenne*
Rewe	Rue	*Ruta graveolans*
Rose	Rose	*Rosa* varieties
Rybwort	Ribwort	*Plantago lanceolata*
Saferowne	Saffroc	*Crocus sativus*
Sage	Garden sage	*Salvia officinalis*
Sanycle	Sanicle	*Sanicula europeae*
Sauerey	Savory	*Satureja hortensis* or *Satureja montana*
Scabyas	Small scabious	*Scabiosa columbaria*
Seueny	Mustard (black, wild or white)	*Sinapsis nigra, arvensis* or *alba*
Sowthrynwode	Southernwood	*Artemisia abrotanum*
Sperewort	Spearwort	*Ranunculus flammula*
Spynage	Spinach	*Spinaca oleracea*
Strowberys	Strawberry	*Fragaria vesca*
Stychworde	Stitchwort	*Stellaria holostea*
Tansay	Tansy	*Tanacetum vulgare*
Totesnay	Tutsan	*Hypericum androsaemum*
Tuncarse	Town cress	*Lepidium sativum*
Tyme	Wild thyme	*Thymus serpylum*
Valeryan	Valerian	*Valeriana officinalis*
Violet	Sweet violet	*Viola odorata*
Warmot	Wormwood	*Artemisia absinthium*
Woderofe	Woodruff	*Asperula odorata*
Wodesour	Woodsour	*Oxalis acetosella* or *Berberis vulgaris*
Wurtys or Wortys	Wild cabbage	*Brassica oleracea*
Wyldresyl	Common teasel	*Dipsacus sylvestris*
Ysope	Hyssop	*Hyssopus officinalis*

(COMMON) IVY

HEDERA HELIX
Family Arialiaceae, Ivy

OTHER NAMES: English ivy, gort, bindwood, lovestone.

DESCRIPTION: Invasive evergreen climber, with dark-green, glossy, angular leaves. The large black berries are eaten by birds in poor winters.

PROPERTIES AND USES: Culpeper: '*About a dram of the flowers (says Dioscorides), drank twice a day in red wine, helps the lask* [diarrhoea], *and bloody flux. It is an enemy to the nerves and sinews, being much taken inwardly, out very helpful to them, being outwardly applied. Pliny says, the yellow berries are good against the jaundice; and taken before one be set to drink hard, preserves from drunkenness, and helps those that spit blood; and that the white berries being taken inwardly, or applied outwardly, kills the worms in the belly. The berries are a singular remedy to prevent the plague, as also to free them from it that have got it, by drinking the berries thereof made into a powder, for two or three days together. They being taken in wine, do certainly help to break the stone, provoke urine, and women's courses. The fresh leaves of Ivy, boiled in vinegar, and applied warm to the sides of those that are troubled with the spleen, ache, or stitch in the sides, do give much ease. The same applied with some Rosewater, and oil of Roses, to the temples and forehead, eases the head-ache, though it be of long continuance. The fresh leaves boiled in wine, and old filthy ulcers hard to be cured washed therewith, do wonderfully help to cleanse them. It also quickly heals green wounds, and is effectual to heal all burnings and scaldings, and all kinds of exulcerations coming thereby, or by salt phlegm or humours in other parts of the body. The juice of the berries or leaves snuffed up into the nose, purges the head and brain of thin rheum that makes defluxions into the eyes and nose, and curing the ulcers and stench therein; the same dropped into the ears helps the old and running sores of them; those that are troubled with the spleen shall find much ease by continual drinking out of a cup made of Ivy, so as the drink may stand some small time therein before it be drank. Cato says that wine put into such a cup, will soak through it, by reason of the antipathy that is between them. There seems to be a very great antipathy between wine and Ivy; for if one hath got a surfeit by drinking of wine, his speediest cure is to drink a draught of the same wine wherein a handful of Ivy leaves, being first bruised, have been boiled.*' In 1597, the British herbalist John Gerard recommended water infused with ivy leaves as a wash for sore or watering eyes. The broad leaves being evergreen afford shelter to birds in the winter, and many prefer ivy to other shrubs, in which to build their nests.

HISTORY: Greek priests presented a wreath of ivy to newly-married persons, and the ivy has throughout the ages been regarded as the emblem of fidelity. Ivy leaves formed the poet's crown, as well as the wreath of Bacchus, to whom the plant was dedicated, probably because of the practice of binding the brow with ivy leaves to prevent intoxication, a quality formerly attributed to the plant. The custom of decorating houses and churches with ivy at Christmas was forbidden by one of the early Councils of the Church, on account of its pagan associations, but the custom remained for centuries. To remove sunburn it was recommended to smear the face with tender ivy twigs boiled in butter, according to the ninth century Anglo-Saxon Leechbook of Bald. English taverns bore over their doors the sign of an ivy bush to indicate the excellence of the liquor supplied within, leading to the old saying *'Good wine needs no bush'* mentioned in Shakespeare's *As You Like It.*

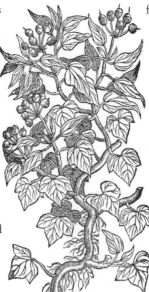

From *Love's Martyr,* 1601

There's Ivy, that doth cling about the tree,
And with her leafy arms doth round
    embrace
The rotten hollow, withered trunk we see,
That from the maiden Cissus took that
    place,
Grape-crowned Bacchus did this damsel
    grace:
Love-piercing windows dazzled so her eye,
That in Love's over-kindness she did die.
A rich-wrought sumptuous Banquet was
    prepared,
Unto the which the Gods were all
    invited:
Amongst them all this Cissus was
    ensnared,
And in the sight of Bacchus much
    delighted:

In her faire bosom was true Love united,
She danced and often kissed him with
    such mirth,
That sudden joy did stop her vital
    breath.
As soon as that the Nourisher of things,
Our Grand-Dame Earth had tasted of
    her blood,
From forth her body a fresh Plant there
    springs,
And then an Ivy-climbing Herb there
    stood,
That for the flux Dysentery is good:
For the remembrance of the God of
    wine,
It therefore always clasps about the Vine.

Robert Chester

JUNIPER

JUNIPERUS COMMUNIS
Family Cupressaceae, Cypress

OTHER NAMES: Culpeper names it Juniper-Bush, as it often only grows to 6 feet (1.8 m) high. Bastard killer, common juniper, gin berry, geneva, gin plant, enegro. There are up to 66 other species of juniper, and *Juniperus communis* has the largest range of any woody plant, being found across Europe, North America and the northern parts of Asia.

DESCRIPTION: The small, slow-growing evergreen has needle-like aromatic leaves, and the conifer can grow to 30 feet (9 m), with berries forming on the female tree.

PROPERTIES AND USES: Culpeper noted its use as a diuretic, against venomous bites, for dropsy, stranguary (difficulty in urinating), wind, colic, stomach aches, coughs, cramps, convulsions, eyesight, gout, sciatica and safe childbirth: '*The ashes of the wood are a special remedy for scurvy in the gums, by rubbing them therewith. The berries stay all fluxes, help the haemorrhoids or piles, and kill worms in children. They break the stone, procure lost appetite, and are very good for palsies and falling sickness. A lye made of the ashes of the wood, and the body bathed therewith, cures then itch, scabs and leprosy.*' Juniper is still used to treat rheumatism, cystitis and kidney inflammation. Juniper oil is used in aromatherapy and for massaging aching muscles. Crushed berries flavour meat dishes and marinades.

HISTORY: Greeks used the berries to increase physical stamina in athletes, and Romans used them as a cheap, domestically produced substitute for the expensive pepper from India. Pliny reported '*Pepper is adulterated with juniper berries, which have the property, to a marvellous degree, of assuming the pungency of pepper.*' Juniper was used to cure snakebites and protect against infectious diseases. It was burnt in homes to ward off the plague. Juniper 'berries', actually black seed cones, give gin its flavour, and its name is the shortened version of *jenever* or *genever*, the Dutch name for the tree, or from the French genièvre. Gin was originally known as *Holland's Gin*, denoting its Dutch origins.

Natural Contraceptive

In his *De Materia Medica*, Dioscorides lists juniper berries, when crushed and put on the penis or vagina before intercourse, as a contraceptive. Native North Americans used juniper berries as a female contraceptive, and in Somerset it was used for abortions and called *bastard killer*.

LADY'S MANTLE

ALCHEMILLA VULGARIS
Family Rosaceae, Rose

OTHER NAMES: Common lady's mantle, Our Lady's mantle, common alchemil, leontopodium, lion's foot, pied-de-lion, bear's foot, nine hooks, woman's best friend, mantell fair (Welsh).

DESCRIPTION: It has rounded, lobed leaves resembling cloaks with yellow-green flowers growing through clumps of soft foliage. (It is similar to *Alchemilla mollis*, but with more potent healing properties). The finely toothed leaves have given it the name of *nine hooks*.

PROPERTIES AND USES: Nicholas Culpeper: '*Lady's Mantle is very proper for inflamed wounds and to stay bleeding, vomiting, fluxes of all sorts, bruises by falls and ruptures. It is also good for some disorders in women's breasts, causing them to grow les and hard, being both outwardly and inwardly applied…a bath…will sometimes prevent miscarriages. It is one of the most singular wound herbs and therefore highly prized and praised by the Germans, used in all wounds inward and outward, to drink a decoction thereof and wash the wounds therewith, or dip tents therein and put them into the wounds which wonderfully dries up all humidity of the sores and abates all inflammations thereof. It quickly heals green wounds, not suffering any corruption to remain behind and cures old sores, though fistulous and hollow.*' 'Green wounds' indicate that they are infected, often with a greenish tinge. It was also used to help control excessive menstrual bleeding or diarrhoea. A noted 'wound herb', cuts, scrapes and burns can be treated with skin washes of lady's mantle to prevent infection. It contains salicylic acid, and has sedative properties that help to alleviate cramps and painful menstruation. Its tannic properties produce a bright green dye for wool.

HISTORY: Jewel-like drops of moisture form on the lobed leaves on humid days, caused by water being forced out of tiny pores, and these were collected by herbalists to cure infertility. The name *Alchemilla* comes from the Arabic '*alkemelych*', alchemist, as early chemists believed that its dewdrops also had magical powers that could really help them in their quest for the *philosopher's stone* capable of turning base metals like lead to precious gold. In Sweden a tradition held that if placed under the pillow at night, the herb would promote a good night's sleep.

Mary's Cloak

Its shapely and pleated leaves look like a lady's cloak (mantle) from medieval times. The cloak was thought suitable for the Virgin Mary, and the original common name of the herb was *Our Lady's mantle* in honour of Mary.

LAVENDER

LAVANDULA ANGUSTIFOLIA
Family Lamiaceae/Labiateae, Mint

OTHER NAMES: Elf leaf, nard, spikenard, spike, English lavender, true lavender, *fleurs de lavande*. It was formerly known as *Lavandula officinalis* and *Lavandula vera*. There are many, many varieties as it crosspollinates freely. What is known as 'Old English lavender' is a cross between L. *angustifolia* and L. *latifolia*, itself known as '*spike lavender*'. French lavender is L. *stoechas*, with camphor-scented leaves and distinctive bracts, or 'ears' of flowers.

DESCRIPTION: This is a wonderfully scented plant, it can grow up to 32 inches (81 cm) high, with richly scented purple-blue flowers and aromatic grey-green leaves.

PROPERTIES AND USES:

Culpeper describes it thus: '*Mercury owns the herb; and it carries his effects very potently. Lavender is of a special good use for all the griefs and pains of the head and brain that proceed of a cold cause, as the apoplexy, falling-sickness, the dropsy, or sluggish malady, cramps, convulsions, palsies, and often faintings. It strengthens the stomach, and frees the liver and spleen from obstruction, provokes women's menses, and expels the dead child and afterbirth... The chemical oil drawn from Lavender, usually called Oil of Spike, is of so fierce and piercing a quality, that it is cautiously to be used, some few drops being sufficient to be* given with other things, either for inward or outward griefs.' Culpeper also says that '*a decoction made with the flowers of Lavender, Horehound, Fennel and Asparagus root, and a little Cinnamon, is very profitably used to help the falling-sickness* [epilepsy] *and the giddiness or turning of the brain.*' William Salmon in his *Botanologia. The English Herbal: or History of Plants* of 1710 says that: '*it is good also against the biting of serpents, mad-dogs and other venomous creature, being given inwardly and applied poultice-wise to the parts wounded. The spirituous tincture of the dried leaves or seeds, if prudently given, cures hysteric fits though vehement and of long standing.*'

Lavender is used to relax muscle spasms, and to relax the body in the presence of pain. It can also be used as an antidepressant, and to ease headaches. Its oil was inhaled to prevent vertigo and fainting. A water solution was used as a gargle for hoarseness or a loss of voice. For restful sleep, drink lavender flower tea or sprinkle a few drops of lavender on sheets and pillowcases. Swollen feet or ankles benefit from a cool footbath with lavender water. For minor scrapes, cuts and abrasions washing the affected area and then applying a few neat drops of lavender will help. Antibacterial lavender is a used for burns, insect bites and most common skin irritations. It kills diphtheria bacteria, streptococcal, pneumococcal and typhoid bacilli. Lavender oil is used in baths, room sprays, toilet waters, perfumes, colognes, massage oils, sachets, salves, skin lotions and oils. It is traditionally used for sachets to place among linens and clothing, both as a perfume and as a moth repellent. Flies and mosquitoes dislike its fragrance, so fresh-cut flowers make a beautiful and practical addition to the dining table. Lavender can be used in cooking, especially in making lavender biscuits. Lavender water is mildly antiseptic and can be used to wipe down kitchen work surfaces. It makes a wonderfully fragrant flower border.

HISTORY: Lavender is derived from the Latin '*lavare*', to wash. It was known by the Greeks as *Nardus*, exported from markets in Naarda, a city in Syria, and used for throat infections and chest complaints. In Roman times the blossoms were sold for 100 denarii per pound, which was about the same as month's wage for a farm labourer. The Romans used lavender flowerheads in their bath water as a fragrance and antiseptic. They introduced it to Britain to heal burns, cuts and wounds, and to repel nits and fleas. In France, since the 17th century the essential oil has been used for perfumes. In medieval times herbalists used lavender to prevent head lice, ease stiff joints and relieve tiredness. '*Who will buy my lavender*' was probably the most famous cry of London street vendors. It was used across Europe for strewing the floors of churches and houses on festive occasions, or to make bonfires on St John's Day, when evil spirits are supposed to be abroad. Traditionally, bundles of lavender were placed in the hands of women during childbirth to bring courage and strength. It is said that planting lavender around the house will help deter evil and protect the people within the household. Putting the flowers between the bed sheets will ensure that a couple will never quarrel.

Cloaking the Smell of Death

During the Great Plague of London (bubonic plague) in 1665, lavender was hung in bunches, so its fragrance would cloak the foul smell of death and decay. In the 17th century huge fields of lavender were grown in France to supply the perfume trade. At this time the glove makers of Grasse in France were scenting their leathers with lavender oil, and many wearers of these gloves in London during the Black Death seemed to stay plague-free. Lavender tends to repel fleas and insects.

LEMON BALM

MELISSA OFFICINALIS
Family Lamiaceae/Labiatae, Mint

OTHER NAMES: Bawm (Culpeper), sweet balm (there are other golden and variegated varieties), melissa, sweet melissa, bee balm (bergamot is also called bee balm), gwenynddail (bee leaves, Welsh – it is one of the greatest attractors of bees to a garden).

DESCRIPTION: It grows in clumps of up to 3 feet (90 cm), with clusters of small cream flowers. The crushed leaves smell of lemon, and it can become invasive. Its lemon scent is lost in cooking.

PROPERTIES AND USES: According to Culpeper, '*It is an herb of Jupiter, and under Cancer, and strengthens nature much in all its actions. Let a syrup made of the juice of it and sugar (as you shall be taught at the latter end of this book) be kept in every gentlewoman's house, to relieve the weak stomachs and sick bodies of their poor sickly neighbour… Serapio said it causes the mind and heart to become merry and revives the heart fainting into swoonings…drives out all troublesome cares and thoughts out of the mind arising from melancholy, or black choler, which Avicenna also confirms. It is very good to help digestion, and open obstructions of the brain; and has such a purging quality, said Avicenna, as to expel those melancholy vapours from the spirits and blood which are in the heart and arteries, though it cannot do so from other parts of the body. Dioscorides said that, if the leaves were steeped in wine, and the wine drunk, and the leaves applied externally, it is a remedy against scorpion stings, and the biting of mad dogs.* [Dioscorides] *commends the decoction thereof for women thereof to bath or sit in, to procure their menses; it is good to wash aching teeth therewith, and profitable for those who have the bloody diarrhoea. Pliny, when writing on balm, informs us that if it be tied to the sword which gave the wound, it instantly stops the blood. The leaves also with a little saltpetre taken in drink are good against a surfeit of mushrooms, help the griping pains of the belly, and, being made into an electuary, are good for them that cannot fetch their breath with ease…A tansy or caudle made with eggs, and the juice thereof when it is young, putting to it some sugar and rose-water, is good for women in child-bed, when the afterbirth is not thoroughly voided, and for their faintings upon and after their sore travail. The herb bruised and boiled in a little wine and oil, and laid upon a boil, will ripen and break it.*' Balm contains tannins and has been found to be antibacterial, antiviral, helping to cure mild depression and aiding digestion. The leaf rubbed into the skin is a natural insect repellent, and can also alleviate pain from stings.

The plant makes one of the best herbal teas, lifting one's spirits, and is thought to be good for the memory. It is popular in France, and known as *'thé de France'*. It is calming, relaxing and releases tension, being beneficial for PMS sufferers. Balm is useful in a range of allergies such as hay fever and eczema. It can relieve cramps and flatulence, and relieve pain caused by irritable bowel syndrome. Melissa oil is used for depression, restlessness, excitement, headache and insomnia. It will seed itself and spread naturally, helping orchard trees become fertilized by bees. Greeks smeared the inside of beehives with its scent.

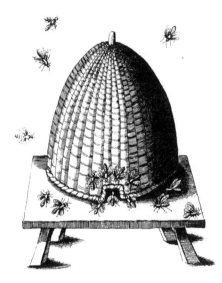

HISTORY: The Greeks called it *Melisphyllon*, honey leaf. Avicenna described balm as cheering and other Arab physicians believed it eased melancholy and heart problems The lemon-scented plant has been valued since antiquity. Pliny and Dioscorides believed

Scientific Research

Research conducted by scientists at Northumbria University suggests that lemon balm increases the activity of acetylcholene, a chemical messenger linked to memory function that is reduced in people with Alzheimer's disease. In 1999 a double-blind German trial studied a topical cream made from dried leaf extract of lemon balm used for the treatment of *Herpes simplex labialis* ('cold sores' on the lips). The lemon balm cream shortened the healing period and had an beneficial effect on associated symptoms such as itching, burning and swelling.

'Balm, being applied, doth close up wounds without any peril of inflammation.' Gerard said *'The juice of Balm glueth together greene wounds, being put in oil, salve or balm for that purpose, makes it of greater efficacy.'* We now know that the hydrocarbons in its oils starve bacteria of oxygen. Culpeper said: *'Used with salt, its takes away wens* [sebaceous cysts], *kernels, or hard swelling in the flesh or throat; it cleanses foul sores, and eases pains of the gout. It is also good for the liver and spleen.'* In the Middle Ages lemon balm dressed wounds, cured rabid dog bites, toothache, boils and skin eruptions, pregnancy sickness, baldness and was a love charm. It was the main ingredient in *Carmelite water*, distilled by Parisian monks from 1611, and still used in France as a digestive and antispasmodic. It was planted by front doors in medieval times to drive away spirits, used as a strewing herb and applied fresh to polish furniture and impart a fragrance to it.

LEMON
CITRUS LIMON
Family Rutaceae, Rue/Citrus

OTHER NAMES: Citrus medica, limone.

DESCRIPTION: The trees are usually around 12–15 feet (3.7–4.6 m) high, with glossy green leaves. Flowers are white with a strong fragrance, and the fruit grows underneath the flowers, so on a healthy lemon tree, flowers and ripe fruits can often be found at the same time.

PROPERTIES AND USES:
In Maud Grieve's *Herbal* we read: *'Locally, it is a good astringent, whether as a gargle in sore throat, in pruritis of the scrotum, in uterine haemorrhage after delivery, or as a lotion in sunburn. It is said to be the best cure for severe, obstinate hiccough, and is helpful in jaundice and hysterical palpitation of the heart. The decoction has been found to be a good antiperiodic, useful as a substitute for quinine in malarial conditions, or for reducing the temperature in typhoid. It is probable that the lemon is the most valuable of all fruit for preserving health. The oil, externally, is a strong rubefacient* [a substance that produces redness of the skin], *and taken internally in small doses has stimulating and carminative properties…A thousand lemons yield between 1 and 2 lb. of oil.'* Because of its high vitamin C content, lemon is used to help build immunity against colds, influenza, to detoxify the body and as a tonic. Drinking diluted lemon juice is proven to help prevent kidney stones.

HISTORY: In Mesopotamia *citrons* were propagated for their beauty and aroma, as they flowered throughout the year. Egyptians used lemons in embalming, and the tribes of Israel brought them to Israel from their captivity in Babylon. Jewish gardeners were responsible for the cultivation of citrus fruits, as Romans commissioned them to develop the orange and lemon, which they did using the citron as grafting stock. As part of his ships' rations, Columbus took citrus seeds to the New World for the first time, where they spread throughout the Caribbean.

The Spanish explorer Ponce de León then took them to Florida in 1513, and required his sailors to plant 100 seeds each wherever they landed, leading to the great Florida citrus industry.

Preventing Scurvy

Lemon juice is probably the best of all antiscorbutics, being used against scurvy. Even though a naval surgeon, James Lind, had proved in 1753 that citrus fruit prevented scurvy, the disease was a major killer of seamen until the early 19th century, when it was at last introduced into naval rations. Not until decades later were merchant seamen given citrus fruit.

LEMON VERBENA

ALOYSIA TRIPHYLLA
Family Verbenaceae, Verbena

OTHER NAMES: Cedron, hierba louisa, lemon louisa, herb louisa, verveine citronelle or odorante, lemon-scented verbena, lemon beebrush.

DESCRIPTION: The pale green leaves are very fragrant, lanceolate, 3 to 4 inches (8 to 10 cm) long, and the many small flowers are pale purple. The plant grows to a height of 6 feet (1.8 m), and gives out a powerful lemon scent, which intensifies when the leaves are rubbed or crushed.

PROPERTIES AND USES: Its uses are similar to those of mint, orange flowers or lemon balm *(Melissa)*, as a stomachic and antispasmodic in dyspepsia, indigestion and flatulence, stimulating skin and stomach. Tea made from dried lemon verbena can be mildly sedative, and it is also good for congestion and can ease indigestion. An infusion of the leaves can be added to your bath water to help calm and soothe, and a compress of the leaves can help to reduce puffiness around the eyes. Its oil is used for massage when diluted with carrier oil, to help ease cramp, indigestion, anxiety, insomnia, nervous tension and stress. The leaves are used for making herbal vinegars. Partnered with lemon thyme, lemon verbena makes superb herb butter. The leaves add a lemon flavour to fish, poultry and white meat dishes, vegetable marinades, salad dressings, jams, jellies, puddings especially fruit salads and fruit-based drinks. The oil has been used in cologne, toilet water, perfume and soap. The leaves can be added to cider vinegar to make a wonderful skin tonic that helps to soften and freshen the skin. Chopped leaves, added to fresh home-made ice-cream, are a particularly refreshing summer treat.

HISTORY: Native to South America, it brought by the Spanish to Europe for its perfume in the 18th century. It was not introduced to England until 1784 and so is missing from Culpeper, and thus not noted in any great depth for medicinal purposes. Some of its names come from Maria Luisa, Princess of Parma (1751–1819), who later became queen of Spain. Her contemporaries described her as an ugly, vicious, coarse woman with no teeth, who completely dominated her husband Carlos IV of Spain. The genus name *Aloysia*, in the Verbenaceae family, was given in her honour.

Freshly Scented

The herb should be included in all herb gardens which are designed for scent, pot-pourris (as the leaves retain their strong scent for years) and culinary uses. The leaves of lemon verbena can be placed between linens or in linen sachets to help keep fabrics smelling sweet. Its citrus scent repels midges, flies and other insects, so is a useful herb to grow underneath windows and near doorways.

LILY OF THE VALLEY

CONVALLARIA MAJALIS
Family Ruscaceae (formerly Liliaceae), Lily

OTHER NAMES: Culpeper also names it conval-lily, May lily and lily constancy. Liricon fancy, male lily, May bells, Our Lady's tears, Mary's tears, ladder to heaven

DESCRIPTION: Around 6 inches (15 cm) high, the small, sweet-scented, nodding, bell-like flowers are most commonly white, but there are also pink varieties and those with variegated leaves. All parts are toxic, and the small plant is difficult to remove, once established. Culpeper noted that it was common on Hampstead Heath in London, but Maud Grieve commented that with the removal of the trees there, the plant also disappeared.

PROPERTIES AND USES:
Culpeper wrote: '*It is under the dominion of Mercury, and therefore without doubt, strengthens the brain, renovates a weak memory, and makes it strong again. The distilled water, dropped into the eyes, helps inflammations thereof, as also that infirmity, which they call pin and web; the spirit of the flower, distilled in wine, restores lost speech, helps the palsy, and is exceedingly good in the apoplexy, comforts the heart and vital spirits.*' It is believed to strengthen memory, to restore speech and as a liquor smeared on the forehead and the back of the neck, to make one have good common

sense. Herbalist John Gerard advocated its use for those who had '*dumb palsie*' (Bell's Palsy, a condition which affects the facial muscles giving them a drooping appearance), and also for those who '*had fallen into apoplexy*'. He also recommended it for heart problems, and wrote: '*Put the flowers of May lilies into a glass and set it into a hill of ants, firmly closed for one month. After which you will find a liquor that when applied eases the pain and grief of gout.*' Even now the plant is used medicinally to treat heart conditions. Its action is effected slowly and steadily unlike foxglove (digitalis) which is released all at once, making it safer.

The leaves and flowers of lily of the valley contain cardiac glycosides, including convallatoxin, which have been used in medicine for centuries. It also contains convallatoxin, which has effects similar to digitalis, so medieval herbalists often used it as a substitute for foxglove in their treatment. The plant strengthens the heartbeat, while slowing and regularizing its rate, without putting extra demand on the pulmonary blood supply. A flower decoction helped to clear urinary canal obstructions and acted as a diuretic.

HISTORY: Apollo is said to have given lily of the valley as a gift to Asclepius, the Greek god of healing. The flowers were once used to make a drink, *'aqua aurea'* (golden water), that was believed to help boost memory and treat heart conditions. This water was so highly prized that it was stored in vessels of gold or silver, and was said to ease vomiting. In 1657, William Coles said that a wine with infused flowers was *'more precious than gold'* and suitable for apoplexy. In the Middle Ages flowers were popular in bridal bouquets, symbolizing purity and modesty. The Elizabethans used it in posies and nosegays to help perfume the air. Carrying a posy of the flowers was also said to improve the memory. The flowers were said to cheer the heart and lift the spirits of all those in their vicinity. The flowers are used as a symbol of humility in religious painting, and considered to be the sign of Christ's second coming. In the 'language of flowers', the lily of the valley signifies the return of happiness. There is a folk tale that describes the affection of a nightingale for lily of the valley, and which did not come back to the woods until the flower bloomed in May. During the First World War, an ointment made from the roots was used to treat burns of the victims of mustard gas. Lily of the valley was the floral emblem of the former Yugoslavia, and became the national flower of Finland in 1967.

Our Lady's Tears

The Latin name *Convallaria majalis* derives from the Latin *convallis* (valley) and *majalis* (May-flowering). In France, it has been used to bring good luck for at least 600 years, and is sold in the streets on May Day. It is one of the flowers associated with the pagan festival of Beltane, which also occurs on 1 May. The flower is also known as *Our Lady's tears*, since traditionally the lily of the valley came into being from Eve's tears after she was driven with Adam from the Garden of Eden. Another Christian legend states that the Virgin Mary's tears turned to lily of the valley when she cried at the Crucifixion of Jesus, and because of this it is also known as *Mary's Tears*. Yet another tradition is that the plant originated from Mary Magdalene's tears when she went to Christ's tomb. Alternatively, the flower sprang from the blood of Saint Leonard of Noblac (or of Limoges) during his sixth-century battles with a dragon in France. The same legend relates to St Leonard fighting a dragon at Horsham in Sussex.

LIQUORICE

GLYCYRRHIZA GLABRA
Family Fabaceae/Leguminosae, Pea/Legume

OTHER NAMES: Licorice, sweet root, sweetwood (its Greek name, *Glycyrrhiza*, means sweet root).

DESCRIPTION: A hardy perennial, growing to 4 feet (1.2 m) with a spread of 3 feet (90 cm). It has feathery pinnate leaves and its spikes of white or pale blue flowers are followed by long pods.

PROPERTIES AND USES:
Nicholas Culpeper: '*It is under the dominion of Mercury. Liquorice boiled in fair water, with some Maiden-hair and figs, makes a good drink for those that have a dry cough or hoarseness, wheezing or shortness of breath, and for all the griefs of the breast and lungs, pthisic or consumptions, caused by the distillation of salt humours on them. It is also good in all pains of the reins, difficulty in passing urine, and heat of urine. The fine powder of liquorice blown through a quill into the eyes of those afflicted with the pin and web, as it is called, or rheumatic distillations into them, cleanses and greatly relieves them. The juice of liquorice is as effectual in all the diseases of the breast and lungs, the reins and the bladder, as the decoction. The juice dissolved in rose-water, with some gum tragacanth, is a fine medicine for hoarseness, wheezing etc.*' Liquorice decreases generation of damaging molecules called free radicals, and inhibits an enzyme which is involved in the inflammatory process. The herb's action as a fast-acting anti-inflammatory agent is due to the compound *glycyrrhizin*, which blocks prostaglandin production and inflammation. It is also a demulcent and expectorant commonly used for throat, stomach, urinary and intestinal irritations. Liquorice has been used in women's formulas for centuries, normalizing and regulating hormone production. Glycyrrhizin has proven helpful in treating adrenal exhaustion, infertility due to hormonal imbalance, menopausal dysfunctions, and Addison's disease. The root inhibits the *Helicobacter pylori* bacterium and is thus used as an aid for healing stomach and duodenal ulcers, and in moderate amounts it may soothe an upset stomach. Liquorice can be used to treat ileitis, leaky gut syndrome, irritable bowel syndrome and Crohn's disease as it is antispasmodic in the bowels. It is said to help with age-related mental decline, and is used in stop-smoking remedies and for hair loss. The root is used to flavour black treacle and stout beers like Guinness. Its dried roots used to be sold as 'sweets' (liquorice sticks) when this author was a child, but they are now generally only found in chemist and herbal shops.

HISTORY: Liquorice was prescribed by early physicians from the time of Hippocrates in cases of dropsy, to prevent thirst. Egyptian physics and Theophrastus recommended liquorice for asthma, dry cough and all diseases of the lungs. Celsus and Scribonius Largus mention liquorice as *Radix dulcis* (sweet root). In 1264, liquorice is accounted for in the *Wardrobe Accounts* of Henry IV, and in 1305, Edward I taxed liquorice imports to pay for the repair of London Bridge. It appears from Turner's *Herbal* that it was cultivated in England in 1562, and Stow says '*the planting and growing of licorish began about the first year of Queen Elizabeth* [1558]'.

Pontefract Cakes

Possibly returning Crusaders first brought liquorice roots to Pontefract in Yorkshire, but more likely it was Dominican monks in the 14th century. They settled at Pontefract Priory close to the Castle, and the plant was known locally as '*Spanish*' or '*Spanish root*', possibly because of the presence of Spanish monks there. Liquorice needs deep soil to grow because the roots can be 4 feet (1.2 m) in length, and the soft loam of Pontefract was perfect. They rarely flowered in the colder English climate, but it was of little importance as the root of the plant provided what was needed. The sap was extracted from the roots and used medicinally by the monks along with other herbs for easing coughs and stomach complaints. Culpeper tells us: '*It is planted in fields and gardens in divers places of this kingdom, greatly to the profit of the cultivators.*' By 1614 the extract of liquorice was being formed into small lozenges and a nobleman called Sir George Saville applied a small stamp to each round 'cake', an early form of what was to become the famous *Pontefract cakes*. Large areas of the town and surrounding areas were turned over to growing liquorice, even the castle courtyard.

In 1760, a Pontefract apothecary, George Dunhill, began adding sugar to the recipe, producing 'Pomfret cakes' commercially as a confectionery, rather than a medicine. More liquorice factories started business in the 19th century, resulting in a shortage of local raw material which created a dependency upon imports. The last liquorice harvest around Pontefract took place sometime in the 1960s. At one time there were 13 liquorice factories in the town, but now there are only two, Dunhill (owned by Haribo of Germany) and Wilkinsons (formerly owned by Cadbury, and now Kraft of the United States). Bassett's famous sweet collection called *Liquorice Allsorts* appeared in 1899 after Wilkinson, a manufacturer of Pontefract cakes, was taken over.

(PURPLE) LOOSESTRIFE

LYTHRUM SALICARIA
Family Lythraceae, Loosestrife

OTHER NAMES: Culpeper calls this *'Loose-Strife, with Spiked Heads of Flowers.'* Blooming Sally, red Sally, long purple, lythrum, purple lythrum, spiked loosestrife, purple willow herb, rainbow weed, sage willow. Welsh llysiau'r milwr coch – bloody, red or gory soldier's herb.

DESCRIPTION: It grows to 6 feet (1.8 m) with a spread of 30 inches (76 cm), with tall spires of small magenta flowers and lance-shaped leaves. A plant can produce 3 million seeds, so although it is a beautiful plant, it has become an invasive problem in the USA, Canada and other countries.

PROPERTIES AND USES: Culpeper recommended it for eye complaints, even types of blindness, and gives a recipe for a salve for wounds. He says *'It likewise cleanses and heals all foul ulcers whatsoever, by washing them with the water, and laying on them a green leaf or two in the summer, or dry leaves in the winter. This water, when warmed, and used as a gargle, or even drunk sometimes, cures the quinsy, or king's evil of the throat. The said water applied warm takes away spots, marks, and scabs, in the skin; and a little of it drunk quenches extraordinary thirst.'* With antibacterial properties, purple loosestrife has been used as an astringent medicinal herb to treat food poisoning, diarrhoea and dysentery, being considered safe to use, even for babies. Medieval herbalists believed the plant to be good for external bleeding, bad menstruation and nosebleeds. As well as stopping bleeding, it is said to brighten eyes, preserve eyesight and soothe sore eyes. An ointment for ulcers and sores can be made, and the herb was used to treat cholera in the 19th century. The whole plant can be made into a gargle for a sore throat. The plant's high tannin content led to it being used as an alternative to oak bark for tanning leather. The tannin, obtained from the roots, was also used to preserve fishing nets. Red dye obtained from the flowers has been used in sweets, and the plant repels flies and gnats.

HISTORY: The Greeks thought that garlands of loosestrife, hung around the necks of oxen, would encourage a team to plough a field in harmony. They used the plant in a hair dye and also burned it to drive away insect pests. For centuries purple loosestrife was used to treat dysentery and diarrhoea, as a gargle and eyewash and to clean wounds.

Gory Herb

Lythrum means 'gore' in Greek, and doctors used loosestrife's leaves to stem bleeding in soldiers' wounds after battle.

(YELLOW) LOOSESTRIFE

LYSIMACHIA VULGARIS
Family Myrsinaceae (formerly Primulaceae), Myrsine (Primula)

OTHER NAMES: Culpeper calls it simply *'Loose-Strife, or Willow-Herb.'* Willow wort, herb willow, yellow willow herb, wood pimpernel, golden loosestrife, yellow rocket, garden loosestrife. Gerard calls it the *'yellow pimpernel'*, but this is also known as *'wood loosestrife'*, another plant in the *Lysimachia* family.

DESCRIPTION: This perennial grows up to 4–5 feet (1.2–1.5 m) with a spread of 3 feet (90 cm), and has bright yellow five-petalled flowers and lance-shaped leaves. It grows in the same damp habitats as purple loosestrife but is not related.

PROPERTIES AND USES: Culpeper: *'This herb is good for all manner of bleeding at the mouth, nose, or wounds, and all fluxes of the belly, and the bloody-flux, given either to drink or taken by clyster* [an enema often involving a syringe]; *it stays also the abundance of women's courses; it is a singularly good wound herb for green wounds, to stay the bleeding, and quickly close together the lips of the wound if the herb be bruised, and the juice only applied. It is often used in gargles for sore mouths, as also for the secret parts. The smoke hereof being burned, drives away flies and gnats, which in the night time molest people inhabiting near marshes, and in the fen countries.'* As it was thought to be a member of the loosestrife family, many of the purple loosestrife's properties were ascribed to it. Fresh young leaves bound around a wound are supposed to stem the flow of blood, and it was used for sore gums. It is used to calm horses and cattle and burning the dried leaves and stems deters insects and snakes. The stem and leaves of the plant were tied around a horse's neck to deter flies.

HISTORY: The first-century Greek medical writer Dioscorides reported that the juice of the leaves, administered as a drink or an enema, was an effective treatment for persons who had dysentery or were vomiting blood. He also called loosestrife a wound herb and stauncher of blood. King Lysimachus of Sicily was said to have promoted its benefits in healing wounds, so *Lysimachia* was named after him. Alternatively, the Greek *lysimachia* means 'loosen strife', possibly from its use to stop insects irritating oxen and horses, which Pliny recounted. William Coles's *Art of Simpling* (1656) relates: *'if loosestrife is thrown between two oxen when they are fighting they will part presently, and being tied about their necks it will keep them from fighting.'*

A Blonde Moment

It is still used by herbalists as a hair dye to highlight blonde hair and restore greying hair to blond.

LOVAGE

LEVISTICUM OFFICINALE
Family Apiaceae/Umbelliferae, Umbellifers

OTHER NAMES: In France, it is called false, or bastard celery *(céleri bâtard)* because of its appearance and flavour. Love parsley, love ache, sea parsley, European lovage, Cornish lovage, Italian lovage, old English lovage.

DESCRIPTION: Its leaves smell of celery when crushed. It grows to 6 feet (1.8 m) tall, with deeply divided large leaves and flat clusters of small greenish-yellow flowers. It is the sole species of the genus *Levisticum*.

PROPERTIES AND USES:
Culpeper: '*It opens, cures, and digests humours, and mightily provokes women's courses and urine…eases all inward gripings and pains, dissolves wind, and resists poison and infection…The distilled water of the herb helps the quinsy in the throat, if the mouth and throat be gargled and washed therewith; and relieves the pleurisy, being drank three or four times. Being dropped into the eyes, it takes away the redness or dimness of them: it likewise takes away spots or freckles in the face. The leaves bruised, and fried with a little hogs-lard, and laid hot to any blotch or boil, will quickly break it.*'
The rhizome and roots have been used in medicine for hundreds of years, especially for their diuretic and carminative (relieving flatulence or colic) properties. Only capers have a higher quercetin content, quercetin being a flavonoid with anti-inflammatory, antioxidant and other beneficial properties. Young leaves spice up salads, and the seeds are used in bread, rice, cheese, cakes, sauces, stews, salad dressings and salads. Phillips of Bristol makes an alcoholic (5.3%) Lovage Cordial, traditionally drunk two parts lovage to one part brandy as a '*winter warmer*' and as a stomach settler. More serious drinkers reverse the proportion. Lovage is a superb companion plant, especially for cucumber and parsley, and is a food plant of hoverflies, wasps and bees.

HISTORY: The Greeks used lovage to cure flatulence and ease digestion. In 1597, John Gerard considered lovage to be one greatest drugs of his day and it was used for jaundice, colic and fever in children. In the Middle Ages, travellers lined their footwear with lovage to help prevent foot odour and for its antiseptic properties. The name 'lovage' meant that it came to be associated with aphrodisiacs, in Chaucer's time becoming known as *love ache* and *love parsley*. Ache was a medieval name for parsley, and *love-ache* transmuted to lovage.

Sweet Smelling

Tudor gentry added lovage seeds to their baths to mask body odour. Later, a lovage root was added to a bath to help with physical cleanliness.

LUNGFLOWER

GENTIANELLA AMARELLA
Family Gentianaceae, Gentian

OTHER NAMES: Autumn gentian, bitterwort, felwort (from field and wort). Culpeper names five types of '*Autumn Gentians*'.

DESCRIPTION: From a rosette of leaves, a 4–8 inch (10–20 cm) flowering stalk bears small, purple trumpet flowers. In sunshine, the lobes of the corolla are spread wide horizontally, forming conspicuous blue stars.

PROPERTIES AND USES:
Culpeper notes: '*They are powerful against putrefaction, venom and poison…it eases pains in the stomach, and helps those that cannot keep or relish their meat, or have lost their appetite. It refreshes those that are fatigued with travelling… the root is likewise help to be good against agues.*' John Gerard, in *The Herball or General History of Plants* 1597 writes of felwort: '*It is excellent good, as Galen says, when there is need of attenuating, purging, cleansing, and removing of obstructions, which quality it takes of his extreme bitterness…This is of such force and virtue, says Pliny, that it helps cattle which are not only troubled with the cough, but are also broken-winded. The root of Gentian given in powder the quantity of a dram, with a little pepper and Herb Grace mixed therewith, is profitable for them that are bitten or stung with any manner of venomous beast or mad dog.*' Gentian's main use is as a digestive tonic, as the plant contains one of the bitterest substances known. In addition to aiding digestion, gentian has antioxidant properties that can help prevent some age-related vision problems, for instance diabetic retinopathy and reducing toxin production that can lead to cataracts.

HISTORY: Gentian's bitters (hence the name *bitterwort*) have been used in herbalism to improve the appetite and digestion for about 3000 years. During the Middle Ages, gentian was commonly employed as an antidote to poison, and in 1552 Tragus noted it as a means of diluting wounds.

Discovery of Gentians

The Illyrian King Gentius (ruled 181–*c*.168 BCE) discovered the medicinal value of these plants, according to Pliny and Dioscorides. Pliny wrote that he '*discovered the gentian, a plant that grows nearly everywhere but does best in Illyria… Gentian grows in great abundance on moist elevations in the Alpine foothills. The root of the plant and its juice are the parts most used. The essential virtue of the gentian root is that it warms the body. However infusions of the root or juice should never be drunk by pregnant women.*'

LUNGWORT

PULMONARIA OFFICINALIS
Family Boraginaceae, Borage

OTHER NAMES: Jerusalem cowslip, soldiers and sailors, Joseph and Mary, llysiau'r ysgyfaint (lung herbs, Welsh), spotted dog, maple lungwort, spotted comfrey, herb of Mary, Virgin Mary's milkdrops, Bethlehem sage.

DESCRIPTION: The evergreen lungwort grows to 1 foot (30 cm) high with five-petalled flowers that extend in clusters as short bells from the green, hairy bracts and stems. The flowers change from pale pink to blue-purple. Its creeping rhizomes help it to spread. The plant, especially its leaves, can act as a skin irritant.

PROPERTIES AND USES: Culpeper states that lungwort is useful for treating diseases of the lungs, for coughs and wheezing and for sores on the private parts, but it appears that he is describing lungmoss, *Lobaria pulmonaria*, a lichen that is referred to as lungwort in some older publications. This is also known as oak moss, and Culpeper also recommended it as '*an excellent remedy, boiled in beer, for broken-winded horses.*' In 1931 Mrs Grieve wrote: '*The Lungwort sold by druggists to-day is not this species, but a Moss, known also as Oak Lungs and Lung Moss. The Lungwort formerly held a place in almost every garden, under the name of 'Jerusalem Cowslip'; and it was held in great esteem for its reputed medicinal qualities in diseases of the lungs.*' Sir J. E. Smith recorded: '*every part of the*

plant is mucilaginous, but its reputation for coughs arose not from this circumstance, but from the speckled appearance of the leaves, resembling the lungs!' Medicinally, only the lungwort leaves were used. They contain saponins, allantoins, silica, flavonoids, tannins, vitamin C and mucilage, and the leaves were used to treat lung diseases such as tuberculosis, asthma and coughs. Lungwort contains antibiotics which act against bacteria in such illnesses. Its silica and allantoin content may be the reason it has been used for healing wounds and for treating eczema, haemorrhoids, varicose veins and burns. The leaves of lungwort are astringent and have been used to help staunch bleeding.

Dr O. Phelps Brown in 1872 published *The Complete Herbalist; or, The People Their Own Physicians*, and wrote: '*Lungwort is a herbaceous perennial, growing in Europe and this country in northern latitudes. In Europe it is a rough-leaved plant, but in this country the entire plant is smooth, which exhibits the peculiar climatic influence. It is showy, and freely cultivated. It flowers in May. The leaves are used for medical purposes. They are without any particular odour. Water extracts their properties. It is demulcent and mucilaginous, and in decoction very useful in bleeding from the lungs, and bronchial and catarrhal affections, and other disorders of the*

respiratory organs. Its virtues seem to be entirely expended upon the lungs, and it is certainly an efficacious remedial agent for all morbid conditions of those organs…'
Lungwort was used in Dr Brown's patent medicine *Acacian Balsam* for all lung illnesses. Made into a tea, the leaves are also used as an expectorant, to relieve congestion and ease a sore throat (often mixed with coltsfoot and cowslip flowers). Recently scientists have discovered that the plant does indeed have anticatarrhal properties. Lungwort may be a good herb to grow in gardens that are plagued with slugs and snails, as they seem to avoid its toxic alkaloids and saponins. The young leaves can be picked and used to make soups and salads. In medieval times, lungwort was a popular pot herb for adding to stews and savoury dishes. The flowers are good for spring floral arrangements and both the flowers and leaves can be dried for adding to pot-pourris. It makes excellent and attractive ground cover in any garden, attracting bumble bees.

HISTORY: From 1348–50 bubonic plague (the 'Black Death') infested Europe, killing possibly 4.2 million people in England alone. Lungwort was one of the herbs used alongside wormwood in attempts to cure the plague. Paracelsus (1493–1541) listed lungwort in his Doctrine of Signatures. Just as goldenrod was said to cure jaundice due to its yellow colouring, lungwort was said to cure pulmonary disease because the spotted leaves resembled diseased lungs. Lungwort became widely used in Europe during the 16th and 17th centuries for treating diseases of the breast and lungs. Lungwort was known by some as the *'herb of Mary'*,

used as proof for revealing if a person was a witch, and worn or used as a protection against witches and evil spirits. It is also called *'Mary's tears'* because the white spots on the leaves resembled teardrops or the Virgin Mary's milk, and the changing colour of the flowers from pink to blue represented blue eyes becoming reddened from weeping.

Elastic Lungs

The leaves actually contain silicic acid, which restores elasticity to the lungs. The name *pulmonaria* is derived from the Latin *pulmo* which means lung. *Officinalis* denotes that it was officially prescribed as a medicine. The word *wort* simply means plant, as in mugwort and soapwort. In German, the plant is called *Gefleckte Lungenkraut*.

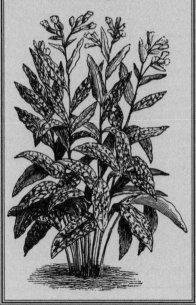

MALLOW and MARSH MALLOW

MALVA SYLVESTRIS
Family Malvaceae, Mallow

OTHER NAMES: Blue mallow, high mallow, tall mallow, cheese-cake, pick-cheese, round dock, country mallow, wild mallow, wood mallow. The common mallow is frequently called marsh mallow, but the true marsh mallow is distinguished from other mallows by the numerous divisions of the outer calyx, by the hoary down which thickly clothes the stems and foliage, and by the numerous panicles of blush-coloured flowers, paler than the common mallow.

DESCRIPTION: Hardy perennial, growing up to 3 feet (90 cm) with a 2-feet (60-cm) spread and large pink flowers which fade to pale blue.

PROPERTIES AND USES: Culpeper includes these under one heading: '*All the mallows are under Venus. The leaves and the roots also boiled in wine or water, with Parsley or Fennel roots, do help to open the body, and are very convenient in hot agues, or other distempers of the body, to apply the leaves so boiled warm to the belly.*' He says these mallows are inferior to marsh mallow, which has more mucilage and therefore is better for treating coughs. In 1931, Maud Grieve agreed that its

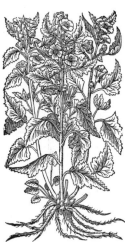

use had been superseded by marsh mallow, but was still '*a favourite remedy with country people where Marsh Mallow is not obtainable*'. Mucilage is present in many of the mallow family, and was employed medicinally, as demulcents, diuretics and emollients. The root was cut into slices to draw out thorns and splinters. The species was used as a natural yellow dye.

HISTORY: Romans thought the young shoots were delicacies. In the Middle Ages, mallow was an antidote to love potions and aphrodisiacs. Celts believed that placing the disc-shaped fruits over the eyes of a dead holy man would stop spirits entering his body, and help him get to the afterlife (the Celts believed in reincarnation). The flowers were used formerly on May Day people for strewing before their doors and weaving into garlands.

Cheese Wheels

It was called *pick-cheese* as, like other mallows, the edible seeds are shaped like wheels of cheese.

MARSH MALLOW
ALTHAEA OFFICINALIS
Family Malvaceae, Mallow

OTHER NAMES: Wymote (USA), mallards, mauls, schloss tea, cheeses, althea root, sweet weed, white mallow, mortification root.

DESCRIPTION: A bushy, leafy plant, 2–4 feet (60–120 cm) high, with soft pink or white flowers, and covered with velvety down which prevents its pores clogging from moisture arising from its wet habitat.

PROPERTIES AND USES: Marsh mallow is added to formulations for the treatment of harsh coughs, acts as a mild expectorant and helps sore throats. Its tannins made it a popular treatment for stomach ulcers, it also acts as a light diuretic. The French ate young leaves in salads to stimulate the kidneys. In cosmetics the mucilage was used as a soothing skin toner and dry hair rinse. Its root is rich in mucilage, paraffin, pectin, lecithin, quercetin, salicylic acid, tannins, amino acids, beta-carotene, calcium, iron, magnesium, manganese, phosphorus, potassium, selenium, zinc, and vitamins B1, B2, B3 and C. It soothes irritated tissue, relieves various forms of inflammation and aids the body in expelling excess fluid and mucus. The generic name *Althaea* is derived from the Greek word for cure, because of the mallow's medicinal properties. The name of the family, Malvaceae, is derived from the Greek word for soft, from the special qualities of the mallows in softening and healing.

HISTORY: The use of marsh mallow originated in traditional Greek medicine and spread to Arabian and Indian Ayurvedic medicine. It was eaten by the Egyptians and Syrians and mentioned by Pythagoras, Plato, Virgil and Dioscorides and Pliny. Pliny wrote: *'Whosoever shall take a spoonful of the Mallows shall that day be free from all diseases that may come to him.'* Arab physicians used the leaves as a poultice to suppress inflammation. The plant was enjoyed as a nutritious food by the Romans in barley soup and in a stuffing for suckling pig, while herbalists praised its gentle laxative properties. Marsh mallow was used in Persia to reduce inflammation in teething babies, and the Holy Roman Emperor Charlemagne insisted that it be planted in his gardens. The root's emulsifying property is still used for cleaning Persian carpets in the Middle East, being thought the best method to preserve the colour of their vegetable dyes. In accordance with the 16th-century Doctrine of Signatures, a potion using the downy 'hair' covering the plant helped promote hair growth.

MUSK MALLOW
MALVA MOSCHATA
Family Malvaceae, Mallow

This is slightly shorter than marsh mallow, with the same 2-feet (60-cm) spread, pale pink flowers but with musk-scented leaves. It has the same medicinal uses as the marsh mallow, but is milder. Mallows, especially the musk mallow, were used to decorate the graves of friends.

MANDRAKE
MANDRAGORA OFFICINARUM
Family Solanaceae, Nightshade

OTHER NAMES: Satan's apple (as it was thought to cause madness), djinn's eggs (in Arabic), love plant (Hebrew), European mandrake, mandragora.

DESCRIPTION: Growing about 1 foot (30 cm) high, with a 12-inch (30-cm) spread of rough leaves, mandrake has small, pretty, bell-shaped, pale blue or purple/white flowers and yellow fruits.

PROPERTIES AND USES: Mandrake has been closely linked with ritual magic and by many is thought an 'evil' plant. The very large brown root is still used in homeopathy for asthma and coughs. Culpeper recorded: *'The root is phlegmatic, and may be eaten with pepper and hot spices…the juice is good in all cooling ointments. The dried juice of the root, taken in a small quantity, purges phlegm and melancholy. In collyriums [eye cleansers], it pain in the eyes. In a pessary, it draws forth the dead child and secundine [afterbirth]. The green leaves, bruised with axungia [goose or pig fat from around the kidneys] and barley-meal, heal all hot swellings and inflammations, and applied to the parts cures hot ulcers and impostumes. A suppository made of the juice, put into the fundament, causes sleep. Infused in wine, and drunk, it causes sleep, and eases pains; the apples smelt to, or the juice taken in a small quantity, also cause sleep. The seed and fruit do cleanse the womb, the leaves heal knots in the flesh, and the roots heal St Anthony's Fire & c. and, boiled with ivy, mollify the same. The oil… may be anointed on the nose and temples of those that have a frenzy. If the patient sleeps too long, dip a sponge in vinegar, and hold it to the nose. Also, it heals vehement pains of the head, and the tooth-ache, when applied to the cheeks and jaws, and causes sleep.'* Mandrake was once placed on mantelpieces to avert misfortune and to bring prosperity to the home.

HISTORY: Plato's student, the philosopher Lucius Apuleius, tells us in his *Herbarium*: *'For witlessness, that is devil sickness or demoniacal possession, take from the body of this said wort Mandrake by the weight of three pennies, administer to drink in warm water as he may find most convenient – soon he will be healed.'* All the parts are now considered toxic, despite Culpeper's advice to eat the root. In Pliny's time a piece of the root was used as an anaesthetic for operations, and it has also been used as an anaesthetic for crucified criminals. In Anglo-Saxon herbals both mandrake and periwinkle are endowed with powers against demoniacal possession. Mandrake was used as an aphrodisiac and for increased fertility in eastern countries. There are many superstitions regarding the root of the mandrake, which resembles a carrot or parsnip. It was supposed to look like the human form as the roots sometime fork like legs. In old herbals we find illustrations of the mandrake as a male with a long beard, and as a female with a very bushy head of hair. The roots of bryony in Tudor times were passed off as mandrake, being trained to grow in moulds to take the desired 'human' shapes. Grains of millet were inserted into the 'face' as eyes, and they fetched high prices, being known as *puppettes* (male effigies) or *mammettes* (female), as they were accredited with magical powers. Italian ladies were known to pay up to 30 golden ducats, a small fortune, for such artificial mandrakes. William Turner, in his 1562 *Niewe Herball* said of these false idols: '*puppettes and mammettes…are so trimmed by crafty thieves to mock the poor people withal and to rob them both of their wit and their money.*' However, he added '*Of the apples of mandrake, if a man smell of them, they will make him sleep and also if they be eaten. But they that smell to much of the apples become dumb…this herb [in] diverse ways taken is very jeopardous for a man and may kill him if he eats it or drinks it out of measure and has no remedy from it… If mandragora be taken out of measure, by and by sleep ensues and a great losing of the strength with a forgetfulness.*'

> ## From *Love's Martyr*, 1601
>
> *In this delightsome country there doth grow,*
> *The Mandrake called in Greek Mandragoras,*
> *Some of his virtues if you look to know,*
> *The juice that freshly from the root doth pass,*
> *Purges all flame like black Helleborus:*
> *Tis good for pain engendered in the eyes;*
> *By wine made of the root doth sleep arise.*
>
> Robert Chester

The plant was said to grow under the gallows of murderers. It was believed to be fatal to dig up the root, which would scream upon being dug up. None might hear its terrible groans and live. Thus, anyone who wanted a plant of mandrake should tie a dog to it for that purpose, who drawing it out would perish, instead of the person.

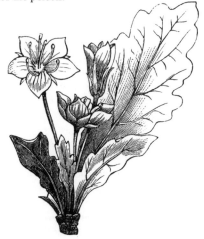

MARIGOLD

CALENDULA OFFICINALIS
Family Asteraeae, Aster

OTHER NAMES: Pot marigold, holigold, bride of the sun, drunkard, husbandman's dial, marybud, margold, Mary gold, Mary gowles, golds, ruddies, summer's bride, sun bride, melyn mair (golden Mary, Welsh), jackanapes-on-horsebacke (Gerard).

DESCRIPTION: It is not a marigold, but a member of the aster family. It should also not be confused with French and African marigolds, which although also members of the aster family, are actually members of the genus *Tagetes* and not *Calendula*. Height and spread up to 2 feet (60 cm), with large orange or yellow flowers.

PROPERTIES AND USES: Culpeper tells us: '*They strengthen the heart exceedingly, and are very expulsive, and a little less effectual in the smallpox and measles than saffron. The juice of Marigold leaves mixed with vinegar, and any hot swelling bathed with it, instantly gives ease, and assuages it. The flowers, either green or dried, are much used in possets, broths, and drink, as a comforter of the heart and spirits, and to expel any malignant or pestilential quality which might annoy them. A plaster made with the dry flowers in powder, hog's-grease, turpentine, and rosin, applied to the breast, strengthens and succours the heart*

infinitely in fevers, whether pestilential or not.' Its phytochemicals mean that it is used as a remedy for skin grazes, wounds, minor burns, nappy rash, sunburn and for fungal conditions such as athlete's foot, ringworm, acne, psoriasis and thrush. Calendula has antibacterial, antifungal, antibiotic and antiseptic properties. An infusion of calendula eyewash can help treat conjunctivitis. A marigold flower tea is good for the digestion, helps to ease colitis and was recommended for female complaints. Marigold salve, preferably cooked in goats lard, was used for burns, bruises and sunburns, just as it is today. There are more than 30 chemical compounds in the flowering plant, including the antirheumatic salicylic acid. Its orange and yellow colours derive from flavonoids and carotenoids, essential for maintaining good eyesight and for skin regeneration. In the garden, marigold deters pests such as tomato horn worms and asparagus beetles. Dried flowerheads can be used in pot-pourris and an infusion of the petals has been used for centuries as a rinse to lighten hair and as a wool dye. The flowers were also used as a natural dye for butter, flour and cheese.

HISTORY: Marigold was prized by the Egyptians for its properties of rejuvenation and healing, and used by the Greeks and Romans for its medicinal and culinary properties. The Romans used the petals as a substitute for expensive saffron. It has been used in Indian and Arab cultures as a dye, food colouring, cosmetic and medicine. In the Middle Ages, the flowers were an emblem of love, and if seen in dreams were a symbol of good luck. Petals, scattered under the pillow, made one's dreams come true. The sap from the stem was used to remove warts, calluses and corns. Garlands of marigolds are said to stop evil from entering the home if hung over the entrance to the doorway, and the plant could strip a witch of her evil will. Charles Stevens, in his 1699 *Maison Rustique, or the Countrie Farme* recommends the marigold for headache, jaundice, red eyes, toothache and ague, and asserts that the dried flowers *'strengthen and comfort the heart… Conserve made of the flowers and sugar, taken in the morning fasting, cures trembling of the heart, and is also given in the time of plague or pestilence. The yellow leaves of the flowers are dried and kept throughout Dutchland against winter to put into broths, physical potions and for divers other purposes, in such quantity that in some Grocers or Spice sellers are to be found barrels filled with them and retailed by the penny or less, insomuch that no broths are well made without dried Marigold.'* Calendula has been a popular garden flower since the Tudor times, the flowers being used to colour and flavour cakes, soups, stews and pot based meals. This is probably how calendula acquired the name *pot marigold*.

A Blooming Fine Day

The Roman Varro said that the term *calends* derived from the priest's practice of calling the citizens together (*calare* = call) on the first day of the month, to inform them of the time of the various sacred days and festivals. At some time, the posting of the calendar in public places replaced this custom, and *calends* came to refer to the whole month, rather than just the first day. Marigold seems to have acquired its botanical name, *Calendula*, either from its reputation for blooming on the first day of every month, or for nearly every month in the year. The word *officinalis* indicates that the plant was an 'official' plant sold in apothecaries' shops as medicine. If the marigold's flowers are open, there will be a fine day ahead, as they are sensitive to temperature variation and dampness. We read in Shakespeare's *A Winter's Tale*, '*Hot lavender, mints, savoury, marjoram; / The marigold, that goes to bed wi' the sun / And with him rises weeping: these are flowers.*'

MARJORAM

ORIGANUM MAJORANA
Family Lamiaceae/Labiatae, Mint

OTHER NAMES: Knotted marjoram, wintersweet, pot marjoram, joy of the mountain, mountain mint. Culpeper calls this *Sweet Marjoram*. (Several edible oreganos are called marjoram – see oregano, dittany of Crete. French oregano *(Origanum x onites)* is also called French marjoram, for instance. For wild marjoram, see oregano.

DESCRIPTION: Half-hardy aromatic perennial, with a height and spread of 10–12 inches (25–30 cm), and tiny white, pink or mauve tubular flowers and oval leaves.

PROPERTIES AND USES: *'It is an herb of Mercury, and under Aries, and therefore is an excellent remedy for the brain and other parts of the body and mind, under the dominion of the same planet. Our common Sweet Marjoram is warming and comfortable in cold diseases of the head, stomach, sinews, and other parts, taken inwardly, or outwardly applied.'* – Nicholas Culpeper. Marjoram tea calms the nerves, and eases insomnia, headaches and colds. Chewing the leaf gives temporary respite from toothache, and is supposed to also calm the libido. Related to the mint family, it is sweeter and more delicate than its relatives oregano and pot marjoram *(Origanum onites)*. The plant tops produce origanum oil, once used as a medicine and later for perfuming soaps. The aroma of the oil is warm and spicy, with a hint of nutmeg. Sweet marjoram is known mainly as a culinary herb and is used to season soups, salads and vegetable sauces. It is the marjoram/oregano most commonly found on pizzas and added to dried herb mixtures, being also an important ingredient in a bouquet garni. It is good used with meat, fish, vegetables and eggs, and complements bay, garlic, onion, thyme, and basil. It can help marinade artichoke hearts, asparagus and mushrooms and is excellent in herb vinegars, oils and butters.

HISTORY: *Origanum* literally means *joy of the mountain*, and it is also known as *mountain mint*. The Greeks believed that if you anointed yourself with marjoram, you would dream of your future spouse. They also believed that planting it on a grave would ensure eternal peace and happiness for the dead. During the Middle Ages its leaves were chewed to relieve indigestion, toothache, coughs and rheumatism. Sweet marjoram was a popular strewing herb in ancient times used for warding off disease and infection, and was put into sachets to keep linens and clothing sweet smelling.

MASTIC TREE
PISTACIA LENTISCUS
Family Anacardiaceae, Cashew/Sumac

OTHER NAMES: Culpeper also calls it the lentisk-tree, and says *'It is called in Latin Lentiscus, and the gum or rosin, resina lentiscina, and mastiche, and mastix, and in English, mastic.'*

DESCRIPTION: A Mediterranean shrub growing to 12 feet (3.6 m) high, in which incisions are cut for drops of resin (mastic) to be harvested.

PROPERTIES AND USES:
Culpeper is effusive about the use of mastic, as it stops fluxes, strengthens the stomach, heals sores, knits broken bones, fastens loose teeth, helps with leprosy and scab, and so on. The liquid is sun-dried when it turns into drops of hard, brittle, translucent resin. When chewed, the resin softens and becomes a bright white and opaque gum. It is a stimulant and diuretic and was used for filling tooth cavities and to sweeten the breath. Mastic contains antioxidants, and also has antibacterial and antifungal properties.

Regular consumption of mastic has been proven to absorb cholesterol, and mastic oil is widely used in the preparation of ointments for skin disorders and afflictions. In Turkey mastic is widely used in desserts such as Turkish Delight.

HISTORY: Mastic has been used as a medicine since antiquity and in Egypt was used in embalming. In its hardened form it was used as incense. The Greeks recommended it for snakebites and healing. Hippocrates believed it was excellent for digestive problems and colds. Galen suggested the plant for treating bronchitis and improving the condition of the blood. It was formerly sold as Arabic gum and Yemen gum. The rarity of mastic made it expensive, with many imitation 'mastics' such as boswellia and gum Arabic (cunningly named to resemble Arabic gum). One of the earliest uses of mastic was as chewing gum, hence our name for the product.

Mastic – Worth Its Weight in Gold

In Greece it is known as the *'tears of Chios'*, being traditionally produced on the island, and even now mastic production in Chios is granted 'Protected Designation of Origin' status because only the mastic trees of southern Chios 'weep' the mastic resin when their bark is incised. When the Ottomans ruled Chios, it was worth its weight in gold, and the sultan's penalty for stealing mastic was execution. In the 1822 Chios Massacre when tens of thousands of Greeks were slaughtered by Ottoman troops in 1822 in reprisal for a revolutionary uprising, the people of the 'mastic villages' were spared to ensure mastic supplies for the sultan and his harem.

MARY GARDENS

These use the herbs and flowers that are related to the Virgin Mary. Mary Gardens are seen in medieval religious art and illustration in which the Virgin and Child are usually depicted in enclosed gardens of symbolic plants. Gardens dedicated solely to plants named after her are known as *Mary Gardens*. St Benedict of Nursia (480–547), the founder of Western Christian monasticism, had a monastic rose garden, known as a *'Rosary'*. The first reference to a garden actually dedicated to Mary is from the life of St Fiacre, the Irish monk who was renowned for growing food and medicinal plants. He is now the patron saint of gardening. (He is also the patron saint of French taxi-drivers, because horse carriages were rented at the Hotel de Saint Fiacre in Paris, and they became known by association as fiacre cabs). Fiacre planted and tended a garden around the oratory and hospice he founded to Our Lady in the seventh century at Breuil in France. There is a legend that after her Assumption, roses and lilies were found in Mary's tomb. In the eighth century St Bede wrote that the translucent white petals of the Madonna lily were a likeness of her pure body as she was assumed into heaven, and its golden anthers symbolized the glorious resplendence of her soul. There are old lists of the flowers, herbs and grains included in the *'Assumption*

bundles' of plants which from the ninth century were associated with Mary through their blessing at the altar on the Feast of the Assumption. In the 12th century St Bernard praised the Virgin Mary as *'The rose of charity, the lily of chastity, the violet of humility… and the golden gillyflower of heaven.'* The first mention of an actual Mary Garden is in a 15th-century record of the purchase of plants *'for S. Mary's garden'* by the sacristan of Norwich Priory, in England.

Some flowers, such as the Madonna lily, are commonly known today by religious names clearly reflecting their association with Mary. Others including the marigold, ladies' mantle, and ladyslipper are held to be named for Mary, with an abbreviation of 'Our Lady'. In some instances plants were given botanical names derived from their popular religious names, e.g. the milk thistle *(Silybum marianum)* named from the legend that the white spots on its leaves (and those of other plants) originated when drops of the nursing Madonna's milk fell on them. Today's Mary Gardens assemble together suitable flowers named for Mary from various countries in a single garden where they can be used together devotionally according to their old names and symbolism.

SOME FLOWERS OF OUR LADY FOR A MARY GARDEN

Botanical Name	Common Name	Religious Name
Alchemilla vulgaris	Lady's mantle	Our Lady's mantle
Allium schoenoprasum	Chives	Our Lady's garlic
Aquilegia vulgaris	Columbine	Our Lady's shoes
Arabis albida	Rock cress	Our Lady's cushion
Begonia fuchsioides	Begonia	Mary's heart
Berberis vulgaris	Barberry	Our Lady's leaf
Calendula officinalis	Pot marigold	Mary's gold
Calluna vulgaris	Heather	Mary's adversary
Campanula rotundifolia	Harebell	Our Lady's thimble
Cerastium arvense	Starry grasswort	Mary's flower
Cheiranthus cheiri	Wallflower	Mary's flower
Chrysanthemum parthenium	Feverfew	Mary's flower
Clematis vitalba	Virgin's bower	Our Lady's bower
Convallaria majalis	Lily-of-the-valley	Mary's tears
Dianthus plumarius	Clove pink	Virgin's pink
Erica carnea	Winter heath	Mary's help
Galanthus nivalis	Snowdrop	Candlemas bells
Galium verum	Lady's or yellow bedstraw	Our Lady's bedstraw
Hosta plantaginea	White day lily	Assumption lily
Hydrangea, var.	Ave Maria	Ave Maria
Hypericum perforatum	St John's Wort	Mary's sweat
Iris, gen.	Iris	Mary's sword of sorrow
Lilium, sp.	Lily, white	Annunciation lily, Madonna lily
Lonicera, gen.	Honeysuckle	Mary's fingers
Malva sylvestris	Purple mallow	Our Lady's cheeses
Myosotis, gen.	Forget-me-not	Eyes of Mary
Narcissus pseudo-narcissus	Daffodil	Mary's star
Oxalis acetosella	Wood sorrell	Our Lady's meat
Potentilla, gen.	Cinquefoil	Mary's hand of pity
Primula elatior	Candelabra primrose	Our Lady's candlestick
Primula polyanthus	Polyanthus	Our Lady's fingers
Primula veris	Cowslip	Our Lady's keys
Pulmonaria officinalis	Lungwort	Mary's milkdrops
Rosa, gen.	Rose	Mary's rose
Rosmarinus officinalis	Rosemary	Rose of Mary
Salix babylonica	Weeping willow	Relates to Mary's sorrow when Christ was scourged
Salvia officinalis	Sage	Our Lady's shawl
Saxifraga umbrosa	London pride	Our Lady's needlework
Thuja occidentalis	Arbor-vitae	Tree of Life
Tulipa, gen.	Tulip	The woman
Vinca minor	Periwinkle	Virgin flower
Viola odorata	Sweet violet	Mary's humility
Viola tricolour	Heartsease; pansy	Trinity; Our Lady's delight

MEADOWSWEET

FILIPENDULA ULMARIA
Family Roseaceae, Rose

OTHER NAMES: Bridewort (formerly bridal wort), queen of the meadows (Culpeper), little queen, lady of the meadow, dolloff, quaker lady, gravel root, meadow wort, meadwort, meadsweet, steeplebush, trumpet weed.

DESCRIPTION: It grows in damp places, 2–4 feet (60–120 cm) tall with a spread of 2 feet (60 cm), with dense clusters of cream-white almond-scented flowers.

PROPERTIES AND USES: '*...It is used to stay all manner of bleeding, fluxes, vomitings, and women's menses...it speedily helps those who are troubled with the colic, being boiled in wine; and, with a little honey, taken warm, opens the belly; but, boiled in red wine, and drunk, it stays the flux of the belly. Being outwardly applied, it heals old ulcers that are cancerous or eaten, or hollow and fistulous, for which it is very much commended, as also for sores of the mouth or secret parts*' – Nicholas Culpeper. Gerard says: '*It is reported that the flowers boiled in wine and drunk take away the fits of a quartain ague* [a fever which returns every fourth day] *and make the heart merry. The distilled water of the flowers dropped into the eyes take away the burning and itching thereof and clear the sight.*' It is good for all digestive problems, and a hot tea will help with colds and flu and relieve head aches. A cool tea soothes inflamed skin or tired eyes. The name is a corruption of *meadwort*, as the leaves and flowers

flavoured mead and beer, and is nothing to do with meadows.

HISTORY: Its virtues have been known since the time of Dioscorides. Meadowsweet, water mint and vervain were three herbs that were said to be most sacred by the Druids, and it has been found in Bronze Age burial cairns in Wales. In 1835, salicylic acid was first synthesized from the stem sap to make acetylsalicylic acid, which is the basis of *aspirin*. The word is probably derived from *spirin*, based on meadowsweet's former name *Spiraea ulmaria*.

Wedding Fragrance

John Gerard writes: '*The leaves and flowers of Meadowsweet far excel all other strewing herbs to deck up houses, to strew in chambers, halls and banqueting-houses in the summer-time, for the smell thereof makes the heart merry and joyful and delight the senses.*' Strangely, the leaves have a different smell to the flowers. It was known as *bridewort* as the fragrant creamy flowers were strewn along church aisles for new brides to walk along, and also used in brides' bouquets as they were thought to bring love, joy, a beautiful wedding day and a happy marriage.

MINT - PEPPERMINT
MENTHA PIPERITA
Family Lamiaceae/Labiatae, Mint

OTHER NAMES: Brandy mint, English mint.

DESCRIPTION: This is a hybrid mint, an accidental cross between spearmint *(Mentha spicata)* and water mint *(Mentha aquatica)*. An invasive perennial, it grows to 12 inches (30 cm) high with pink to mauve flowerswhich attract honey bees.

PROPERTIES AND USES: Culpeper: *'It is an herb of Venus. This herb has a strong, agreeable, aromatic smell, and a moderate warm bitterish taste, it is useful for complaints of the stomach, such as wind, vomiting, for which there are few remedies of greater efficacy.'* Peppermint is the most widely used mint, owing to its higher menthol content. Its antispasmodic effect soothes stomach aches, and is effective for colic and flatulence. Externally peppermint oil is used in pain-relieving ointments and massage oils, increasing blood flow to the affected area. Peppermint oil contains azulene, with anti-inflammatory and ulcer-healing effects. The plant seems to have antibacterial and antiviral properties. Rats dislike peppermint; you can prevent them from using outhouses by scenting cardboard, cotton balls or rags with the oil and placing them where the rats are probably getting in.

HISTORY: Mint was used by the ancient Assyrians in rituals to their fire god. Pliny states that Greeks and Romans crowned themselves with peppermint at feasts and adorned their tables with its sprays, and that its essence was used in sauces and wines. Peppermint was possibly first cultivated by the Egyptians, but was first included in the *London Pharmacopeia* in 1721, after which it was used extensively in medicine. Peppermint oil capsules have been proven to help sufferers of indigestion and irritable bowel syndrome. The smell of peppermint is being pumped into a primary school in Liverpool in an experiment to see if the smell improves memory and alertness.

Helps in a Stinking Breath

Culpeper also describes *'wild or horse-mint'*, known to us as the familiar water mint *(Mentha aquatica)*: *'to dissolve wind in the stomach, to help the colic...an effectual remedy against venereal dreams and pollutions in the night, being outwardly applied to the testicles. The juice dropped into the ears eases the pains thereof and destroys the worms that breed therein. They are good against the venomous bites of serpents. The juice, lid on warm, helps the king's evil, or kernels in the throat. The decoction, or distilled water, helps in a stinking breath proceeding from the corruption of the teeth; and snuffed up the nose, purges the head...Mints are extremely bad for wounded people; it being asserted, that whoever eats mint, when wounded, will never be cured.'*

MINT - SPEARMINT

MENTHA SPICATA
Family Lamiaceae/Labiatae, Mint

OTHER NAMES: Garden mint, lamb mint, mackerel mint, hart mint, fish mint, Our Lady's mint, sage of Bethlehem, menthe de Notre Dame, green mint, spire mint, silver mint, menthol mint. There are hundreds of other varieties of mint.

DESCRIPTION: A hardy invasive perennial which grows up to 2 feet (60 cm), with small mauve flowers in spikes. The leaves are lighter green than those of peppermint. The strong mint taste of the leaves varies according to soil conditions and climate.

PROPERTIES AND USES: Culpeper lists nearly 40 distinct illnesses for which mint is singularly recommended: '*Being smelled into, it is comfortable for the head and memory, and a decoction when used as a gargle, cures the mouth and gums, when sore…Garden Mint is most useful to wash children's heads when the latter are inclined to sores, and Wild Mint, mixed with vinegar is an excellent wash to get rid of scurf. Rose leaves and mint, heated and applied outwardly cause rest and sleep.*' Culpeper thought it was '*an incentive to venery and bodily lust*', but among its virtues: '*it stays bleeding… stays the hiccough, vomiting and allays choler. It dissolves imposthumes…it is good to repress milk in women's breasts; and for such that have swollen, flagging or large breasts…it helps the bite of a mad dog…it eases the pains of the ears…helps digestion…The decoction thereof, when used as a gargle, cures the mouth and gums…and helps stinking breath…*' Mint is aromatic, carminative, diuretic, antiseptic, antispasmodic, anti-inflammatory, antibacterial, antiparasitic, restorative and is also a stimulant. A mint infusion or tea can be used internally for nausea, headaches, indigestion, colds, flu, hiccoughs, flatulence, or insomnia. Externally it can be used for chapped skin, as a rinse for oily hair, a facial tonic or in a refreshing and stimulating bath. Spearmint can relieve heavy colds when drops of the essential oil are inhaled or sprinkled on a handkerchief. Both spearmint and peppermint can be used when diluted in carrier oil in massages for the relief of migraine, facial neuralgia and rheumatic and muscular aches.

Spearmint is the best-known and most commonly used culinary mint. The leaves were chewed to relieve toothache. The oil is a mosquito repellent and used as an antiseptic for itching skin. Five tablespoons of peppermint leaves can be added to half a pint of water and the same amount of cider vinegar to make a rinse for greasy hair. Mint is also used for a cleansing and soothing face pack for greasy skin. The leaves make an excellent addition to pot-pourris and herbal bath bags. It is moth repellent so sachets are hung in wardrobes or added to drawers. Traditionally, in England, mint complements roast lamb, and the fresh leaves are added to potatoes and peas while cooking. Mint grown near roses will deter aphids and will deter ants from entering a house. Mice are also averse to the smell of mint, either fresh or dried.

HISTORY: Around

1000 BCE Egyptians used mint as part of the funerary process, and its spread paralleled the Roman empire's growth. The smell of mint in Roman houses was a symbol of hospitality. Pliny the Elder advised scholars to wear a crown of mint to aid concentration, but he also warned that it did not help procreation. Greeks believed the opposite, however. Their soldiers were warned to avoid mint during a war as it was feared that increased love-making would diminish their courage. Mint is said to bring luck and helps to increase prosperity if a few leaves are rubbed into the purse. Headaches were cured by rubbing a few mint leaves on the forehead. In the Middle Ages, mint cured mouth sores, dog bites and insect stings, it helped to whiten teeth and prevented milk from curdling. Mint has

been used in baths since Roman times, and was also strewn to sweeten the smell of churches. Its distilled oil is still used to flavour toothpastes, confectionery, chewing gums, and also to perfume soap. Spearmint has been found to have some antifungal properties and has excellent antioxidant activity, and recent studies find that spearmint tea may be useful for mild female hirsutism, as the tea reduces levels of male sex hormones. The leaves and stems contain the essential oil menthol, but spearmint does not contain high amounts of menthol (0.5 per cent compared to the 40 per cent in peppermint), making it the least pungent herb in the mint family. Spearmint also contains minerals like potassium, calcium, manganese, iron and magnesium. It is also rich in many antioxidant vitamins including vitamin A, beta carotene, vitamin C, folates, vitamin B-6, riboflavin and thiamin.

The Fate of Menthe

Menthe was the name of a beautiful water nymph pursued by Pluto, Roman god of the underworld. When his wife Persephone found out, she turned Menthe into a plant that would be trodden underfoot. Pluto could do nothing but accept his wife's vengeance, but he altered the plant so that when it was trodden on, it would release a beautiful fragrance.

MISTLETOE

VISCUM COLORATUM, V. ALBUM
Family Santalaceae, Parasitic Plants

OTHER NAMES: European mistletoe, common mistletoe, white-berried mistletoe, birdlime mistletoe, loranthus, mulberry mistletoe, bird-lime, all-heal, druid's herb, witch's broom, thunderbesem, wood of the cross, lignum crucis, holy wood, golden bough, all heal, devil's fuge.

DESCRIPTION: Parasitic evergreen shrub with sticky, round, white berries and leathery, green, tongue-like leaves, growing on the branches of trees in bushes 2–5 feet (60 cm to 1.5 m) across. The plant prefers apple trees as hosts.

PROPERTIES AND USES: *'This is under the dominion of the Sun, with something of the nature of Jupiter, the leaves and berries do heat and dry, and are of subtle parts. Bird-lime,* [the sticky juice] *made thereof, mollifies hard knots, tumours and imposthumes, ripens and discusses them, and draws forth thick as well as thin humours from the remote parts of the body, digesting and separating them; and being mixed with equal parts of rosin and wax, mollifies the hardness of the spleen, and heals old ulcers and sores...Some hold it so highly in esteem, that it is called lignum sanctae crucis, or wood of the holy cross, believing it to cure falling sickness, apoplexy and palsy, very speedily, not only when taken inwardly, but applied externally, by hanging it around the neck. Tragus says, that by bruising the green wood of any mistletoe, and dropping the juice so drawn into the ears of those who are troubled with imposthumes, it heals the same in a few days.'* – Nicholas Culpeper. The Physicians of Myddfai, the legendary 12th-century Welsh herbalists, wrote on the use of mistletoe: *'In any case of bodily debility, whether in the nerves, joints, back, head, or brain, stomach, heart, lungs or kidneys, take three spoonfuls of the decoction, and mix with boiling water, ale, mead or milk; then add to a good draught thereof a spoonful of the powder, which should be drunk in the morning fasting. Half as much should be taken the last thing at night. It is good for any kind of disease of the brain, nerves, and back, epilepsy, mania or mental infirmity of any kind, paralysis, all weakness of joints, sight, hearing, or senses. It will promote fruitfulness, the begetting of children, and restrain seminal flux. The man who takes a spoonful thereof daily in his drink will enjoy uninterrupted health, strength of body, and manly vigour.'* The herb was

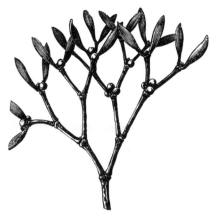

used extensively in the 16th and 17th centuries for treatment of epilepsy and other convulsive nervous disorders. The plant is a nervine, and a narcotic, affecting the nervous system. Today, mistletoe is used medicinally for headaches, dizziness, energy loss, irritability, vertigo and other symptoms connected with raised blood pressure. Eating the berries can cause convulsions in children.

HISTORY: The Druids and other pagan groups revered mistletoe and celebrated the beginning of winter by collecting it (by a high ranking priest who cut it with a golden knife) and hanging branches in their homes. It is also said to be the legendary *Golden Bough* that saved Aeneas from the underworld in Virgil's poem.

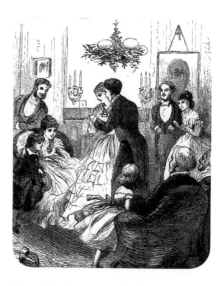

Romans, Celts and Germans believed that mistletoe was a key to the supernatural, and the plant also represented sex and fertility. Kissing under the mistletoe at Christmas is traced to the Greeks who used mistletoe in the Cronia festival. Mistletoe also features in the Scandinavian legend of Balder, god of peace, who was killed with an arrow of mistletoe, the only plant in creation that had not sworn to his mother Frigg that it would not harm him. He was restored to life, mistletoe was then given into the keeping of the goddess of love, and it was ordained that everyone who passed under it should receive a kiss, to show that the branch had become an emblem of love, and not of hate. With each kiss, a berry should be removed, and when all are gone, the mistletoe is said to have lost its powers. In Brittany, where the mistletoe grows abundantly, it is called *herbe de la croix*, because, according to legend, the Cross was made from its wood, on account of which it was degraded to be a parasite. It was believed that life could spring spontaneously from dung, and it was observed in ancient times that mistletoe would often appear on a branch where birds had left droppings. '*Mistel*' is Anglo-Saxon word for dung, and '*tan*' is the word for twig, so mistletoe possibly means dung-on-a-twig. By the 16th century, botanists discovered that the stickiness of the berries caused propagation. The berries would stick to the bills of birds and they consequently rubbed their beaks on barks of trees to try to get rid of the berries which would this fall to the ground. It was also discovered that seeds survive the passage through the digestive tracts of birds and are excreted together with their droppings, another source of propagation. Mistletoe extracts have been extensively studied in Europe as a supplemental treatment in cancer therapy. Clinical studies show that injections of mistletoe boost the body's immune systems, helping it attack malignant melanoma.

THE MODERN HERB GARDEN

Most readers can quite easily plant and develop a herb garden, either by dedicating a part of the kitchen garden to it, or simply using containers or even window boxes in which to grow herbs. Once flower production begins, leaf production ceases. Therefore, in annuals and herbaceous varieties, harvesting the foliage consistently before the plant flowers can extend leaf production somewhat if care is taken to cut consistently. Some herbs can be used as flavourings, others as dyes, teas, cooking spices, companion plants or for herbal medicine, or even simply for their appearance and fragrance. If you have space, your herb garden will be home to five major families of plants.

Apiaceae or **Umbelliferae** – Parsley family. This family is made up of plants with 'umbrella-shaped' flowerheads e.g. chervil, fennel, parsley, dill, hemlock, anise, cumin, coriander, caraway etc.

Asteraceae – Aster/Sunflower family. The family is recognizable by its daisy-shaped flowers, and it includes daisy, thistle, calendula, dandelion etc.

Brassicaceae – Mustard family. Taste is an indicator of this family which includes cabbage, kale, mustard, broccoli, Brussels sprouts, rape seed, mustard seed, turnip, horseradish etc.

Lamiaceae or **Labiatae** – Mint family. Generally has a squared stem, opposing leaves and often wrinkly or hairy leaf types; includes all the mints, pennyroyal, lavender, rosemary, sage, savory, marjoram, oregano, thyme, basil etc.

Liliaceae – Lily family. The lily family has long, tapered leaves and a bulbous body stalk. Recently this group has undergone a good deal of taxonomic change and while it still includes lilies and fritillaries, historically the group included onion, garlic (both now Aliaceae), asparagus (now Asparagaceae), hyacinth (now Hyacinthaceae), daffodil (now Amaryllidaceae) etc.

Evergreen varieties of herb, e.g. sage, rosemary and thyme, do not die back over the winter, but remain green year-round. They will still require pruning to maximize their production of new tender and flavourful growth, and should be pruned at least once a year.

Herbaceous herbs include oregano, mints, tarragon, chives, lemon balm, winter savory etc. These plants will die back to the ground at wintertime. There is no need to prune these plants with care, as they can be chopped right to the ground and will come back strong and healthy. For some, an annual mowing is an easy solution.

Annual herbs, unlike evergreens and herbaceous herbs, do not live for more than one season. While evergreens and herbaceous herbs are perennials, and grow for two years or longer, annuals produce flowers and then seeds before dying off at the end of each growing season. Therefore, annuals require new plantings each spring, although some like nasturtium, fennel and poppy often seed themselves. Examples of annual herbs are coriander, basil, dill, summer savory and chervil.

MONKSHOOD

ACONITUM NAPELLUS
Family Ranunculacae, Buttercup

OTHER NAMES: Common monkshood, monk's blood, blue wolf's-bane, aconite, women's bane, leopard's bane, devil's helmet, blue rocket, friar's cap, auld wife's huid.

DESCRIPTION: This monkshood grows to 3 feet (90 cm) with a slim stem and a spike of beautiful blue-purple hooded blossoms.

PROPERTIES AND USES: The common monkshood is one of the most poisonous plants of European flora. According to Culpeper, this *'blue wolf's-bane is very common in many gardens... if inwardly taken they inflame the inward parts and destroy life itself. Dodonaeus reports of some men of Antwerp, who unawares did eat some of the monks'-hood in a salad, instead of some other herb, and died forthwith; this I write that people who have it in their gardens might beware of it.'* If it is carefully dosed, aconitine can be applied externally as an effective painkiller for neuralgia and in cases of rheumatism, headache, gout, migraine and colds accompanied with high body temperature.

HISTORY: The Greeks called aconite *'the Queen of Poisons'*, believing that it was created by the goddess Hecate from the saliva of the three-headed dog Cerberus. The witch Medea used aconite to try and kill Theseus. Since ancient times, people have known that it is poisonous and have used it as a weapon by coating their spears and arrowheads with its strong toxin. The plant was used for hunting wolves, panthers and other carnivores with poison-tipped arrows. The Ancient Roman naturalist Pliny describes *friar's cap* under the name *'plant arsenic'*, and it has been used throughout history both as a poison and to put criminals to death.

Powerful Poison

Aconitine, present in monkshood, is one of the strongest plant poisons. At first, it acts as a stimulant but then it paralyzes the nervous system. After eating, burning and tingling sensations in the mouth lead to numbness and paralysis, blindness, vomiting and intense pain before death from respiratory failure and cardiac arrest. Children may get poisoned if they hold tubers in their hands for a long time. In 1881 Dr George Lanson fed monkshood to his brother-in-law in a slice of Dundee cake, hoping thereby to get a share of his inheritance, but he was convicted of murder and hanged.

MOTHERWORT

LEONURUS CARDIACA
Family Lamiaceae/Labiatae, Mint

OTHER NAMES: European motherwort, lion's tail, lion's ear, lion's tart, throw-wort, heart-wort.

DESCRIPTION: A bushy perennial that can grow to 3–4 feet (90–120 cm), with small pink, pale purple or white flowers and a pungent smell.

PROPERTIES AND USES: Culpeper wrote of motherwort: *'Venus owns this herb and it is under Leo. There is no better herb to drive melancholy vapours from the heart, to strengthen it and make the mind cheerful, blithe and merry. May be kept in a syrup, or conserve, therefore the Latins call it cardiaca…It cleanses the chest of cold phlegm, oppressing it and kills worms in the belly. It is of good use to warm and dry up the cold humours, to digest and disperse them that are settled in the veins, joints and sinews of the body and to help cramps and convulsions.'* Gerard commended it for: *'infirmities of the heart. Moreover the same is commended for green wounds; it is also a remedy against certain diseases in cattle, as the cough and murrain, and for that cause divers husbandmen oftentimes much desire it.'* The herb is said to have a relaxing and toning effect on the uterus and can be taken a week or two before childbirth to stimulate labour. It is claimed to have a calming effect on palpitations and irregular heart beat, and to help lower blood pressure

HISTORY: Since ancient times, motherwort has been used to treat palpitations and rapid heart beat, especially when associated with anxiety. The Greeks and Romans used it for a remedy for both physical and emotional heart troubles. Because of its use to treat palpitations and cardiac problems, it was given the scientific name *cardiaca*. In the Middle Ages it treated female disorders, particularly those related to childbirth. In Maud Grieve's *Herbal* we read: *'Motherwort is especially valuable in female weakness and disorders (hence the name), allaying nervous irritability and inducing quiet and passivity of the whole nervous system. Old writers tell us that there is not better herb for strengthening the heart.'* Recently, it has been found to have sedative properties, and acts as a tonic without making one feverish.

Healthy Heart

Motherwort regulates the menses, promotes blood circulation and stimulates the development of new tissue. In traditional Chinese medicine, motherwort was used to promote longevity and strengthen the heart, and scientists now are studying motherwort's application for heart-related conditions.

MUGWORT

ARTEMISIA VULGARIS
Family Asteraceae/Compositae, Sunflower

OTHER NAMES: Artemisia, St John's plant, St John's girdle, muggons, naughty man, old uncle Henry, felon herb, artemis herb, witch herb, sailor's tobacco, old man, felon herb, chrysanthemum weed, wild wormwood.

DESCRIPTION: A perennial, with a height of about 3 feet (90 cm) and a spread of about 18 inches (46 cm), with long aromatic leaves, tiny clusters of whitish-green to yellow flowers and a strong sage fragrance.

PROPERTIES AND USES: *'This is an herb of Venus. Its tops, leaves and flowers are full of virtue, they are aromatic, and most safe, and excellent in female disorders.'* – Nicholas Culpeper. As a 'herb of Venus', it is most widely used to treat the female reproductive system, used as a uterine stimulant that can bring on delayed menstruation and help restore a woman's natural monthly cycle. It is mildly sedative and useful in calming nerves and easing stress. It has been used as a digestive stimulant, being effective taken before or after heavy meals to alleviate flatulence and bloating. The Japanese use its leaves to make a cure for rheumatism, and the Germans to season a roasting goose. It was traditionally used as a 'dream herb', as one of the main ingredients of sleep pillows, being said to bring the dreamer more lucid dreams.

HISTORY: It is accounted as one of the nine sacred herbs of the Druids, and was often used as a ceremonial smoking or burning herb. Roman soldiers placed it in their sandals to prevent fatigue. In the Middle Ages, the plant was known as *cingulum Sancti Johnnis*, it being believed that John the Bapist wore a girdle of it in the wilderness. Mugwort was believed to preserve the wayfarer from fatigue, sunstroke, wild beasts and evil spirits generally. A crown made from its sprays was worn on St John's Eve to gain security from evil possession. It was also used in medieval times to flavour beer.

From Love's Martyr, 1601

First of this Mugwort it did take the name,
Of Artemisia wife to Mausoleus,
Whose sun-bred beauty did his heart inflame,
When she was Queen of Halicarnassus,
Diana gave the herb this name to us:
Because this virtue to us it hath lent,
For women's matters it is excellent.
And he that shall this herb about him bear,
Is freed from hurt or danger any way...

Robert Chester

MULBERRY

MORUS NIGRA
Family Moraceae, Mulberry/Fig

OTHER NAMES: Common mulberry, black mulberry.

DESCRIPTION: An ornamental tree up to 30 feet (9 m) high with large, juicy, blackberry-like fruits, with the gnarled branches of older specimens often spreading wider than the tree's height.

PROPERTIES AND USES: Culpeper relates: '...*the ripe berries, by reason of their sweetness and slippery moisture, opening the body, and the unripe binding it, especially when they are dried, and then they are good to stay fluxes, lasks, and the abundance of women's courses... The juice, or the syrup made of the juice of the berries, helps all inflammations or sores in the mouth, or throat, and palate of the mouth when it is fallen down. The juice of the leaves is a remedy against the biting of serpents, and for those that have taken aconite...The leaves of Mulberries are said to stay bleeding at the mouth or nose, or the bleeding of the piles, or of a wound, being bound unto the places. A branch of the tree taken when the moon is at the full, and bound to the wrists of a woman's arm, whose courses come down too much, doth stay them in a short space.'* Mulberries are refreshing but have laxative properties, and the bark was used to expel tapeworm and roundworm.

HISTORY: The poet Horace recommended that mulberries should be gathered before sunset, and they were eaten at Roman feasts. It may have been brought to Britain by the Romans, and was known to be in cultivation in the early 16th century. In Ovid's *Metamorphoses*, Pyramus and Thisbe were slain beneath its shade, and the fruit changed from white to deep red through absorbing their blood. Pliny wrote of its use in medicine in Egypt, Cyprus and Rome. In the ninth century, Charlemagne ordered its cultivation upon imperial farms. In 1608 King James I tried to encourage the silk industry by issuing an edict encouraging the cultivation of mulberry trees, but the attempt to rear silkworms in England proved unsuccessful, apparently because the black mulberry was cultivated instead of the white, which is preferred by the silkmoth caterpillars.

Here We Go Round...

Many of us will recall the children's song and game, with its subsequent verses and actions, and this chorus:

Here we go round the mulberry bush,
The mulberry bush,
The mulberry bush.
Here we go round the mulberry bush
On a cold and frosty morning.

MULLEIN

VERBASCUM THAPSUS
Family Scrophulariaceae, Figwort

OTHER NAMES: White mullein (Culpeper). Great mullein, common mullein, woolly mullein, blanket mullein, velvet mullein, verbascum flowers, flannel, flannel leaf, flannel flower, Adam's flannel, blanket herb, woollen blanket herb, beggar's blanket, poor man's blanket, Our Lady's blanket, old man's blanket, feltwort, bullock's lungwort, cow's lungwort, pig taper, hare's beard, mullein dock, Aaron's rod, Adam's rod, ice-leaf, hag's taper, hedge taper, high taper, candlewick plant, candlewick herb, torches, velvet plant, velvet back, shepherd's club, shepherd's staff, mullein dock, Jupiter's staff, Jacob's staff, Peter's staff, Virgin Mary's candle, old man's fennel, lady's foxglove, shepherd's herb, blanket leaf, graveyard dust, velvet plant, pannog melyn (cloth plant, Welsh), torches, Our Lady's flannel, velvet dock, velvet plant, woollen, rag paper, wild ice leaf, clown's lungwort, shepherd's staff, beggar's stalk, Adam's flannel.

DESCRIPTION: There are bright yellow, saucer-shaped flowers on a silver-grey stem reaching 6 feet (1.8 m) high. The leaves appear grey-green because of their felt-like covering which irritates browsing animals and protects the plant.

PROPERTIES AND USES: '*It is under the dominion of Saturn. A small quantity of the root given in wine, is commended by Dioscorides, against lasks and fluxes of the belly. The decoction hereof drank, is profitable for those that are bursten* [ruptured], *and for cramps and convulsions, and for those that are troubled with an old cough, and when used as a gargle it eases toothache.*' – Nicholas Culpeper. A fresh poultice of the mashed leaves makes an excellent antimicrobial, astringent first aid for minor burns and insect bites. It is made into a tea, and is frequently combined with other herbs in mixtures for treating cough.

HISTORY: It was called *Aaron's rod* from the Old Testament story of the staff that sprouted with blooms, and in mythology was the plant which Ulysses took to protect himself against the machinations of Circe. Pliny wrote of it, and *verbascum* is thought to be a corruption of *barbascum* (with beards), an allusion to the hairy filaments covering the leaves.

Up in Flames

Many folk-names allude to its use for candle-wicks, tapers and funeral torches in the Middle Ages. The stems were used as flares, and the fluffy hairs scraped from the soft leaves and made into tapers (wax-coated wicks).

MUSHROOM

AGARICUS CAMPESTRIS
Family Agaricaceae, Mushroom

OTHER NAMES: Field mushroom, common mushroom, meadow mushroom (North America), true meadow mushroom.

DESCRIPTION: The cap is white, up to 4 inches (10 cm) in diameter, and the gills are initially pink, turning dark brown, as is the spore print. Mild-tasting, it is the mushroom that many of us used to gather as children, but is becoming very much rarer. Fields in late summer after rainfall used to be covered in 'white-outs' of the fungus. It is solitary, or appears in small circular groups of 'fairy rings'. It is very closely related to the edible button mushroom *Agaricus bisporus* which we buy in shops, but is difficult to cultivate commercially. It needs organic meadows grazed by sheep, cattle or especially horses.

PROPERTIES AND USES: Culpeper praises the mushroom: '*Mushrooms are plants more perfect than many people imagine…*' before describing the edible common mushroom. In the past, slices of field mushrooms were applied to scalds and burns in parts of Scotland, and research into fungal dressings for the treatment of ulcers, and bed sores, using fungal mycelial filaments, is ongoing. Culinary uses of the field mushroom include eating it sautéed or fried, in sauces, soups, stews or sliced raw and included in salads. Mushrooms contain more of the immune-boosting antioxidant *ergothioneine* than any other food, so they are an excellent defence against colds. Mushrooms fried with olive oil and garlic – garlic mushrooms – is far more healthy than it sounds.

HISTORY: From 4600 years ago, hieroglyphics show us that Egyptians thought the plant bestowed immortality, with no commoner being allowed to even touch them. Across cultures, they are associated with being a powerful aphrodisiac. In the 11th century, the Normans traditionally prepared a wedding dish consisting of a pound of mushrooms, to be fed to the groom only.

Poisonous Fungi

There is no clear-cut delineation between edible and poisonous fungi, so that a mushroom may be edible, poisonous or unpalatable. While the similar *Agaricus arvensis*, (horse mushroom) is edible, unfortunately several poisonous species resemble the field mushroom. *Amanita virosa* (the European destroying angel) is morbidly toxic, and *Agaricus xanthodermus* (the yellow stainer) causes gastrointestinal problems. Most of the white *Clitocybe* species that often grow on lawns and fields can be dangerous.

MUSHROOMS AND TOADSTOOLS

There are about 3600 species of fungi in the United Kingdom alone, of which between 50 to 100 are dangerous. Culpeper refers to some different types, and the following shows the variety of wonderful names for these fungi.

Edible Fungi: Beefsteak fungus; brittlegills – powdery, greencracked, common yellow, yellow swamp; fairy ring champignon; mushrooms – field, oyster, macro, St George's, horse, wood, blushing wood, hedgehog; puffballs – common, stump, meadow, giant; charcoal burner; chanterelle; porcelain fungus; saffron milkcap; oak milkcap; the blusher; the deceiver; parasol; shaggy parasol; waxcaps – crimson, scarlet, meadow; tawny grisette; trumpet chanterelle; wood blewit; field blewit; shaggy inkcap; oak milkcap; horn of plenty, the prince; boletes – bay, orange birch, orange oak, scarletina; velvet shank; the miller; morels; summer truffle; jelly ear; chicken of the woods; cauliflower fungus and slippery Jack (or sticky bun).

Poisonous Fungi: Devil's bolete; sickener; beechwood sickener; panthercap (can kill); destroying angel; livid pinkgill; splendid webcap (deadly poisonous, smelling of pepper); deadly webcap (deadly poisonous, but similar to edible chanterelles); fool's and other webcaps; funeral bell (can kill); deadly fibrecap; fool's funnel (seriously poisonous, can be deadly); fenugreek milkcap; the dapperlings including the star, deadly and fatal dapperling; fly agaric; the sickeners; silky pinkgill; poisonpies; common inkcap;

inky mushroom; bitter bolete; false morel (can kill); sulphur tuft; inky mushroom; brown roll rim (can kill if eaten uncooked, but sometimes edible if cooked. It killed the great German mycologist Julius Schaeffer in 1940). The yellow stainer is the most likely to cause stomach upsets as it is similar in appearance to some of the edible agaric mushrooms. Liberty caps are also now known as magic mushrooms for their hallucinogenic properties, but they are classed as poisonous and are the only fungi which it is illegal to pick, being considered a class-A drug. The common inkcap is edible, but poisonous if taken with alcohol. Deathcap is aptly named, as if untreated there is a 50-90 per cent mortality rate. Even with expert hospital care, there is only a 20 per cent survival rate. It is responsible for 90 per cent of all fungus deaths, and is not uncommon, being found in mixed woods and looking similar to agaric mushrooms. However, the '*trumpet of death*', also called the black trumpet, black chanterelle and horn of plenty, the evil-looking *Cratellerus fallax* is edible. Strangely, its French name is also '*trompette de la morte*'.

The Strange World of Fungi: One of the strangest fungi is the powdercap strangler, which takes over the earthy powdercap, its own cap and stipe (stalk) replacing those of its host. Equally, the snaketongue truffleclub parasitizes the subterranean false truffle, and the parasitic bolete grows on the common earthball. Many fungi are named after where they are found, e.g. near pine, hazel, larch, willow, oak, alder, birch, beech – in heaths, meadows, bogs, swamps etc. St George's mushroom is supposed to begin fruiting upon St George's Day (23 April).

Strangely Named Fungi: The pretender; lurid bolete; deceiving bolete; old man of the woods; foxy bolete; ghost bolete; slippey Jack; ugly milkcap; blackening brittlegill; charcoal burner; the flirt; parasol; shaggy parasol; skullcap dapperling; blusher; persistent waxcap; spangle waxcap; herald of winter; deceiving knight; girdled knight; booted knight; prunes and custard; plums and custard; spring cavalier; common cavalier;

trooping funnel; the goblet; club foot; spindleshank; crazed cap; snapping bonnet; powdery piggyback; elastic oysterling; the miller; deer shield; variable webcap; bitter bigfoot webcap; the gipsy; bog bell; dung roundhead (grows in cowpats); blueleg brownie; the prince; weeping widow; lawyer's wig (shaggy inkcap); horn of plenty; handsome club; wood cauliflower; devil's fingers; common jellyspot; artist's bracket; fluted bird's nest; pepperpot; leopard earthball; winter stalkball; barometer earthstar; ear pick fungus; glue crust; leafy brain; jelly rot; earthfan; wood hedgehog; bog beacon; jellybaby; common eyelash; semi-free

---

Magic Mushrooms

The beautiful vivid red *Amanita muscaria* or fly agaric is covered with white spots – the essence of a fairy toadstool. It is mildly poisonous, and also contains ibotenic acid, which transmutes into the powerful psycho-active drug *muscimol* when digested. Symptoms include euphoria, sickness, difficulty in speaking, a wish to sleep and confusion, similar to an overdose of alcohol. There can be a feeling of floating and it has been used by shamans over the years. In Siberia, mushroom users had no other intoxicants, until the Russians introduced alcohol. The Siberian Koryak people dried the mushrooms in the sun and ingested them either on their own or as an extract in water, reindeer milk, or the juice of several sweet plants. When the mushroom was swallowed as a solid, it was first moistened in the mouth,

or women rolled it in their mouths into a moistened pellet for the men to swallow. The ceremonial use of the *fly agaric* developed a ritualistic practice of urine drinking, since the tribesman learned that the psychoactive *muscimol* of the mushroom passes through the body only partially metabolized, or in the form of still active metabolites. An early account reported that the Koryak people '*pour water on some of the mushrooms and boil them. Then they drink the liquor, which intoxicates them; the poorer sort, who cannot afford to lay in a store of the mushroom, post themselves on these occasions round the huts of the rich and watch for the opportunity of the guest coming down to make water and then hold a wooden bowl to receive the urine, which they drink off greedily, as having still some virtue of the mushroom in it, and by this way, they also get drunk.*'

morel; hare's ear; toad's ear; midnight disco; alder goblet; dead man's fingers; dead moll's fingers;.

Coloured Fungi: *Boletes* – Inkstain, scarletina, ruby, sepia, orange birch, orange oak, saffron; *Milkcaps* – Lemon, yellow bearded, lilac, sooty, orange; *Brittlegills* – Scarlet, ochre, yellow swamp, golden, gilded, greencracked, greasy green, copper, primrose, coral, purple, purple swamp, yellowing, bloody; *Dapperlings* – Freckled, green, chestnut, lilac, blushing, pearly; orange grisette; *Waxcaps* – Golden, crimson, scarlet, blackening, butter, pink, parrot, snowy; ivory woodwax; *Knights* – Yellow, sulphur, grey, ashen, yellowing, blue spot; *Domecaps* – Violet, pink, white; frosty funnel; *Deceivers* – Amethyst, bicoloured, russet, redleg; *Bonnets* – Bleeding bonnet, lilac, blackedge, yellowedge, pinkedge; orange, scarlet, milky; orange mosscap; olive oysterling; indigo pinkgill; yellow shield; *Webcaps* – Violet, sepia, orange, yellow, sunset, cinnamon, blood red; lilac leg fibrecap; sulphur tuft; blue roundhead; lilac oysterling; rosy spike; copper spike; yellowing curtain crust; violet coral; yellow club; red cage; yellow stagshorn; cowberry redleaf; witches' butter; white brain; jelly tongue; hen of the woods, chicken of the woods; purplepore bracket; *Porecrusts* – Bleeding, green, pink; cobalt crust; yellow cobweb; yellow brain; *Tooths* – Black, blue, orange; scarlet caterpillarclub; green earthtongue; yellow fan; lemon disco; purple jellydisc; green elfcup; orange cup; scarlet elf cup; ochre cushion.

Aromatic Fungi: Iodine bolete; coconut milkcap; curry milkcap; fenugreek milkcap; geranium brittlegill; stinking brittlegill; crab brittlegill; stinking dapperling; honey waxcap; cedarwood waxcap; soapy knight; aniseed funnel; fragrant funnel; mealy funnel; chicken run funnel; cucumber cap; cabbage parachute; rancid greyling; garlic parachute; foetid parachute; flowery blewit; iodine bonnet; mealy bonnet; aromatic pinkgill (peardrops); mousepee pinkgill; pelargonium webcap; earthy webcap; goatcheese webcap; gassy webcap (smells of acetylene gas or over-ripe pears); honey webcap; sweet poisonpie; bitter poisonpie (radishes); pear fibrecap; aniseed cockleshell; stinkhorn; dog stinkhorn; anise mazegill; stinking earthfan (putrid garlic); peppery bolete; bitter bolete; fiery milkcap; bitter almond brittlegill; burning brittlegill; burnt knight; aromatic knight; bitter oysterling.

Textured Fungi: Suede bolete; woolly milkcap; velvet brittlegill; snakeskin grisette; slimy waxcap; dark honey fungus; warty knight; velvet shank; twisted deceiver; butter cap; wood woolly-foot; porcelain fungus; dripping bonnet; dewdrop bonnet; silky rosegill; velvet rollrim; wrinkled peach; angel's wings; haresfoot inkcap; slimy spike; starfish fungus; greasy bracket; hairy bracket; turkeytail; beeswax bracket; daisy earthstar; spiny puffball; coral tooth; jelly ear; tripe fungus; hairy earthtongue; pig's ears; orange peel fungus; bonfire cauliflower; King Alfred's cakes (cramp balls, resembling burnt cakes).

MUSTARD

BRASSICA NIGRA
Family Brassicaceae/Cruciferae, Cabbage

OTHER NAMES: Black mustard, mustard seed, brown mustard, white mustard. *Brassica alba* is a similar, but more hairy, plant, with slightly larger yellow flowers.

DESCRIPTION: There are small, bright yellow flowers, fading to pale, followed by narrow, upright four-sided seed pods about ½ inch (1.25 cm) long, on a plant which can grow to 6 feet (1.8 m) high.

PROPERTIES AND USES: Culpeper suggests it to remove foreign bodies in the flesh, and *'for the Falling sickness or Lethargy, drowsy forgetful evil, to use it both inwardly and outwardly to rub the Nostrils, Forehead, and Temples, to warm and quicken the Spirits, for by the fierce sharpness it purges the Brain by sneezing, and drawing down Rheum and other Viscous Humours, which by their Distillations upon the Lungs and Chest procure coughing, and therefore with some Honey added thereto doth much good therein.'* He prescribes a decoction of mustard in wine for poisoning and venom, as well as agues. *'The Seed taken either by itself or with other things either in an Electuary or Drink, doth mightily stir up Bodily lust, and helps the Spleen and pains in the sides, and gnawing in the Bowels.'* Mustard can make a gargle for sore throats and a poultice for toothache, sciatica, gout and other joint aches. *'It is also used to help the falling of the Hair: The Seed bruised, mixed with Honey and applied, or made up with Wax, takes away the Marks, and black and blue spots of Bruises or the like, the roughness or scabbedness of the Skin, as also the Leprosy and lousy evil…'* He states, *'It is an excellent Sauce for such whose Blood wants clarifying and for weak Stomachs being an Herb of Mars, but naught for Choleric people, though as good for such as are aged or troubled with cold Diseases, Aries claims something to do with it, therefore it strengthens the heart and resists poison, let such whose Stomachs are so weak, they cannot digest their meat or appetite it, take of Mustard Seed a dram, Cinnamon as much, and having beaten them to Powder add half as much Mastic in Powder, and with Gum Arabic dissolved in Rose Water, make it up into Troches* [lozenges that dissolve in the mouth, like cough drops], *of which they may take one of about half a dram weight an hour or two before meals, let old men and women make much of this medicine, and they will either give me thanks, or manifest ingratitude.'* Richard Mabey, in his 1988 The New Age Herbalist gives us the following: *'Pungent mustard oil is antibacterial and antifungal, warm and stimulating. Mustard not only* adds a spicy tang to food, but it eases digestion. Mustard can be applied externally in poultices, or added to foot baths in the treatment of stubborn chest congestion and coughs, arthritis, and poor circulation.' Mabey also tells us that when mixed with a soothing substance such as slippery elm powder, the seeds make a stimulating poultice. Mustard footbaths have been used for centuries for chilblains, poor circulation and upper respiratory mucus. Thomas Tusser (1524–80) tells us that in February we should: '*Sow mustard seed, And help to kill weed / Where sets do grow, See nothing ye sow.*'

HISTORY: The Greek physicians held mustard in such esteem that they attributed its discovery to Asclepius, the pioneer of medicine and healing. The seeds have been ground and used as a condiment for thousands of years, and the leaves used in liniments. C. Anne Wilson wrote: '*Probably the cheapest spice of all*

was native-grown mustard seed. It was purchased for less than a farthing a pound for the household of Dame Alice de Bryene in 1418–19; and in the course of a year eighty-four pounds were consumed. Mustard was eaten with fresh and salt meat, brawn, fresh fish and stockfish, and indeed was considered the best sauce for any dish. As in Roman times mustard seed was pounded in the mortar and moistened with vinegar.'

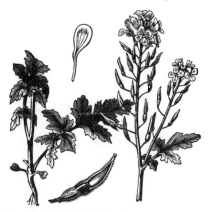

NETTLE

URTICA DIOICA subsp. *DIOICA*
Family Urticaceae, Nettle

OTHER NAMES: Stinging nettle, European stinging nettle, common nettle, burn nettle, burn weed, burn hazel.

DESCRIPTION: It grows to 6 feet (1.8 m) tall and its soft green leaves are strongly serrated and covered with fine 'stinging' hairs. Tiny hairs break off when it is touched, and release acid into the skin. The irritation can be relieved by applying dock leaf, rosemary, mint, sage or the juice of the nettle itself.

PROPERTIES AND USES: *'The roots or leaves boiled, or the juice of either of them, or both made into an electuary with honey and sugar, is a safe and sure medicine to open the pipes and passages of the lungs, which is the cause of wheezing and shortness of breath, and helps to expectorate tough phlegm… The decoction of the leaves in wine, being drank, is singularly good to provoke women's courses, and settle the suffocation, strangling of the mother, and all other diseases thereof; it is also applied outwardly with a little myrrh. The same also, or the seed provokes urine, and expels the gravel and stone in the reins or bladder, often proved to be effectual in many that have taken it. The same kills the worms in children, eases pains in the sides, and dissolves the windiness in the spleen,*

as also in the body, although others think it only powerful to provoke venery. The juice of the leaves taken two or three days together, stays bleeding at the mouth. The seed being drank, is a remedy against the stinging of venomous creatures, the biting of mad dogs, the poisonous qualities of hemlock, henbane, nightshade, mandrake, or other such like herbs that stupefy or dull the senses; as also the lethargy, especially to use it outwardly, to rub the forehead or temples in the lethargy, and the places stung or bitten with beasts, with a little salt…The juice of the leaves, or the decoction of them, or of the root, is singularly good to wash either old, rotten, or stinking sores or fistulous, and gangrenes, and such as fretting, eating, or corroding scabs, manginess, and itch, in any part of the body, as also green wounds, by washing them therewith, or applying the green herb bruised thereunto, yea, although the flesh were separated from the bones; the same applied to our wearied members, refresh them, or to place those that have been out of joint, being first set up again, strengthens, dries, and comforts them, as also those places troubled with aches and gouts, and the defluxion of humours upon the joints or sinews; it eases the pains,

and dries or dissolves the defluxions.'
Culpeper's remedy for joint aches has a
contemporary resonance in that the
plant is used for rheumatism
today. Nettles are high in
boron, and the Rheumatoid
Disease Foundation
recommends that people
should take 3 milligrams
of boron every day.
Stinging nettles contain
antihistamines and anti-
inflammatories (including
quercetin), which open up
constricted bronchial and
nasal passages, helping
to ease hay fever, and
nose and sinus problems.
Extracts of nettle roots
are diuretics that encourage excretion
of uric acid, but simultaneously
discourage night-time visits to the
bathroom urges, making it useful for
gout, bed-wetting, and benign prostate
enlargement. Nettles were used as a tonic
by Native North American women who
used it throughout pregnancy, and as a
remedy to stop haemorrhaging during
childbirth. It tastes a little like spinach
and makes herbal teas and a wonderful
soup. Strongly brewed nettle tea and the
powdered plant itself are noted for having
power to stop haemorrhaging, internal
bleeding and excessive flow from wounds
and cuts. Leftover nettle tea also makes
nutritious houseplant water and leaves or
dregs can be sprinkled on potted plant soil
to boost mineral content. Finely crushed,
dried nettles can be used in place of dried
parsley for adding colour to soups, stews
and other dishes. Flies dislike nettles and
a bunch hung by the kitchen door may
keep them out.

HISTORY: Nettle stings prevented
sorcery, and the presence of plants
prevented milk from being soured by
witches. Their presence often
denotes a former human or
animal habitation, probably
because of the elevated levels
of phosphate and nitrogen
in the soil. One remedy for
hay fever is to strip off and roll
in a bed of stinging nettles,
or preferably to take a
concoction of stinging
nettle root. If a horse
cuts its leg and is ridden
through a large patch
of nettles, the bleeding
seems to stop, which may
be the origin of the belief of nettles
helping with heavy menstrual periods.

Eating Nettles

The Stinging Nettle Eating
Championship draws thousands
of people to Dorset's Bottle Inn at
Marshwood near Bridport every
June, where competitors attempt
to eat as much of the raw plant as
possible. They are given 20-inch
(50-cm) stalks of the plant, from
which they must strip the leaves
and eat them. Whoever strips and
eats the most leaves in an hour
is the winner. An accumulated
stem length of 76 feet (23.2 m)
is the world record so far. The
championship has separate men's
and women's sections and attracts
competitors from as far afield as
Canada and Australia.

NUTMEG TREE and MACE

MYRISTICA FRAGRANS
Family Myristicaceae, Nutmeg

OTHER NAMES: Nutmeg, mace, nux moschata.

DESCRIPTION: A tropical evergreen which grows to a height of around 45 feet (14 m), producing up to 2000 nuts per year. The stone of the fruit is enclosed in a husk, and the seed covering when dried is known as *mace*. This fibrous, branched aril wraps itself around the nutmeg seed. The blossoms are wonderfully fragrant, and its name comes from *nux* (nut) and *muscat* (musky).

PROPERTIES AND USES: The *pit*, or stone, contains the brown nutmeg kernel. Nutmeg and mace have been used to treat many illnesses ranging from those affecting the nervous system to ailments of the digestive system. Nutmeg has been used as the active ingredient in commercial cough and congestion preparations such as Vicks Cough Syrup and in herbal pain-relieving ointments. Culpeper recommended both for coughs and to '*dry up distillations of rheum falling upon the lungs*'. Culinary uses vary around the world. In the USA it is used in hot dogs, in sausages and processed luncheon meats. The Dutch and Scandinavians use it with vegetables, including mashed potatoes and spinach, and even with pineapple. In France, it is added to béchamel sauce. Nutmeg and mace are widely used in drinks, cosmetics and in flavourings in dental pastes.

HISTORY: Pliny the Elder writes of a tree bearing nuts with two flavours. In the sixth century, nutmegs were brought by Arab traders to Constantinople. In the 12th century, Crusaders found a whole new world of taste in the Holy Land, and nutmeg became the most expensive spice in the world. At one time, the trees were only grown on the island of Banda in the Moluccas, and the Dutch massacred and enslaved all its inhabitants to ensure a monopoly in the product and to keep prices high. In 1760, the price of nutmeg in London was 85 to 90 shillings per pound, a price kept artificially high by the Dutch deliberately burning full warehouses of nutmegs in Amsterdam. The Dutch held control of the 'Spice Islands' until the Second World War. Frenchman Pierre Poivre ('Peter Pepper') transported nutmeg seedlings to Mauritius where they flourished, which helped to break the Dutch monopoly of the spice. The British East India Company spread the nutmeg tree across the empire, most notably to Grenada in the Caribbean, where it is the national emblem on the country's red, yellow and green flag. At the height of its value in Europe, nutmeg was carried around by the upper classes as a demonstration of wealth. Diners would flourish tiny graters and grate their own nutmeg in restaurants and at each

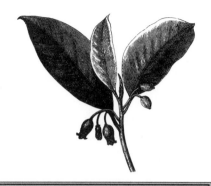

other's houses. Connecticut is sometimes referred to as the 'Nutmeg State', with G.E. Shankle in 1941 writing that it *'...is applied to Connecticut because its early inhabitants had the reputation of being so ingenious and shrewd that they were able to make and sell wooden nutmegs...Some claim that wooden nutmegs were actually sold, but they do not give either the time or the place.'*

How the English Obtained Manhattan

'In Elizabethan times it was believed that nutmeg could ward off the plague (35,000 died in England in 1603), and it was also used in perfumes and oils. As the world's only source of nutmeg and mace, the Banda islands had attracted traders from China, Asia and the Middle East for over 3000 years, ever since the Persians first traded cloves from Moluccas. The Roman empire's spices also came from these islands. By the 1600s, the spices were more widely available due to the new sea routes used by Portuguese traders. The Dutch, British and Portuguese began to battle to control the islands. During the 'Spice Wars' of the Middle Ages, the Dutch took control of nutmeg importation from the Portuguese, who had discovered nutmeg in the Moluccas of Indonesia a century previously. The profit on a ship successfully carrying nutmeg to Europe was around 3200 per cent, such was the popularity and scarcity of the spice. Run is one of the smallest of the Banda Islands, only about 2 miles (3 km) long and less than 0.6 miles (1 km) wide, but of immense value because of its nutmeg trees. The English had occupied Run

Island, but were driven out by the Dutch. Initially the Dutch had traded amicably with the Bandanese, but 6000 islanders were then killed in a spice war. Banda was so rich that merchants joked that when they shook a nutmeg tree, golden guilders would fall down. After the war, the Banda Islands were run as a series of plantation estates, with the Dutch mounting annual expeditions in local war-vessels to eliminate nutmeg trees planted elsewhere. Desperate to keep a monopoly on the nutmeg, the Dutch only allowed nutmeg trees to grow on islands such as Run, which they could easily guard with their forces. In addition, they limed each kernel that left the islands to ensure that it was its sterile, and thus to prevent anyone from growing their own trees. The death penalty was pronounced on anyone caught smuggling the seeds. Eventually the English gave up their claim to the Spice Islands in return for Manhattan. They had already smuggled nutmeg seeds to Grenada and other possessions, breaking the Dutch monopoly on the spices.' (From T.D. Breverton, *The Book of the Sea – Breverton's Nautical Curiosities*, 2010.)

OAK

QUERCUS ROBUR
Family Fagaceae, Beech

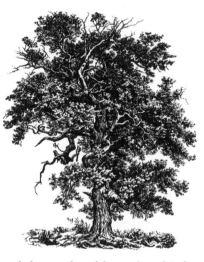

OTHER NAMES: English oak, pedunculate oak, gospel oak. There are several hundred species of trees that have the common name oak. The genus *Quercus* is native to the northern hemisphere, and includes deciduous trees and evergreens such as holly.

DESCRIPTION: A long-lived deciduous tree which can grow well over 100 feet (30 m) tall, with lobed leaves and familiar nut-like fruit known as acorns. Its wood is particularly tough and hard, leading to its name of *robur*, robust.

PROPERTIES AND USES: Culpeper relates: '*Jupiter owns the tree. The leaves and bark of the Oak, and the acorn cups, do bind and dry very much. The inner bark of the tree, and the thin skin that covers the acorn, are most used to stay the spitting of blood, and the bloody-flux. The decoction of that bark, and the powder of the cups, do stay vomiting, spitting of blood, bleeding at the mouth, or other fluxes of blood, in men or women; lasks [diarrhoea] also, and the nocturnal involuntary flux of men. The acorn in powder taken in wine, provokes urine, and resists the poison of venomous creatures. The decoction of acorns and the bark made in milk and taken, resists the force of poisonous herbs and medicines, as also the virulence of cantharides [Cantharis vesicatoria – 'blister beetles' or 'Spanish flies'], when one by eating them hath his bladder exulcerated, and voids bloody urine. Hippocrates says, he used the fumes of Oak leaves to women that were troubled* with the strangling of the womb; and Galen applied them, being bruised, to cure green wounds. The distilled water of the Oaken bud, before they break out into leaves is good to be used either inwardly or outwardly, to assuage inflammations, and to stop all manner of fluxes in man or woman. The same is singularly good in pestilential and hot burning fevers; for it resists the force of the infection, and allays the heat. It cools the heat of the liver, breaking the stone in the kidneys, and stays women's courses. The decoction of the leaves works the same effects. The water that is found in the hollow places of old Oaks, is very effectual against any foul or spreading scabs. The distilled water (or concoction, which is better) of the leaves, is one of the best remedies that I know of for the whites [fluor albus – vaginal discharges] in women.'* Oak bark is a powerful astringent, and has been used by herbalists for thousands of years. Decoctions of oak bark are used for throat infections, acute diarrhoea and bleeding, and have been studied for use in kidney infections and stones. The juice from crushed oak leaves can be applied directly onto wounds and the leaves can be soaked in boiling water, allowed to cool and the liquid used to relieve tired and inflamed eyes. The same liquid can ameliorate cuts and burns, be used as a mouthwash for bleeding gums, a gargle for sore throats and for bathing haemorrhoids and varicose veins. A decoction of the bark can be used for reducing fevers, diarrhoea, dysentery, tonsillitis, pharyngitis and laryngitis. The bark also yields a tannin which was used extensively for preparing leather and twine. Oak galls (formed by larvae of the gall wasp) yield a black ink, and a coffee substitute can be made from acorn kernels.

HISTORY: Of all the trees in prehistoric times, the oak was the most widely venerated, as it was believed that the oak was the first tree created and that man sprang from it. It was sacred to the Hebrews. The Greeks dedicated it to Zeus, to the Romans the oak was the tree of Jupiter, and to the Teutonic tribes, it was the Tree of Life, sacred to Thor. It was the most sacred tree of the Celtic Druids, who collected rainwater from hollows in the trunk and branches to ritually cleanse themselves. Until men devised iron cutting tools, the oak resisted all attempts to fell it, but then became the main construction material for houses, churches and ships. Its elasticity and strength made it particularly advantageous in shipbuilding, and the oaks of the Forest of Dean in Gloucestershire provided much of the raw material for the Royal Navy's '*wooden walls of England*'. Philip of Spain gave special orders to the Armada to burn and destroy every oak in the forest. In England, the oak has assumed the status of a national emblem, since the future King Charles II hid from Parliamentarians in an oak tree at Boscobel House in 1651 after his defeat at the Battle of Worcester during the English Civil War.

Life in an Oak Tree

The pedunculate oak supports the highest biodiversity of insect herbivores of any British plant, with over 400 species recorded in a single tree. The acorns also are a valuable food resource for several small mammals such as squirrels and some birds, notably jays. Jays were the primary propagators of oaks before humans began planting them commercially, because of their habit of taking acorns from the umbra of a parent tree and burying them undamaged elsewhere.

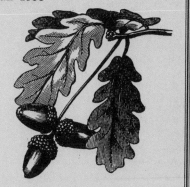

OATS

AVENA SATIVA
Family Poaceae, True Grasses

OTHER NAMES: Groats, oatmeal, oatstraw, wild oats.

DESCRIPTION: An annual grass growing 2–4 feet (60–120 cm), with narrow pale green leaves and seeds borne on nodding heads, which thrives in damper climates.

PROPERTIES AND USES:
Culpeper tells us that they are principally used as food for man and beast, but: '… *fried with bay salt, and applied to the sides as warm as can be endured, take away the pains of stitches and wind in the sides and colic in the belly. A poultice made of the meal of Oats, and some oil of Bay helps the itch, leprosy, fistulas of the fundament, and dissolves hard imposthumes* [abscesses]. *The meal of Oats boiled with vinegar, and applied, takes away freckles and spots in the face, and other parts of the body. It is also used in broth or milk, to bind those who have a lask* [diarrhoea], *or other flux; and with sugar is good for them that have a cough or cold.'* Oats have always had a reputation as a wholesome, healthy food, being a rich source of complex sugars needed to fuel a working body, some of which are also important for immune system stimulation. Its B vitamins help fight stress and build body tissue, and it is one of the best foods if not pre-packaged and refined. Oats help to regulate the thyroid, soothe nervous and digestive systems, stabilize blood sugar levels and are said to reduce cigarette cravings. Oat extract is often used in skin lotions to soothe skin conditions. Oat grass has been used traditionally to help balance the menstrual cycle, treat dysmenorrhoea, and for osteoporosis and urinary tract problems. Oat straw baths are used for rheumatic problems, lumbago, paralysis, liver ailments and gout, kidney, eczema and neuralgia problems. Porridge, oatcakes and muesli are especially beneficial meals, with detoxifying and cholesterol-lowering properties.

HISTORY: In the 1800s doctors advocated oat straw tea, made from young oat stalks and unripe grain, as a nerve tonic, which is sold commercially today for mild anxiety. Samuel Johnson included this celebrated entry for oats in his *A Dictionary of the English Language*: '*a grain, which in England is generally given to horses, but in Scotland supports the people.*' The Scottish riposte was '*England is known for the quality of its horses, and Scotland for its men*'.

Wild Oats

It is believed that horses that eat oats are more likely to mate. Old sayings like '*feeling one's oats*' or '*sowing wild oats*', refer to the belief in oats act as an aphrodisiac. Recent studies show that its consumption does indeed raise testosterone levels.

OREGANO

ORIGANUM VULGARE
Family Lamiaceae/Labiatae, Mint

OTHER NAMES: Culpeper calls it *'Wild or Field Marjoram…Called also origane, origanum, eastward marjoram… and grove marjoram.'* Maud Grieve notes: *'In the older herbals oregano is referred to as Wild Marjoram, which can be confused with the herb known today as wild marjoram, Thymus mastichina, which is a wild-growing species of thyme.'*

DESCRIPTION: Height and spread of 18 inches (46 cm), with clusters of tiny mauve flowers and hairy aromatic leaves.

PROPERTIES AND USES: Culpeper: *'It strengthens the stomach and head much, there being scarce a better remedy growing for such as are troubled with a sour humour in the stomach; it restores the appetite being lost; helps the cough, and consumption of the lungs; it cleanses the body of choler, expels poison, and remedies the infirmities of the spleen; helps the bitings of venomous beasts, and helps such as have poisoned themselves by eating Hemlock, Henbane, or Opium. It provokes urine and the terms in women, helps the dropsy, and the scurvy, scabs, itch, and yellow jaundice. The juice being dropped into the ears, helps deafness, pain and noise in the ears. And thus much for this herb, between which and adders, there is a deadly antipathy.'* It has also been used to relieve fevers, diarrhoea, vomiting and jaundice. Oregano tea is still used for indigestion, bloating, flatulence, sore throats, coughs, urinary problems, bronchial problems, headaches, swollen glands, and to promote menstruation.

Unsweetened tea is also used as a gargle or mouthwash. Its rosmarinic acid and thymol content have strong antioxidant and antibacterial properties, and oregano is thought to be effective against *Heliobacter pylori*, the stomach bacteria that cause ulcers. For tired joints and muscles, or rheumatic conditions, put a handful of leaves in a cheesecloth bag in a hot bath. An attractive spreading border plant, it attracts butterflies.

HISTORY: In myth Venus was the first to grow the herb in her garden. The Greeks used it extensively, both internally and externally, as a remedy for narcotic poisons, convulsions and dropsy. The Greeks believed it was a cure-all, and Aristotle said it was an antidote to poison, after seeing a tortoise eat a snake and then some oregano.

Pizza Herb

Oregano is sometimes known as the *'pizza herb'*, being widely used in Italian cuisine. The cultivated species, *Origanum onites* (pot marjoram), *Oreganum majorana* (sweet or knotted marjoram), and *Oreganum heracleoticum* (winter marjoram) are those varieties which are generally used in cookery as a seasoning. Culpeper's wild marjoram, *Oreganum vulgare* was more used for medicinal purposes.

OLIVE TREE

OLEA EUROPAEA
Family Oleaceae, Olive

OTHER NAMES: Olivier, cultivated olive, European olive.

DESCRIPTION: Evergreen, this long-lived, gnarled and twisted tree grows up to 30 feet (9 m) tall, with silvery green leaves, creamy fragrant small flowers, and green fruits which ripen to black. There are records of 1500-year-old trees still producing olives. All fresh olives are bitter and tough, whether green and unripe or black and ripe. When harvested, they must be processed to be edible, with a ton needed to make 50 gallons (227 litres) of olive oil. Olives are only properly edible after being soaked in brine, salt or oil, so they cannot be eaten straight off the trees. Olives have to be rinsed in fresh water once a day for ten days before being placed in salt water for eight or nine weeks after which they are edible. There are around 800 million olive trees growing around the world, with Spain, Italy, Greece and Turkey being the main olive producers.

PROPERTIES AND USES: Culpeper: '*This is a tree of the Sun. The fruit of this tree has a bitter, austere, disagreeable taste; but when pickled, as they come from abroad, they are less ungrateful, and promote appetite and digestion; it also cuts and attenuates tough phlegm in the stomach and first passages. The Lucca Olives are smaller than the others, and have the weakest taste; and the Spanish, or larger, the strongest; those brought from Provence, which are of a middling size, are most esteemed. But the principal consumption of this fruit is in making the common salad-oil, which is obtained by grinding and pressing them when ripe; the finer, and most pure oil, issues first on their being gently pressed, and the inferior sorts on heating the mass, and pressing it more strongly. This oil, in its virtues, does not differ materially from the other tasteless expressed oils, but it is preferred to all of them for esculent purposes; and is chiefly used in the preparation of plasters, ointments, &c. Oil is moderately healing and mollifying, rendering the body lax and soluble; it is good for disorders of the breast and lungs, tempering the sharp choleric humours in the bowels. What is drawn from the unripe Olives is called omphacinum, and is accounted drying and restringent, and fitter for some external remedies; what is pressed out of the ripe fruit is called Oil of Olives, being what is generally eaten, and made use of in medicines: the different fineness being from the different care and management in the making it; the sweetest, and what we esteem most, comes from Florence.*' The oil is a safe laxative, good for circulation and improves digestion. The leaves have been traditionally used to disinfect wounds. The monounsaturated oil is used widely in cooking and as skin care oil. Olive leaf teas have been used in traditional herbal medicine to lower fevers, and olive leaf poultices are among the oldest therapies for infections of the skin, cuts and bruises. Olives contain antibacterial and antifungal properties. The main compound of olive oil, *oleocanthal*, has the same properties as painkillers used to treat heart conditions. The healthy, life-prolonging 'Mediterranean Diet' relies upon olive oil.

HISTORY: Olives have been cultivated since prehistoric times in Asia Minor. Moses exempted from military service men who would work at their cultivation, and in almost all early writings olive oil is a symbol of goodness and purity, with the tree representing peace and happiness. In the Old Testament, the dove returned to the Ark with a sprig of olive, showing that the flood waters had abated. The oil,

in addition to its wide use in diet, was burned in the sacred lamps of temples, and winners of events in the Olympic Games were crowned with olive leaves. Homer called olive oil *'liquid gold'*. In Greece, the dead were anointed with the oil the mask the smell, and the Romans used it to prevent stretch marks on the bodies of pregnant women.

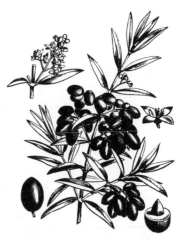

The Gift of an Olive Tree

The first king of Attica (the region of Greece around Athens) was said to have been Cecrops I. There was a competition between Athena, the goddess of wisdom, war, the arts, industry, justice and skill, and Poseidon, the god of the sea to become patron of his new city. They agreed that each would give his people one gift, and Cecrops would choose whichever gift was better. Poseidon struck the rock of the Acropolis with his trident and a spring sprang from it. The water was salty and was not thought very useful,

but Athena struck the rock with her lance and an olive tree sprung up. Cecrops judged the olive tree as the superior gift, for the olive tree brought wood, oil and food, and thus accepted Athena as the patron of the new city, which was then called Athens in her honour. Poseidon decided to grant his gift anyway. The Athenians had misunderstood that he was offering them sea power, not fresh water, and the power of the Athenian navy ensured domination over the rest of Greece.

ONION and LEEK

ALLIUM CEPA and *ALLIUM AMPELOPRASUM VAR. PORRUM*
Family Alliaceae, Onion

OTHER NAMES: Onion – garden onion, bulb onion. Leek – tree onion, Egyptian onion, lazy man's onion.

DESCRIPTION: The bulbous onion only shows one shoot above the ground. The leek grows to 3 feet (90 cm), producing a long cylinder of bundled leaf sheaths.

PROPERTIES AND USES: Culpeper tells us: '*Mars owns them, and they have gotten this quality, to draw any corruption to them, for if you peel one, and lay it upon a dunghill, you shall find it rotten in half a day, by drawing putrefaction to it; then, being bruised and applied to a plague sore, it is very probable it will do the like. Onions are flatulent, or windy; yet they do somewhat provoke appetite, increase thirst, ease the belly and bowels, provoke women's courses, help the biting of a mad dog, and of other venomous creatures, to be used with honey and rue, increase sperm, especially the seed of them. They also kill worms in children if they drink the water fasting wherein they have been steeped all night. Being roasted under the embers, and eaten with honey or sugar and oil, they much conduce to help an inveterate cough, and expectorate the tough phlegm. The juice being snuffed up into the nostrils, purges the head, and helps the lethargy, (yet the often eating them is said to procure pains in the head). It hath been held by divers country people a great preservative against infection to eat Onions fasting with bread and salt. As also to make a great Onion hollow, filling the place with good treacle, and after to roast it well under the embers, which, after taking away the outermost skin thereof, being beaten together, is a sovereign salve for either plague or sore, or any other putrefied ulcer. The juice of Onions is good for either scalding or burning by fire, water, or gunpowder, and used with vinegar, takes away all blemishes, spots and marks in the skin: and dropped in the ears, eases the pains and noise of them. Applied also with figs beaten together, helps to ripen and break imposthumes [abscesses], and other sores. Leeks are as like them in quality, as the pomme-water [apple juice] is like an apple. They are a remedy against a surfeit of mushrooms, being baked under the embers and taken, and being boiled and applied very warm, help the piles. In other things they have the same property as the Onions, although not so effectual.*'

Earache could be relieved by holding a roasted onion to the ear, and a mixture of honey, salt and bruised onion rubbed into a bald patch would encourage hair growth. As a cosmetic aid a mixture of onion juice and vinegar was applied to freckles and spots in the Middle Ages. European herbalists recommended onion and onion juice for healing burns, sores and ulcers, treating the symptoms of various epidemics experienced in medieval times, curing chilblains and removing warts. The juice was also used to ease swellings, to treat not only children's coughs and colds but also patients with diphtheria, and it was believed to be a helpful remedy for insect bites too. When cutting an onion, a chemical is released that irritates the eyes and nose, causing us to shed tears. Onion skins yield a yellow dye, and onion juice was used by children to make a 'secret ink', which would reappear when the paper was warmed. Both onions and leeks are invaluable in cooking, and amongst the healthiest of vegetables to consume.

HISTORY: Onions were cultivated in Egypt from at least 3200 BCE. It is claimed that along with garlic *(Allium sativum)* or leeks *(Allium ampeloprasum* var. *porrum)*, or garden parsley *(Petroselinum crispum)*, the onion formed part of labourers' wages when the pyramids were built by Cheops, *c.*2600 BCE. Alexander the Great (356–23 BCE) is traditionally said to have introduced the onion to Greece, and provisioned his armies with it for its war-like properties. Onions were popular in England in the early 13th century when Abbot Neckham of Cirencester (1157–1217) listed the onion as a vegetable that could be cultivated successfully for the tables of the wealthy. An old country adage is: '*Onion skin very thin, / Mild winter coming in, / Onion skin thick and tough, / Coming winter cold and*

rough.' King Cadwaladr of Gwynedd in Wales fought the Saxons in a leek field in the seventh century, and he ordered his soldiers to wear leeks so that they could recognize each other during the fighting. The leek became, along with the daffodil, the national symbol of Wales. Raw onion seems to be helpful in reducing swelling from bee stings, and in Malta a popular remedy for painful sea urchin wounds is to tie half a baked onion to the afflicted area overnight.

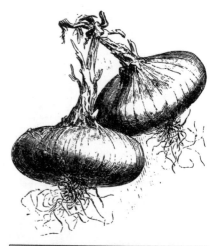

Bone Hardener

Inulin is a soluble fibre found in some fruit and vegetables, and is a food source for 'good' probiotic bacteria in the gut, i.e. it acts as a 'probiotic'. It also helps bodies absorb calcium, so is good for women as a defence against osteoporosis. Just one 100g leek provides 10g inulin, more than the amount from 14 medium-sized bananas of 100g each.

THE ORIGIN OF PARADISE AND THE BEGINNING OF HERB GARDENS

The Greeks wrote of fine pleasure parks all over the lands of the Medes and Persians, of such size and beauty that there was a saying that they had been founded by the legendary Assyrian Queen Semiramis. The soldier and historian Xenophon (*c.*430–354 BCE) wrote that Socrates told his pupils: '*Everywhere the Persian king is zealously cared for, so that he may find gardens wherever he goes; their name is Paradise, and they are full of all things fair and good that the earth can bring forth. It is here that he spends the greatest part of his time, except when the season forbids.*' This is the first recorded mention of '*paradise*' in any Greek narrative. The Persian Prince Cyrus the Younger (*c.*424-401 BCE) showed the Greek Lysander the paradise of his palace at Sardis. Lysander marvelled at the beautiful 'shade trees' and fruit trees, the prettiness of the rows of flowers and the many sweet fragrances around the pathways. Cyrus, the son of Emperor Darius, then told Lysander that he himself had designed the paradise, and had even planted some of the trees himself. As part of their education, young Persian princes and nobles were taught the art of gardening and horticulture.

From accounts and monumental inscription we find that these Persian paradises were originally hunting-parks, with fruit-trees grown for food, just as in their Babylonian-Assyrian predecessors. They were in fact 'garden palaces', with vast colonnades open to walled green spaces surrounding them, and 'throne rooms' overlooking reflecting pools and groves of trees. They were thus fertile, cultivated, enclosed areas in a wilderness. Indeed, in Old Persian *pairi-daeza* means 'a walled space'. The Greeks adapted the word as *paradeisos* to describe the gardens of the Persian empire, and Greek translations of the Bible used this same word as the term for both the Garden of Eden and Heaven. For the course of much of human history, the entire natural world has been charged with meaning, with gods being identified everywhere: in the water, flowers, trees, sky etc. Human existence had come to depend upon agriculture, so particularly powerful gods and goddesses resided in water, the sun, trees and plants. The Mesopotamian idea of an everlasting, ever-fruitful paradise was already old by the times of the Achaemenid kings of Persia (559–329 BCE). Fragments of the earliest known writing, from Sumer in Mesopotamian around 2800 BCE, include a poem describing the creation of such a paradise, ordered by the god of water and provided by the sun god. The Sumerian *Epic of Gilgamesh* (c.2150 BCE) describes an 'immortal' garden centred on a sacred tree standing by a holy fountain. King Sennacherib (c.705–681 BCE) built a garden with canals, ponds, vines, fruits and spices at Assyria's capital of Nineveh. *The Hanging Gardens of Babylon* (also in modern Iraq) were sometimes called the *Hanging Gardens of Semiramis*, and were probably built by Nebuchadnezzar II around 600 BCE. He may have built this tiered paradise for his homesick wife, Amytis of Media, who was missing the fragrant flowers and plants of Persia. The gardens were destroyed by several earthquakes after the second century BCE, but in 50 BCE Diodorus Siculus recorded this Wonder of the Ancient World, '*built up in tiers, so it resembled a theatre*'.

Alexander the Great's conquest of Egypt found more 'paradises', with Egyptian gardeners being honoured individuals. From this time on, both public and private garden and park design became important in Greece, and later in Rome and across Europe. A quarter of the city of Alexandria in Egypt was given over to gardens, and Pliny recorded Italian gardens '*set out with beds of flowers and sweet-smelling herbs*'. Charlemagne in 802 issued a list of the herbs to be grown in his royal estates in a famous *Capitulary*. He owned a number of villas which were planned on the Roman model. Since he spent most of

his life pursuing military campaigns, his possessions were transported in wagons and arranged in whichever villa he chose to stay in. Charlemagne specified in each villa garden: *Flowers*: lily, rose, flag iris. *Physical Herbs*: fenugreek, costmary, sage, rue, southernwood, gourd, cumin, rosemary, caraway, squills, dragons, anise, colocynth, ammi, black cumin, burdock, lovage, savin, dill, fennel, centaury, poppy, asarabacca, marshmallow, coriander, caper spurge, clary, houseleek. *Salads*: cucumber, melon, lettuce, rocket, cress, alexanders, parsley, celery, dittander, mustard, chives, radish, chervil. *Pulses*: kidney bean, chickpea, broad bean, pea. *Pot-herbs*: chicory, pennyroyal, endive, savory, horse mint, mint, wild mint, tansy, catmint, beet, mallow, orach, blite, kohl-rabi, colewort. *Roots*: skirret, carrot, parsnip, onion, leek, shallot, garlic. *Industrial plants*: madder, teasel. *Fruit trees*: apple, pear, plum, service, medlar, peach, quince, mulberry, fig, cherry. *Nut trees*: chestnut, hazel, almond, pine, walnut.

The first monastery garden we know dates from around 825 and was established at St Gall Benedictine monastery in France. It contained the following plants: *Vegetable garden*: onions, shallots, garlic, leek, celery, parsley, coriander, chervil, dill, lettuce, poppy, savory, radishes, parsnip, carrots, colewort (cabbage), beet, black cumin. *Orchard*: apple, pear, mulberry, peach, plum, service tree, medlar, laurel, chestnut, fig, quince, hazelnut, almond, walnut. *Physic garden*: kidney bean, savory, rose, horsemint, cumin, lovage, fennel, tansy, lily, sage rue, flag iris, pennyroyal, fenugreek, mint, rosemary.

PARSLEY

PETROSELINUM CRISPUM
Family Apiaceae/Umbelliferae, Umbellifer/Carrot

OTHER NAMES: Common parsley, garden parsley, rock parsley, curly leaf parsley, persil, devil's oatmeal.

DESCRIPTION: A hardy biennial which reaches 16 inches (40 cm) with a 12-inch (30 cm) spread, and bright green leaves with curly serrated edges.

PROPERTIES AND USES:
Culpeper: *'It is under the dominion of Mercury; is very comfortable to the stomach; helps to provoke urine and women's courses, to break wind both in the stomach and bowels, and doth a little open the body, but the root much more. It opens obstructions both of liver and spleen, and is therefore accounted one of the five opening roots. Galen commended it against the falling sickness, and to provoke urine mightily; especially if the roots be boiled, and eaten like Parsnips. The seed is effectual to provoke urine and women's courses, to expel wind, to break the stone, and ease the pains and torments thereof; it is also effectual against the venom of any poisonous creature, and the danger that comes to them that have the lethargy, and is as good against the cough. The distilled water of Parsley is a familiar medicine with nurses to give their children when they are troubled with wind in the stomach or belly which they call the frets; and is also much available to them that are of great years.*

The leaves of Parsley laid to the eyes that are inflamed with heat, or swollen, doth much help them, if it be used with bread or meal; and being fried with butter, and applied to women's breasts that are hard through the curdling of their milk, it abates the hardness quickly; and also takes away black and blue marks coming of bruises or falls. The juice thereof dropped into the ears with a little wine, eases the pains. Tragus sets down an excellent medicine to help the jaundice and falling sickness, the dropsy, and stone in the kidneys, in this manner: Take of the seed of Parsley, Fennel, Anise and Caraway, of each an ounce; of the roots of Parsley, Burnet, Saxifrage, and Caraway, of each an ounce and an

Packed With Goodness

Parsley contains more vitamin C than oranges, more calcium than milk, more iron than steak and more potassium than bananas. It has been traditionally used to lower blood pressure, before it was known scientifically that its high potassium content counteracts sodium, lowering blood volume and hence blood pressure. Studies have also proved its diuretic qualities.

Anyone for Parsley?

For an interesting and highly unusual example of early genetic engineering, look no further than the works of the German botanist and physician Leonhart Fuchs, specifically as noted in his *Historia Stirpium* [*The New Herball*], 1543: 'If you will have the leaves of the parcelye grow crisped, then *before the sowing of them stuffe a tennis ball with the seedes and beat the same well against the ground whereby the seedes may be a little bruised or when the parcelye is well come up go over the bed with a weighty roller whereby it may so press the leaves down or else tread the same downe under thy feet.'*

half; let the seeds be bruised, and the roots washed and cut small; let them lie all night to steep in a bottle of white wine, and in the morning be boiled in a close earthen vessel until a third part or more be wasted; which being strained and cleared, take four ounces thereof morning and evening first and last, abstaining from drink after it for three hours. This opens obstructions of the liver and spleen, and expels the dropsy and jaundice by urine.' Parsley is a wonderful digestive aid, so is a good addition to a salad. It is high in iron content and rich in vitamins A, B, C, iodine and trace minerals. Leaves, seeds and root all have been used in the treatment of diseases of the bladder and kidneys, rheumatism, arthritis and sciatica. Nowadays we know through scientific research that parsley has a lot to offer us. As well as being a wonderful breath-freshener after eating curry or garlic or chilli dishes, it is effective in reducing depression. A hair rinse made from the seeds is said to kill head lice.

HISTORY: In Greece, the herb was held sacred to oblivion and to the dead, having sprung from the blood of the Greek child Archemorus, which means the forerunner of death. The herb was dedicated to Persephone and to funeral rituals. Romans used it to disguise strong smells, to curb drunkenness, and believed that the seeds had to go to the devil and back seven times before they would germinate. It is used as a symbol of spring and rebirth in the Hebrew celebration of Passover. Hippocrates documented that parsley was used to cause an abortion, and Pliny the Elder (23–79 CE) stated that parsley was used to cause sterility. In the Dark Ages parsley was known as the *devil's herb*, and people were convinced that moving the plant would lead to certain death.

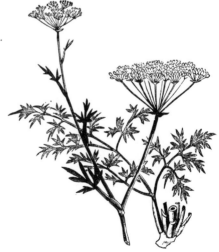

PARSNIP

PASTINACA SATIVA
Family Apiaceae, Umbellifer

OTHER NAMES: Culpeper calls it the Parsnep, and the Common Garden Parsnep.

DESCRIPTION: Similar to a carrot, with the root being generally pale cream.

PROPERTIES AND USES: Culpeper wrote: '*Parsneps are more used for food than medicine, being a pleasing nourishing root, though somewhat windy, are though to be provokers to venery...The wild Parsnip differs little from the garden, but grows not so fair and large, nor has so many leaves, and the root is shorter, more woody and not so fit to be eaten and, therefore, more medicinal. The Garden Parsnip nourishes much and is good and wholesome, but a little windy, and it fattens the body if much used. It is good for the stomach and reins and provokes urine. The wild Parsnip hath a cutting, attenuating, cleansing and opening quality therein. It eases the pains and stitches in the sides and expels the wind from the stomach and bowels, or colic. The root is often used, but the seed much more, the wild [Pastinaca sativa subsp. sylvestris] being better than the tame.*' In 1931 Maud Grieve noted: '*The food value of Parsnips exceeds that of any other vegetable except potatoes. It is easy of production and should be more extensively grown.*' A strong decoction of the root is a good diuretic, and it has been employed as a remedy for jaundice and gravel. Along with radish, parsnip seems to be the easiest garden crop to cultivate, and can be roasted, steamed or mashed for eating.

HISTORY: According to Pliny, the Emperor Tiberius believed that parsnips were so beneficial that he had them annually brought to Rome from the banks of the Rhine, where they were then successfully cultivated. Pliny also tells us it was grown either from the root transplanted or else from seed, but that it was impossible to get rid of the pungent flavour, and not until the 19th century were plants grown which were significantly better than the wild parsnip.

Sweet Parsnips

They taste sweeter after the first frosts, as Joseph Pitton de Tournefort, in *The Compleat Herbal* (1716), wrote: '*...they are commonly boiled and eaten with butter in the time of Lent; for that they are the sweetest, by reason the juice has been concocted during the winter, and are desired at that season especially, both for their agreeable Taste and their Wholesomeness. For they are not so good in any respect, till they have been first nipped with Cold...*'

PASSION FLOWER

PASSIFLORA INCARNATA
Family Passifloraceae, Passion Flowers

OTHER NAMES: Passion vine, purple passion flower, granadilla, maypops.

DESCRIPTION: This fast-growing climber with a pineapple-orange scent is native to the southern United States, Mexico and Central America. It was not included in earlier editions of Culpeper. *Passiflora incarnata* is the most common form of the edible passion fruit that is grown worldwide, producing egg-shaped fruits which are filled with a tart, fruity, bright orange pulp.

PROPERTIES AND USES: This is the variety commonly used medicinally, recommended for its soothing properties and as a general nerve tonic. Used together in an extract, the alkaloids and flavonoids in passion flower are stronger sedatives and relaxants that any one constituent used on its own, reminding us of the wisdom of using the whole herb, instead of isolated extracts. It is used in herbal treatments for withdrawal from opiates, alcohol and painkillers, and may help lessen reliance on drugs such as Valium and Librium. Passion flower contains *passiflorine*, which has been likened to morphine, thus it is also used to help treat neuralgia and insomnia. Other uses included lessening the pain of herpes and neuralgia, treating nervous tension, epilepsy and irritable bowel syndrome. The plant has a calming and antispasmodic effect but causes less drowsiness that many prescription drugs. The flowers can be dried and used in pot-pourris, and the fruit oil is used in cosmetics and as scent in bath products. Dried leaves and flowers can be combined with hops, chamomile and lavender to make a fragrant and soothing sleep pillow. The dried leaves can be added to lavender and rose petals in bath water. The orange fruit of *Passiflora incarnata* is edible, although it is not as tasty as the purple fruiting variety *Passiflora edulis*, which we see in supermarkets. The purple passion fruit makes refreshing fruit sorbet, smoothies and drinks, either on its own or when added to other fruits. Passion fruit can be made into jams, chutneys, syrups, jellies and a purée, used as cake filling. It is also a source of potassium and vitamins A and C.

HISTORY: It was first discovered in Peru in 1569 by the Spanish physician and botanist Nicolás Monardes. In the 1800s *Passiflora* became popular with the Victorians when hybridization began to give us hundreds of different forms. Passion flower leaves were used by Native North Americans to heal bruises and cuts.

PEACH

PRUNUS PERSICA
Family Rosaceae, Rose

OTHER NAMES: Dudgeon, Persian apple, eirinen wlanog (Welsh for woolly plums).

DESCRIPTION: It can grow to 30 feet (9 m) in height and bears light purple blossoms and the familiar fruit.

PROPERTIES AND USES: Culpeper notes: *'Lady Venus owns this tree, and by it opposes the ill effects of Mars, and indeed for children and young people, nothing is better to purge choler and the jaundice, than the leaves or flowers of this tree being made into a syrup or conserve. Let such as delight to please their lust regard the fruit; but such as have lost their health, and their children's, let them regard what I say, they may safely give two spoonfuls of the syrup at a time; it is as gentle as Venus herself. The leaves of peaches bruised and laid on the belly, kill worms, and so they do also being boiled in ale and drank, and open the belly likewise; and, being dried, is a far safer medicine to discuss humours. The powder of them strewed upon fresh bleeding wounds stays their bleeding, and closes them up. The flowers steeped all night in a little wine standing warm, strained forth in the morning, and drank fasting, doth gently open the belly, and move it downward…* [kernel] *oil put into clysters, eases the pains of the wind colic: and anointed on the lower part of the belly, doth the like, and dropped into the ears, eases pains in them; the juice of the leaves doth the like. Being also anointed on the forehead and temples, it helps the megrim, and all other pains in the head. If the kernels be bruised and boiled in vinegar, until they become thick, and applied to the head, it marvellously procures the hair to grow again upon bald places, or where it is too thin.'* This last point owes its reference to the Doctrine of Signatures. The furry down on a peach resembles fine growing hair.

HISTORY: It has been cultivated from time immemorial in most parts of Asia, probably coming originally from China, and appears to have been introduced into Europe as *Malus persica*, or Persian apple. The expeditions of Alexander the Great probably brought it to the attention of the Greek philosopher Theophrastus, 392 BCE, who speaks of it as a Persian fruit. By the mid-16th century, John Gerard had several varieties of peach growing in his garden in England.

Peach Stones

Cultivated peaches are divided into clingstones and freestones, depending upon whether the flesh sticks to the stone or not. Either can have white or yellow flesh. The nectarine is a cultivar group of peach with a smooth skin.

PEAR

PYRUS COMMUNIS
Family Rosaceae, Rose

OTHER NAMES: European pear.

DESCRIPTION: Pear trees resemble apple trees but grow more erect and have glossier leaves.

PROPERTIES AND USES: Culpeper tells us: *'The tree belongs to Venus, and so doth the apple-tree. For their physical use they are best discerned by their taste. All the sweet and luscious sorts, whether manured or wild, do help to move the belly downwards, more or less. Those that are hard and sour, do, on the contrary, bind the belly as much, and the leaves do so also. Those that are moist do in some sort cool, but harsh or wild sorts much more, and are very good in repelling medicines; and if the wild sort be boiled with mushrooms, it makes them less dangerous. The said Pears boiled with a little honey, help much the oppressed stomach, as all sorts of them do, some more, some less: but the harsher sorts do more cool and bind, serving well to be bound to green wounds, to cool and stay the blood, and heal up the green wound without farther trouble, or inflammation, as Galen says he hath found by experience. The wild Pears do sooner close up the lips of green wounds than others. Schola Salerni advises to drink much wine after Pears, or else (say they) they are as bad as poison; nay, and they curse the tree for it too; but if a poor man find his stomach oppressed by eating Pears, it is but working hard, and it will do as well as drinking wine.'* They can be made into perry, the pear equivalent of cider, and eaten in much the same way as apples, either raw or sliced and used in tarts, baked, stewed or puréed. The trees can produce fruit for up to 100 years.

HISTORY: Archaeological evidence shows that pears were collected from the wild long before their introduction into cultivation. Homer referred to pears as 'gifts from the gods' and Theophrastus, Cato the Elder and Pliny the Elder all wrote about their cultivation and grafting. Pears have been cultivated for about 4000 years, and there are now more than 5000 varieties. The leading pear producers, in order, are China, Italy and the United States.

Healthy Skin

Most of the vitamin C is in the skin, so never peel pears before you eat them. As a 'health food', pears contain no cholesterol, sodium or saturated fat. They offer a quick source of energy, due to their high amounts of two monosaccharides: fructose and glucose, plus levulose, the sweetest of natural sugars, found to a greater extent in fresh pears than in any other fruit.

PENNYROYAL

MENTHA PULEGIUM
Family Lamiaceae/Labiatae, Mint

OTHER NAMES: Penny royal, upright pennyroyal, royal thyme, pulegium, run-by-the-ground, lurk-in-the-ditch, pudding grass, piliolerial.

DESCRIPTION:
The smallest mint, it grows to 6 inches (15 cm), and can be invasive like all mints. There are small, fragrant, purple flowers in globular clusters around the stem, and small aromatic rounded leaves.

PROPERTIES AND USES: Culpeper says of pennyroyal: *'This herb is under Venus. Dioscorides says that penny-royal makes tough phlegm thin, warms the coldness of any part that it is applied to, and digests raw and corrupt matter. Being boiled and drunk, it removes the menses, and expels the dead child and afterbirth; being mixed with honey and salt, it voids phlegm from the lungs. Drunk with wine, it is good for venomous bites, and applied to the nostrils with vinegar revives those who faint and swoon. Dried and burnt, it strengthens the gums, helps the gout, if applied of itself to the place until it is red, and applied in a plaster, it takes away spots or marks on the face; applied with salt, it profits those that are splenetic, or liver grown. The decoction does help the itch, if washed therewith; being put into the baths for women to sit in, it helps the swelling and hardness of the womb. The green herb bruised and put into vinegar, cleanses foul ulcers and takes away the marks of bruises and blows about the eyes, and burns in the face, and the leprosy, if drank and applied outwardly. Boiled in wine, with honey and salt, it helps the tooth-ache. Pliny adds, that pennyroyal and mint together help faintings or swoonings, infused in vinegar, and put to the nostrils, or a little thereof put into the mouth. It eases the headache, and the pains of the breast and belly, stays the gnawings of the stomach, and inward pains of the bowels…One spoonful of the juice sweetened with sugar-candy is a cure for hooping-cough.'*

Flee, Fleas!

This native of most parts of Europe and parts of Asia is the *pulegium* of the Romans, named by Pliny for its power of driving away fleas, *pulex* being the Latin for flea. The name pennyroyal is a corruption of the old herbalists' name '*Pulioll-royall*' (*Pulegium regium*).

It was traditionally used for cases of spasms, hysteria, diarrhoea, flatulence and sickness, and disorders caused by sudden chill or cold. *Pennyroyal water* was distilled from the leaves and given as an antidote to spasmodic, nervous and hysterical complaints, and the herb was used against '*affections of the joints*'. The oil is highly toxic and can cause serious kidney damage. A hot infusion was used for colds as it promotes sweating. Cold pennyroyal tea was used as a gargle or throat wash. Persistent drinking of the tea can lead to organ failure because of the toxicity of its oil element. Pennyroyal is still used in European cuisine, but in Britain is now out of favour, as it is the most aromatic of mints but is too pungent for most tastes. However, it makes a strong mint sauce. It is a sting relief for horseflies, mosquitoes and wasps, and an insect repellent which particularly deters both mosquitoes and ants. Pennyroyal was used for getting rid of fleas, with the crushed leaves being rubbed on dogs and cats. The herb was also burned to dispel fleas, and a strong decoction was used for mopping floors.

HISTORY: Pennyroyal has been used historically since the time of Pliny to stimulate suppressed menstruation, alleviate cramps and tension during a woman's monthly cycle and facilitate childbirth. Pliny gave a long list of disorders for which pennyroyal was a remedy, recommending it for hanging in bedrooms, and physicians said it was even more conducive to health than roses. Its dried leaves were said to purify water, with Gerard telling us: '*If you have Pennyroyale in great quantity dry and cast it into corrupt water, it helpeth it much,*

neither will it hurt them that drink thereof.' As well as water, it was said to cleanse the blood: '*Penny-royale taken with honey cleanseth the lungs and cleareth the breast from all gross and thick humours.*' The famous herbalist John Gerard wrote: '*A garland of Penny-royale made and worn about the head is of great force against the swimming in the head and the pains and giddiness thereof.*' The Royal Society in 1665 published a paper on the use of pennyroyal to kill rattlesnakes. It was also used to stimulate abortions, this use being first noted by the dramatist Aristophanes, and so acquired an unsavoury reputation. It was called *pudding grass*, as it was used in stuffings for hog's puddings (*grass*, like *wort*, is a word which simply meant herb or plant in earlier times).

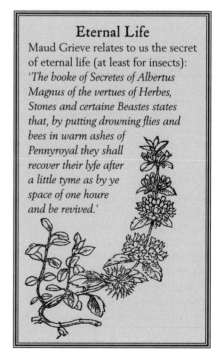

Eternal Life

Maud Grieve relates to us the secret of eternal life (at least for insects): '*The booke of Secretes of Albertus Magnus of the vertues of Herbes, Stones and certaine Beastes states that, by putting drowning flies and bees in warm ashes of Pennyroyal they shall recover their lyfe after a little tyme as by ye space of one houre and be revived.*'

PEPPER

PIPER NIGRUM
Family Piperaceae, Pepper

OTHER NAMES: Black pepper.

DESCRIPTION: An evergreen vine native to Asia with long racemes of flowers which produce the pungent fruit seeds, 'peppercorns'.

PROPERTIES AND USES: *'All peppers are under the dominion of Mars, and of temperature hot and dry, almost to the fourth degree, but the white is the hottest…It comforts and warms the stomach, consumes crude and moist humours, and stirs up the appetite. It helps to dissolve wind in the stomach or bowels, to provoke urine, to help the cough and other diseases of the breast, and is effective against the bitings of serpents…'* – Culpeper. Pepper stimulates the taste buds and helps to promote digestion, because of the compound piperine. Scientific studies indicate that it also boosts the immune system and helps fight cancer.

HISTORY: Pepper, like cinnamon and cloves is one of the oldest known spices and was being used in India over 4000 years ago. Hippocrates prescribed it as a medicine, and pepper was used as a currency during the siege of Rome in 408 CE. It is said that Attila the Hun demanded 3000 pounds (1360 kg) of pepper in ransom for the city. The Venerable Bede, on the point of death in 735, carefully divided his greatest treasure amongst his friends – it was a handful of pepper. Pepper's ability to spice up the bland European diet made it an item of extreme luxury, worth its weight in gold, because overland traders from India exerted a monopoly on the supply. (Hot capsicum peppers from the New World were then unknown). Columbus and other European explorers set off across the Atlantic to try and find a direct route to India for such spices. The term *'peppercorn rent'* is derived from the high price of black pepper during the Middle Ages, when it was accepted in lieu of money or as a dowry. Today the term means exactly the opposite of its original use.

Peppercorn Colours

The pea-sized berries of the pepper shrub are bright red when ripe. When the skin and fleshy parts are removed from the fully ripe berry, the remaining hard seed is white, our familiar 'white pepper'. Black, white, and green peppercorns all come from the same plant, but they are harvested at different times and handled in different ways. Black peppercorns are the sun-dried red berries, which are picked before they are ripe, then dried. Green peppercorns are the soft under-ripe berry, usually preserved in brine, but also sold dried.

PIGNUT

CONOPODIUM MAJUS
Family Apiaceae/Umbelliferae, Umbellifers

OTHER NAMES: Culpeper calls this plant the Earth Chestnut, '*called also Earth-Nuts, Ground-Nuts, Cipper-Nuts, and in Sussex they are called Pig-Nuts.*' Kipper nut, hog nut, St Anthony's nut.

DESCRIPTION: A perennial herb with umbels of tiny white flowers, up to 18 inches (46 cm) high, whose underground part resembles a chestnut and is sometimes eaten as a wild or cultivated root vegetable. This root has a sweet, aromatic flavour compared to that of the chestnut, hazelnut, sweet potato and Brazil nut. Palatable and nutritious, its eating qualities are widely praised, and it is popular among wild food foragers, but it remains a minor crop, due in part to its low yields and difficulty of harvest. The plant was widespread in meadows, pastures, woods and roadside verges, but now is only common in national parks, untouched woodlands or where organic farming is practised. Its dainty clusters of flowers appear during June and July and can cause a meadow or woodland to appear white from a distance.

PROPERTIES AND USES: Culpeper says: '*A description of them were needless, for every child knows them. Government and virtues: They are something hot and dry in quality, under the dominion of Venus; they provoke lust exceedingly, and stir up those sports she is mistress of; the seed is excellent good to provoke urine; and so also is the root, but it does not perform it so forcibly as the seed doth. The root being dried and beaten into powder, and the powder being made into an electuary, is a singular remedy for spitting and pissing of blood, as the former chestnut are for coughs.*'

HISTORY: Pigs used to be used to unearth them, just as they do when truffle-hunting, but with the loss of grassland these 'earth chestnuts' are becoming rare. It is now illegal to dig them up without the landowner's permission. From its popularity with pigs come the names pignut, hognut, and more indirectly Saint Anthony's nut, named for Anthony the Great or Anthony of Padua, both patron saints of swineherds.

Among the Bluebells

Pignuts often grow among bluebells, which have poisonous white bulbs. One has to follow the stalk down carefully to the pignut (root), which lies at a 90 degree angle to the stalk, having evolved to break free if pulled up out of the ground. Larger than bluebell bulbs, the pignut's brown skin is peeled and they can be eaten raw, or cooked.

PLANT NAMES IN FOLKLORE

One of the most fascinating areas that I uncovered while researching this book was the discovery of the different names given to plants in different regions. At least 22 separate varieties of plant are called *bachelor's button* across different parts of Britain alone. Elizabeth Mary Wright, in *Rustic Speech and Folklore* (1913) tells us: '*Even a common name like Honeysuckle is not restricted to the fragrant climber Lonicera peryclymenum with which we of the standard speech always associate it. The following plants may all be called Honeysuckle:*
1. The purple clover, Trifolium pratense.
2. The white clover, T. repens.
3. The bird's-foot trefoil, Lotus corniculatus. 4. The dwarf cornel, Cornus suecica. 5. The great bindweed, Convolvulus sepium. 6. The white dead-nettle, Lamium album. 7. The louse wort, Pedicularis sylvalica.
8. The blossoms of the willow.'
She also gives some of the names of plants associated with Biblical subjects. *Virgin Mary*, *Virgin Mary's honeysuckle*, *Virgin Mary's milkdrops* and *Lady's Milk-sile* are names of the lungwort *Pulmonaria officinalis*, referring to the legend that during the flight into Egypt some of the Blessed Virgin's milk fell on its leaves as she nursed the infant Jesus. The same legend is also told to account for similar spots on the leaves of the blessed thistle, Our Lady's thistle, *Carduus marianus*. Another legend says that the Virgin Mary, when thirsty, met a cow and after using the broad leaf of the thistle as a drinking-cup for its milk, willed that the plant should ever after be called by her name, and bear the stains of the milk on its leaves. The lungwort is also called *Mary's tears*, and the spots which decorate the plant's leaves are traced to the tears shed by her at the Crucifixion.

Tradition also tells us that once the Virgin Mary plucked up a root of the crab's claw, *Polygonum persicaria*, and then threw it away, saying '*That's useless*', hence *useless* has been its name in Scotland ever since, and the blotches on its leaves are the marks of her fingers. *Gethsemane* is a folk name for the early purple orchid, *Orchis mascula*, said to have been growing at the foot of the Cross, and to have received drops of blood on its leaves, the marks of which it has never lost. The same legend is attached also to the *Calvary clover, Medicago echinus*, the leaves of which are marked with dull red, irregular blotches exactly like real bloodstains. *Saint Peter's herb* is the cowslip, the flowerhead suggesting a bunch of keys; *Abraham, Isaac, and Jacob* is a name of the garden comfrey, *Symphytum officinale*, as well as of other plants having flowers of different shades of colour on the same stem. The *Alleluia plant* is the wood sorrel, *Oxalis acetosella*, so called because it blossoms between Easter and Whitsuntide, when in the Catholic Liturgy psalms ending with '*Alleluia*' were sung in churches.

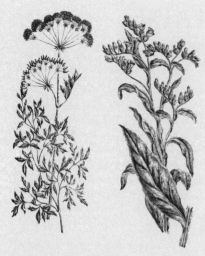

Wright also relates that the smell of the common buttercup was formerly supposed to induce madness, hence its nickname *crazy*. In the same way poppies are called *headaches*, because it is believed that the smell of them will cause a headache. *Pick-pocket*, the shepherd's purse, *Capsella bursa-pastoris*, is so named because it impoverishes the farmer's land. Children gathered it and repeated: '*Pick-pocket, penny nail, Put the rogue in the jail.*' The same plant is also called *pick your mother's heart out*, or simply *mother's heart*. Children played a kind of game with the heart-shaped seedpods. They used to get one another to pick one of these off, and there followed the accusing cry: '*You've picked your mother's heart out.*' In parts of Yorkshire the derisive cry was '*Pick packet to London, You'll never go to London.*' In Dorsetshire '*Break your mother's heart*' is the hemlock, *Conium maculatum*; and '*pick your mother's eyes out*' was the field speedwell, *Veronica agrestis*. In the Lake District certain curative properties were attributed to

Solomon's seal, *Polygonatum officinale*, so it was called the *vagabond's friend* as it was thought to be a remedy for black eyes, bruises, and broken noses.

Courtship and matrimony was the name of the meadowsweet, *Filipendula ulmaria*, so called from the scent of the flower before and after bruising, which is thought to be typical of the two states in life. Names for the common pansy included: *jump up and kiss me; meet her in the entry kiss her in the buttery; kiss me behind the garden gate, kiss me at the garden gate; kiss me John at the garden gate; meet me love behind the garden door; kiss behind the garden gate;* and *meet me love*, names also given to London pride, *Saxifraga x urbium*. *Kiss me quick and go* was a name for lad's love or southernwood, *Artemisia abrotanum; lift up your head and I'll kiss you* was the bleeding heart, *Dicentra spectabilis; Kitty come down the lane jump up and kiss me* was the cuckoo-pint, *Arum maculatum*. *Granny jump out of bed* was another name for the monkshood; *Welcome home husband tho' never so drunk* was the yellow stonecrop, *Sedum acre*. The alternative names for plants open up a new world of understanding of the past.

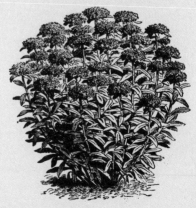

PLANTAIN

PLANTAGO MAJOR
Family Plantaginaceae, Plantain

OTHER NAMES: Psyllium, common plantain, greater plantain, rat tail plantain, broad-leaved plantain, ripple grass, waybread, snakeweed, white man's foot, Englishman's foot (it is supposed to appear in every country where the English have settled).

DESCRIPTION: A familiar perennial weed which is found by roadsides and in meadowland. There is a large, radial rosette of leaves and a few long, slender, densely-flowered green spikes around 6 inches (15 cm) long.

PROPERTIES AND USES:
'*It is true, Misaldus and others, yea, almost all astrology-physicians, hold this to be an herb of Mars, because it cures the diseases of the head and private parts, which are under the houses of Mars, Aries, and Scorpio. The truth is it is under the command of Venus, and cures the head by antipathy to Mars, and the private parts by sympathy to Venus; neither is there hardly a martial disease but it cures*'. – Nicholas Culpeper. William Salmon's *Herbal* (1710) gives the following uses: '*The liquid juice clarified and drunk for several days helps distillation of rheum upon the throat, glands, lungs, etc…An especial remedy against ulceration of the lungs and a vehement cough arising from same. It is said to be good against epilepsy, dropsy, jaundice and opens obstructions of the liver, spleen and reins. It cools inflammations of*

the eyes and takes away the pin and web (so called) in them. Dropped into the ears, it eases their pains and restores hearing much decayed…Powdered seeds stop vomiting, epilepsy, lethargy, convulsions, dropsy, jaundice, strangury, obstruction of the liver, etc. The liniment made with the juice and oil of Roses eases headache caused by heat, and is good for lunatics.'

Plantain leaves are best used fresh, mashed with the roots to put on bee stings and used for skin irritations, ulcers, burns, and to stop bleeding in minor cuts. When combined with water, the seed husk swells up to 14 times its volume, and research shows that the seed reduces high cholesterol and triglyceride levels, binding with dietary cholesterol to prevent its absorption. Wild plantain leaves, yarrow and watercress can be combined with a dressing for a tasty salad.

HISTORY: The plantain is one of the nine plants invoked in the Anglo-Saxon Nine Herbs Charm intended for treatment of poison and infection through the preparation of nine herbs, and was later used to cure the bite of rabid dogs.

Snakebite Remedy
Native North American Indians used the herb as the chief remedy for the bite of the rattlesnake.

POLYPODY OF THE OAK

POLYPODIUM VULGARE
Family Polypodiaceae, Polypod Ferns

OTHER NAMES: Common polypody, wall fern, brake root, rock brake (break), rock of polypody, polypody, female fern, sweet fern, wood liquorice, rock cap fern, adder's fern, rock polypod, fern root.

DESCRIPTION: A delicate perennial fern growing to a height of 12 inches (30 cm).

PROPERTIES AND USES: Culpeper says it is *'good for those troubled with melancholy. It is also good for the hardness of the spleen, and for prickings or stitches in the sides, and also for the colic…is good against the cough, shortness of breath and wheezing…The fresh roots beaten small, or the powder of the dried roots mixed with honey and applied to any of the limbs out of joint, does much help them. Applied to the nose, it cures the disease called polypus, which is a piece of fungous flesh growing therein, which in time stops the passage of breath through that nostril; and it helps those clefts or chops which come between the fingers and toes.'* Polypody stimulates bile secretion and is a gentle laxative. Traditionally, polypody has been used as a treatment for hepatitis and jaundice, and as a remedy for indigestion and loss of appetite. The rhizome is also expectorant, having a stimulating effect on the respiratory system. It was taken for the relief of congestion, bronchitis, pleurisy and dry irritable coughs.

HISTORY: The Greeks and Romans prescribed preparations derived from this fern as a mild laxative, purgative, and remedy for coughs and chest complaints. Herbalists also recommended preparations of the dried and powdered rhizome for internal use to expel tapeworms and for external use as a liniment. Because polypody is often found clinging to oak trees, herbalists believed it absorbed its vigour and strength. Fern plants that grew upon the roots of an oak, which this fern frequently does, were deemed to have special medicinal powers, in the same way the mistletoe that grew (rarely) on the oak was thought by the Druids to have special powers. The name polypody comes from a Greek word meaning 'many-footed', and alludes to the appearance of the plant's branching rhizomes, which some think look like many feet.

Sweeter Than Sugar

The liquorice-flavoured rhizome, or underground stem, of polypody has been prized since ancient times, not so much for its sweetness as for its medicinal powers. It was also used in confectioneries such as nougat. In 1971 a saponin was found in the roots, which makes the root 500 times sweeter than sugar by weight.

(OPIUM) POPPY

PAPAVER SOMNIFERUM
Family Papaveraceae, Poppy

OTHER NAMES: Garden poppy, black poppy, white poppy, cwsglys (Welsh for sleep herb).

DESCRIPTION: The plant is an erect annual, varying in the colour of its flowers from pure white to reddish purple. All parts of the plant, but particularly the walls of the capsules, or seed vessels, contain a system of vessels filled with white, sticky latex.

PROPERTIES AND USES: Culpeper wrote: *'The Garden Poppy Heads with Seeds made into a Syrup, is frequently and to good effect used to procure rest and sleep in the sick and weak, and to stay Catarrhs and Defluxions of hot thin Rheums from the Head into the Stomach, and upon the Lungs, causing a continual Cough, the Fore-runner of a Consumption: It helps also Hoarseness of the Throat, and when one hath lost their voice, which the Oil of the Seed doth likewise. The black Seed boiled in Wine and drunk, is said also to stay the Flux of the Belly and Women's Courses...'* The plant's opium is the source of morphine, codeine and other opiate-based painkillers. The botanical name *somniferum* means sleep-bringing, referring to the sedative properties of some of these opiates.

HISTORY: Poppy seeds have been found in Egyptian grain stores dating from 4500 years ago, and the Romans held the plant sacred to the corn goddess Ceres. Hildegarde of Bingen, the German religious visionary and polymath, wrote, *'Its seed, when eaten, brings sleep and prevents prurigo. The seeds check hungry lice and nits. They can be eaten after being steeped in water, but are better and more useful eaten raw rather than cooked. The oil which is expressed from them does not nourish or refresh a person, nor does it bring him health or sickness.'*

Extracting Opium

Culpeper did not believe that opium was produced from the seedheads of *Papaver somniferum*, as he writes *'...of the juice of it is made opium, only for lucre of money they cheat you, and tell you it is a kind of tear, or some such like thing that drops from Poppies when they weep, and that is somewhere beyond the sea, I know not where, beyond the moon.'* Opium is extracted from the poppy heads before they have ripened. When the petals have fallen from the flowers, incisions are made in the wall of the unripe capsules. The exuded juice, partially dried, is collected by scraping and formed into cakes, which are wrapped in poppy leaves and dried in the sun.

(WILD) POPPY

PAPAVER RHOEAS
Family Papaveraceae, Poppy

OTHER NAMES: Corn poppy, corn rose, field poppy, Flanders poppy, red poppy, red weed, headache.

DESCRIPTION: Found growing in fields and waste places, it has petals of a rich scarlet colour when fresh, and is often nearly black in its centre.

PROPERTIES AND USES:
Culpeper notes: *'The wild poppy, or corn rose, as Mathiolus says, is good to prevent the falling sickness. They syrup made with the flowers is given with good effect to those that have the pleurisy. The dried flowers also, either boiled in water, or made into powder, and drunk, either in the distilled water of them, or in some other drink, has the same effect. The distilled water of the flowers is held to be much good against surfeits, being drunk evening and morning. It is also more cooling than any of the other poppies, and therefore cannot be as effective in hot agues, frenzies and other inflammations.'* It has been used in traditional medicine to relieve pain, to treat coughs and insomnia and to aid digestion. The petals have been used to colour medicines.

HISTORY: The poppy was the symbol of love in Persia. Because of the blooming of countless red poppies in the disturbed ground of the battlefields of the First World War, the flower has come to symbolize the remembrance of war. Armistice Day is remembered by wearing artificial poppies on the 11th hour of the 11th day of the 11th month every year, which is when peace was declared in the First World War in 1918.

In Flanders Fields

Dr John McCrea was serving in the Royal Canadian Army Medical Corps when his poem *In Flanders Fields* was published anonymously in *Punch* on 8 December 1915.

In Flanders fields the poppies blow
Between the crosses, row on row,
That mark our place; and in the sky
The larks, still bravely singing, fly
Scarce heard amid the guns below.

We are the Dead. Short days ago
We lived, felt dawn, saw sunset glow,
Loved, and were loved, and now we lie
In Flanders fields.

Take up our quarrel with the foe:
To you from failing hands we throw
The torch; be yours to hold it high.
If ye break faith with us who die
We shall not sleep, though poppies grow
In Flanders fields.

QUINCE

CYDONIA OBLONGA
Family Rosaceae, Rose

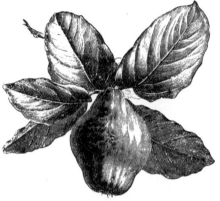

OTHER NAMES: Honey apple, Cydonian apple, quince pear, quoyne. Coine (Old French) became the Middle English quin, and hence quince from its plural, quins.

DESCRIPTION: Small trees with white or pink flowers resembling apple blossom and yellow, irregularly shaped, pear-like fruits which smell of honey. This pretty tree will benefit from underplanting of chives and garlic as companion plants.

PROPERTIES AND USES: Today we regard quince as an inconvenient fruit. In these colder climes it cannot be eaten raw, it sometimes has a light fur on the skin and its flesh is hard and tannic. It needs long, slow cooking to make it palatable. Culpeper says: '*Quinces when they are green, help all sorts of fluxes in men or women, and choleric lasks* [diarrhoea], *casting, and whatever needs astriction, more than any way prepared by fire; yet the syrup of the juice, or the conserve, are much conducible, much of the binding quality being consumed by the fire; if a little vinegar be added, it stirs up the languishing appetite, and the stomach given to casting; some spices being added, comforts and strengthens the decaying and fainting spirits, and helps the liver oppressed, that it cannot perfect the digestion, or corrects choler and phlegm… To take the crude juice of Quinces, is held a preservative against the force of deadly poison; for it hath been found most certainly true, that the very smell of a Quince hath taken away all the strength of the poison of white Hellebore. If there be need of any outwardly binding and cooling of hot fluxes, the oil of Quinces, or other medicines that may be made thereof, are very available to anoint the belly or other parts therewith; it likewise strengthens the stomach and belly, and the sinews that are loosened by sharp humours falling on them, and restrains immoderate sweating. The mucilage taken from the seeds of Quinces, and boiled in a little water, is very good to cool the heat and heal the sore breasts of women. The same, with a little sugar, is good to lenify the harshness and hoarseness of the throat, and roughness of the tongue. The cotton or down of Quinces boiled and applied to plague sores, heals them up: and laid as a plaster, made up with wax, it brings hair to them that are bald, and keeps it from falling, if it be ready to shed.*' From the Doctrine of Signatures, it was concluded that the light down on the skin suggests that the fruit will restore hair to the head. Quince syrup was added to drinks in times of sickness, especially looseness of the bowels, which it was said to restrain by its astringency. The seeds were used medicinally for the sake of their mucilage. One of their main uses today is as grafting rootstock for pears and apples, to restrict the height of the trees. The fruits perfume a room and can be used as bases for pomanders. In a Spanish tapas bar, you will come across *membrillo*, the jelly-like paste served with Spanish cheeses such as manchego. The word marmalade originally meant a quince jam, *marmelo* being the Portuguese for quince.

HISTORY: Cultivation of quince probably preceded apple culture, originating in Persia and Turkestan, and the 'apple' of the Biblical Song of Solomon may have been a quince. Quince was a ritual offering at Greek weddings, for Aphrodite (Venus) had brought it from the Levant. Plutarch reported that before entering the bridal chamber, a Greek bride would eat a piece of quince, '*in order that the first greeting may not be disagreeable nor unpleasant*'. Elsewhere, Plutarch noted that the dictator Solon decreed that '*bride and bridegroom shall be shut into a chamber, and eat a quince together*'. The Greeks obtained the tree from Cydon in Crete, from which we derive the genus name *Cydonia*. The Romans also treasured the quince, calling it melimelum, honey apple, because its flavour and fragrance are honey-like. Venus is often depicted with a quince in her right hand, the gift she received from Paris. Virgil's 'Golden Apples' were probably quinces, as oranges did not arrive in Italy until the time of the Crusades. Charlemagne in 812 encouraged their

planting across his empire, and Chaucer refers to them as *coines*. Quinces were associated with love from the earliest times, and used in wedding feasts – we read in Dr John Case's book *The Praise of Musicke* (1586): '*I come to marriages, wherein as our ancestors did fondly and with a kind of doting, maintain many rites and ceremonies, some whereof were either shadows or abodements* [abodings] *of a pleasant life to come, as the eating of a Quince Pear to be a preparative of sweet and delightful days between the married persons.*'

Tempting Quince

Genesis does not mention the specific fruit that Adam and Eve took from the Tree of Knowledge, but it is thought that the fruit of temptation was a quince. Throughout the Scriptures, the Hebrew word *tappauch* is translated as apple, but many scholars believe that the fruit was a quince.

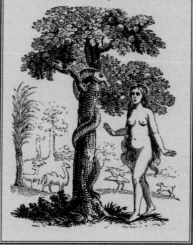

RHUBARB

RHEUM RHABARBARUM
Family Polygonaceae, Knotweed

OTHER NAMES: Culpeper also names it Great Monk's Rhubarb, Great Garden Patience and English Rhubarb. Garden rhubarb.

DESCRIPTION: Grown in the vegetable plot, it is prized as a fruit, growing around 2 feet (60 cm) high with edible red stalks and large dark green leaves. Rhubarb is usually considered to be a vegetable, but a New York court adjudicated in 1947 that as it was used as a fruit, it was to be counted as a fruit for the purpose of regulations and duties.

PROPERTIES AND USES: Culpeper writes profusely on the plant: '...*It purges the body of choler and phlegm, being either taken of itself, made into powder, and drank in a draught of white wine, or steeped therein all night, and taken fasting, or put among other purges, as shall be thought convenient, cleansing the stomach, liver and blood, opening obstructions, and helping those griefs that come thereof, as the jaundice, dropsy, swelling of the spleen, tertian and daily agues, and pricking pains of the sides; and also stays spitting of blood. The powder taken with cassia dissolved, and washed Venice turpentine, cleanses the reins and strengthens them afterwards, and is very effectual to stay the gonorrhea. It is also given for the pains and swellings in the head, for those that are troubled with melancholy, and helps the sciatica, gout, and the cramp. The powder of the Rhubarb taken with a little mummia and madder roots in some red wine, dissolves clotted blood in the body, happening by any fall or bruise, and helps burstings and broken parts, as well inward as outward. The oil likewise wherein it hath been boiled, works the like effects being anointed. It is used to heal those ulcers that happen in the eyes or eyelids, being steeped and strained; as also to assuage the swellings and inflammations; and applied with honey, boiled in wine, it takes away all blue spots or marks that happen therein.'* Rhubarb is grown primarily for its fleshy petioles, commonly known as rhubarb sticks or stalks.

HISTORY: Not until the 17th century, when sugar from the Caribbean plantations became affordable, was rhubarb used widely as food. In the 19th century it was realized that oxalic acid is found in both docks and rhubarb, with rhubarb also containing large quantities of nitric and malic acid. The combination gives an agreeable taste when cooked but can cause digestive problems for sufferers of gout and other ailments.

(WILD) ROCKET

DIPLOTAXIS MURALIS
Family Brassicaceae, Brassica

OTHER NAMES: Rucola.
Culpeper says that salad rocket,
or garden rocket (*Eruca vesicaria*
subsp. *sativa*) is only used for
salads, so does not include it.
Salad rocket is also known as
rocket or arugula.

DESCRIPTION: Height
12 inches (30 cm) and spread
6 inches (15 cm), with yellow,
four-petalled flowers and green,
deeply divided aromatic leaves.

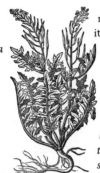

rocket is a digestive stimulant, and
its high sulphur content benefits
hair, nails and skin.

HISTORY: Pliny the Elder
writing of its strong aphrodisiac
qualities: *'Three leaves of wild
rocket plucked with the left hand,
beaten up in hydromel, and then
taken in drink, are productive of a
similar effect.'*

PROPERTIES AND USES: Culpeper:
*'The wild Rocket is more strong and
effectual to increase sperm and venerous
qualities, whereunto all the seed is more
effectual than the garden kind. It serves
also to help digestion, and provokes urine
exceedingly. The seed is used to cure the
biting of serpents, the scorpion, and the
shrew mouse, and other poisons, and expels
worms, and other noisome creatures that
breed in the belly. The herb boiled or stewed,
and some sugar put thereto, helps the cough
in children, being taken often. The seed also
taken in drink, takes away the ill scent of
the arm-pits, increases milk in nurses, and
wastes the spleen. The seed mixed with
honey, and used on the face, cleanses the
skin from morphew* [scurfy eruptions], *and
used with vinegar, takes away freckles and
redness in the face, or other parts; and with
the gall of an ox, it mends foul scars, black
and blue spots, and the marks of the smallpox.'* It can be used in salads, with a more
peppery flavour than salad rocket. Wild

From *Love's Martyr*, 1601

O School-boys I will teach you such
  a shift,
As will be worth a Kingdom when you
  know it,
An herb that hath a secret hidden drift,
To none but Truants do I mean to
  show it,
And all deep read Physicians will
  allow it:
O how you play the wags, and fain
  would hear
Some secret matter to allay your fear.

There's garden Rocket, take me but
  the seed,
When in your Master's brow your
  faults remain,
And when to save your selves there is
  great need,
Being whipped or beaten you shall feel
  no pain...

               Robert Chester

ROSE

*ROSA CENTIFOLIA, R. DAMASCENA, R. GALLICA, R.
EGLANTERIA, R. CANINA*
Family Rosaceae, Rose

OTHER NAMES: *Rosa gallica
officinalis* was called *The Apothecary's Rose*
in the *British Pharmacopoeia*, an annual
publication listing quality standards
for medicines.

DESCRIPTION: *Rosa gallica* was
hybridized so much that any
scented roses of a deep red
or deep pink colour came
to be used in medicine,
as long as they yielded
a strongly coloured and
fragrant infusion in hot
water. The Provence rose
(Rosa gallica), damask rose
(Rosa damascena), and
eglantine *(Rosa eglanteria)*
are the three oldest roses
in cultivation, and all are
strongly scented. The cabbage
rose *(Rosa centifolia)*, is also known as
the *hundred-petalled Rose*, and along with
the tea rose *(Rosa indica)*, is commonly
grown for scent and beauty. The dog rose
(Rosa canina) is commonly seen growing
in country hedges.

PROPERTIES AND USES: Culpeper:
'*It is under the dominion of Venus. Botanists
describe a vast number of roses, but this
(Damask), and the common red rose, and
the dog rose, or hip, are the only kinds
regarded in medicine...*[the oil] *is used
to cool hot inflammation or swellings and
to bind and stay fluxes of the humours, to
sores and is also put into ointments and
plasters that are cooling and binding.*' John

Gerard writes: '*The conserve of roses taken
in the morning fasting, and last at night,
strengthens the heart, and takes away the
shaking and trembling thereof, strengthens
the liver, kidneys, and other weak entrails,
comforts a weak stomach that is moist
and raw.*' The oil is used on the
skin because of its antiseptic,
cooling, moisturizing and
nourishing properties.
The 'hips' or rosehips of
the dog rose are valued
because they contain
high levels of vitamin
C and also flavonoids,
tannins and vitamins A,
B1, B2, B3 and K. In the
Middle Ages, the dog rose
was recommended as a
marvellous cure for chest
complaints. The apothecary rose is used
today more for its aromatherapy and
cosmetic properties than its medicinal
properties, but it is known to have

The Rosary

In Renaissance art, the apothecary
rose was the most painted of all
roses. Its deep pink colour was said to
represent the blood of the Christian
martyrs. Its petals were dried and
rolled into beads, then strung into
beaded chains for religious use.
These beads later became known
as the '*rosary*'.

Otto of Roses

Maud Grieve informs us: '*It was between 1582 and 1612 that the oil or OTTO OF ROSES was discovered, as recorded in two separate histories of the Grand Moguls. At the wedding feast of the princess Nour-Djihan with the Emperor Djihanguyr, son of Akbar, a canal circling the whole gardens was dug and filled with rose-water. The heat of the sun separating the water from the essential oil of the Rose, was observed by the bridal pair when rowing on the fragrant water. It was skimmed off and found to be an exquisite perfume. The discovery was immediately turned to account and the manufacture of Otto of Roses was commenced in Persia about 1612 and long before the end of the seventeenth century the distilleries of Shiraz were working on a large scale.'*

sedative and antidepressant properties, and is an astringent and useful for lowering cholesterol. The petals and hips are often found in pot-pourris and dried dog rose hips are particularly useful because of their ability to hold scent, making them ideal for using as a fixative. The petals are also sold as biodegradable wedding confetti.

HISTORY: The cultivation of roses originated in Persia, where an extensive rose-water trade began in the eighth century. Sappho, the Greek poetess, writing *c.*600 BCE, crowned the rose *Queen of Flowers*. Roses were held to be sacred to the goddess of love, Venus to the Romans and Aphrodite to the Greeks, and were symbolic of protection and rebirth. During funeral ceremonies, the Romans scattered rose petals to symbolize resurrection. The Romans placed a rose over the door of a public or private banquet hall, and each citizen who passed under it bound himself not to disclose anything said or done in the meeting. It then became the custom across Europe to suspend a rose over the dinner table as a sign that all confidences were to be held secret (hence the phrase *sub rosa*, under the rose), and the plaster ornament in the centre of a ceiling is still known as the ceiling rose. Nostradamus prescribed '*rose petal pills*' to guard against the plague. Roses were grown in monastery gardens in the Middle Ages in Europe and used by the monks for medicinal purposes. In 1798, Napoleon's wife, Empress Josephine, created one of greatest rose gardens outside Paris at her Château de Malmaison, with every known variety cultivated there. Today roses are used primarily in the perfume industry. The oil from the Bulgarian Kazanlik rose *(Rosa damascena forma trigintipetala)* is considered to be the best in the world and is used by Chanel and Christian Dior in their perfumes. It takes 4 tons of roses (or approximately two million flowers) to make 2lb (900 g) of rose *attar* (another Persian word for oil, like *otto* and *ottar*), which explains why pure rose oil is so expensive.

ROSEMARY

ROSMARINUS OFFICINALIS
Family Lamiaceae/Labiatae, Mint

OTHER NAMES: Compass weed, compass plant, dew of the sea, sea dew, elf leaf, guardrobe, incensier, polar plant, rose of Mary. There are many varieties of rosemary.

DESCRIPTION: A hardy evergreen perennial with a height and spread of 36 inches (90 cm), short, needle-shaped and aromatic leaves and pretty pale blue flowers.

PROPERTIES AND USES:
'The Sun claims dominion over it. It helps a weak memory, and quickens the senses. The leaves are used much in bathing and made into ointments or oil are good to help cold benumbed joints, sinews, or members...a remedy for the windiness in the stomach, bowels, and spleen and expels it powerfully.' – Culpeper. Rosemary is one of the most useful herbs, not only being a wonderfully attractive plant in the garden but also with many culinary, medicinal and aromatherapy uses. The leaf is said to alleviate hangovers, indigestion and stress, cure plague and stop bad dreams. Rosemary stimulates the central nervous system and circulation, making it beneficial for low blood pressure and sluggishness. The essential oil is distilled from the fresh flowering tops and the upper part of the herb, and can be diluted for topical use to alleviate the pain of sprains, arthritis, sciatica and neuralgia. Burning a sprig of rosemary will freshen the room and also freshen the mind, being said to increase circulation to the brain. Its principal commercial use was as *Spiritus Rosmarini*, an ingredient in hair lotions, for its odour and effect in preventing premature baldness. A cold infusion of the antiseptic plant is one of the best hair rinses, helping to prevent scurf and dandruff.

HISTORY: The Virgin Mary, in her flight to Egypt, is reputed to have thrown her blue cloak over a white rosemary bush, which turned its flowers blue for ever, hence the name *rose of Mary*. Legend compares the growth of a rosemary plant with the life of Jesus, and declares that after 33 years it increases in breadth, but never in height. Hippocrates, Galen and

---

From *Love's Martyr*, 1601

There's Rosemary, the Arabians justify,
(Physicians of exceeding perfect skill,)
It comforteth the brain and Memory,
And to the inward sense gives strength at will,
The head with noble knowledge it doth fill.
Conserves thereof restores the speech being lost,
And makes a perfect Tongue with little cost.

Robert Chester

Affecting the Heart

In Maud Grieve's *Herbal*, we read the following extract: *Miss Anne Pratt (Flowers and their Associations) says: 'But it was not among the herbalists and apothecaries merely that Rosemary had its reputation for peculiar virtues. The celebrated Doctor of Divinity, Roger Hacket, did not disdain to expatiate on its excellencies in the pulpit. In a sermon which he entitles "A Marriage Present", which was published in 1607, he says:*

"Speaking of the powers of rosemary, it overtoppeth all the flowers in the garden, boasting man's rule. It helpeth the brain, strengtheneth the memory, and is very medicinable for the head. Another property of the rosemary is, it affects the heart. Let this rosmarinus, this flower of men, insignia of your wisdom, love and loyalty, be carried not only in your hands, but in your hearts and heads."'

Dioscorides all prescribed rosemary for liver problems. The plant was said to bring eternal youth, and rosemary oil was rubbed on the temples to ease headaches. It is traditionally associated with helping to cure poor memory, and is being researched for senility treatment. In Ancient Greece, students wore garlands of rosemary braided into their hair or around their necks in order to improve their memory when taking exams. A British study has found that inhaling rosemary oil boosted memory compared to a control group of people not exposed to the oil. Rosemary was an essential plant for every apothecary during the Renaissance, with the French regarding it as a cure-all. Rosemary was regarded as a preventive to plague. In 1665–6, the Great Plague killed 100,000 people in London alone, a fifth of the population, and the price of rosemary rose from 12 pence for an armful to 72 pence for a handful. Rosemary was burned in sick chambers, and in French hospitals was burned with juniper berries to purify the air and prevent infection. With rue, it was placed in the dock of courts of justice, the prevent the spread of contagious gaol-fever. A sprig of rosemary was carried in the hand at funerals, being distributed to the mourners before they left the house, to be cast on to the coffin when it had been lowered into the grave. Sir Thomas More wrote: *'As for rosemary I let it run all over my garden walls, not only because my bees love it, but because it is the herb sacred to remembrance and to friendship, whence a sprig of it hath a dumb language.'* Sprigs of rosemary are worn on Anzac Day (25 April) in remembrance of the Australian and New Zealand servicemen who died at Gallipoli during the First World War. Australian soldiers spoke of rosemary growing wild on the battlefield of Gallipoli, and how the perfume of its crushed leaves evoked memories of their lost friends.

RUE

RUTA GRAVEOLENS
Family Rutaceae, Rue/Citrus

OTHER NAMES: Herb of grace, herb of repentance, garden rue, mother of the herbs, herbygrass.

DESCRIPTION: Hardy evergreen with a height and spread of 24 inches (60 cm). It bears small yellow flowers, and lobed, musk-scented, blue-green leaves. The symbol in playing cards for the suit of clubs is said to be modelled on a leaf of rue.

PROPERTIES AND USES: *'It is an herb of the Sun, and under Leo. It provokes urine and women's courses, being taken either in meat or drink. The seed thereof taken in wine, is an antidote against all dangerous medicines or deadly poisons. The leaves taken either by themselves, or with figs and walnuts, is called Mithridate's counter-poison against the plague, and causes all venomous things to become harmless'* – Nicholas Culpeper. Used in small amounts rue can ease headaches, and the leaves can be applied externally in a poultice to relieve sciatica. Rue makes a lovely low hedge in a knot garden, but has declined in popular use as it is poisonous in large amounts and can cause violent stomach upset, skin irritation and photosensitivity.

HISTORY: One of the oldest garden plants cultivated for medicinal use was introduced into England by the Romans. Since earliest times rue was used to ward off contagion (often combined with rosemary) and the attacks of fleas and other insects. Herb of grace reflects the time when a twig of rue was used to sprinkle the holy water in the ceremony on the Sunday before High Mass. Brides carried a sprig in their wedding bouquet. It was thought to be an antidote to snakebites and poisonous fungi. Gerard wrote: *'If a man be anointed with the juice of rue, the poison of wolf's bane, mushrooms, or todestooles, the biting of serpents, stinging of scorpions, spiders, bees, hornets and wasps will not hurt him.'* Rue is one of the ingredients in the *'Vinegar of the Four Thieves'*, a mixture of vinegar and herbs that was popular during the plague years in Europe as it was thought to protect against the pestilence. In the Middle Ages and later, rue was considered a powerful defence against witches, and was also thought to bestow second sight. Rue was once believed to improve the eyesight and creativity, and Michelangelo and Leonardo da Vinci were said to regularly use it for these benefits.

Pest Repellent

It is a fly and ant repellent, and can be tied to a horse's mane to keep the flies away. Most cats dislike the smell of it and therefore it can be used as a cat deterrent in one's garden.

RUPTUREWORT

HERNIARIA GLABRA
Family Caryophyllaceae, Pink/Carnation

OTHER NAMES: Glabrous, smooth rupturewort, rupturewort, green carpet.

DESCRIPTION: The garden nursery industry is now marketing the plant as *green carpet*. The bright green creeper spreads effortlessly in all directions occupying up to 2 feet (60 cm) per plant, and growing only about 2 inches (5 cm) high, so it is excellent for rockeries.

PROPERTIES AND USES:

Culpeper says this about it: '...*Rupture-wort...is found by experience to cure the rupture, not only in children but also in elder persons, if the disease be not too inveterate, by taking a dram of the powder of the dried herb every day in wine, or a decoction made and drank for certain days together. The juice or distilled water of the green herb, taken in the same manner, helps all other fluxes either of man or woman; vomiting also, and the gonorrhoea, being taken any of the ways aforesaid. It doth also most assuredly help those that have the stranguary, or are troubled with the stone or gravel in the reins or bladder. The same also helps stitches in the sides, griping pains of the stomach or belly, the obstructions of the liver, and cures the yellow jaundice; likewise it kills also the worms in children. Being outwardly applied, it conglutinates wounds notably, and helps much to stay defluxions of rheum from the head to the eyes, nose, and teeth, being bruised green and bound thereto; or the forehead, temples, or the nape of the neck behind, bathed with the decoction of the dried herb. It also dries up the moisture of fistulous ulcers, or any other that are foul and spreading. The whole plant has a salty taste, and is somewhat astringent, but it increases the urinary discharge; and the juice dropped into the eyes, takes away specks and films from them.'* The whole plant together with its long root, gathered when it is in flower, is astringent, diuretic and expectorant.

HISTORY: Maud Grieve stated that rupturewort was *'successful in the treatment of dropsy, whether of cardiac or nephritic origin...It is recommended for catarrh of the bladder.'* Its active constituent herniarin is believed to have diuretic properties, and the leaves have been emulsified for use in hand cleansers. It has been used for treating bladder problems, dropsy, cystitis and kidney stones. It has also gained a reputation for treating hernias. Rupturewort also has been used as a poultice to speed the healing of ulcers.

Sheep's Favourite

Sheep seem to relish the plant; cattle and horses eat it, while pigs and goats reject it, according to tradition.

SAFFRON

CROCUS SATIVUS
Family Iridaceae, Iris

OTHER NAMES: Spanish saffron, hay saffron, karkom, Persian saffron.

DESCRIPTION: Lilac to pale mauve in colour, its three orange stamens distinguish it from other crocuses.

PROPERTIES AND USES:
Culpeper: '*It quickens the brain…it helps consumptions of the lungs, and difficulty of breathing: it is excellent in epidemical diseases, as pestilence, small-pox, and measles. It is a notable expulsive medicine, and a good remedy for the yellow-jaundice…It is said to be more cordial, and exhilarating than any of the other aromatics, and is particularly serviceable in disorders of the breast in female obstructions, and hysteric depressions. Saffron is endowed with great virtues, for it refreshes the spirits, and is good against fainting-fits, and the palpitation of the heart: it strengthens the stomach, helps digestion, cleanses the lungs, and is good in coughs. It is said to open obstructions of the viscera, and is good in hysteric disorders. However, the use of it ought to be moderate and seasonable; for when the dose is too large, it produces a heaviness of the head, and sleepiness; some have fallen into an immoderate convulsive laughter, which ended in death.*' Saffron has been used to reduce fever, to regulate the menstrual cycle, to combat epilepsy and convulsions and to treat digestive disorders. Modern research confirms it is an antidepressant. It yields a deep, rich yellow dye used to colour the robes of Buddhist monks. Just a single thread can flavour a whole meal, as it contains more than 150 volatile and aroma-yielding compounds. Saffron is used as a flavouring agent for butter, cheese, pastry and confectionery, and is an essential ingredient of paella and bouillabaisse. It needs heat to release its flavour.

HISTORY: *Krokos* is Greek and saffron comes from the Arabic *zafaran*, meaning yellow. In mythology Krokos was a mortal so unhappy from his unrequited love for Smilax that the gods turned him into the saffron flower. From earliest times, the best quality saffron came from Cilicia (Armenia) in the Persian empire, so that '*Crocum in Ciliciam ferre*' became a common expression, equivalent to '*carrying coals to Newcastle*'.

Wanton Delights

Cleopatra was supposed to bathe in saffron water as an aphrodisiac. The Greek dramatist Aristophanes, in *The Clouds*, writes of a character who wants a woman '*redolent with saffron, voluptuous kisses, the love of spending, good cheer and of wanton delights*'. Saffron was also used to dye the hems of the robes of prostitutes in ancient Greece.

Highly Prized Saffron

There are three stigmas per flower, and unbelievably it takes the stigmas from 50,000–75,000 flowers to yield 1 pound (450 g) of dry saffron. This represents an area the size of a football field densely packed with plants, which flower only for about two weeks and have to be picked in the morning before the flowers wilt. It takes about 20 hours' labour to pick enough flowers to produce a pound of dry saffron. Once extracted, the stigmas must be dried quickly, lest decomposition or mould ruin the batch's marketability. Because the cost of the labour-intensive picking is reflected in the high price, it is very often adulterated with turmeric or safflower, yet still sold as saffron. Sealed in airtight glass containers, retail saffron prices are around $1000 per pound, which may comprise between 70,000 and 200,000 orange-crimson flower threads. Iran, even now, accounts for around 80 per cent of the world's saffron production.

To the nations of eastern Asia, its yellow dye embodied the perfection of beauty, and its odour made a perfect ambrosia. Saffron yellow shoes formed part of the dress of the Persian kings. Non-Persians feared the Persians usage of saffron as a drugging agent and aphrodisiac. During his Asian campaigns, Alexander the Great used Persian saffron in his infusions, with rice, and in baths as a curative for battle wounds. Alexander's troops imitated the practice learned from the Persians and brought saffron-bathing to Greece. Saffron was first documented in the seventh century BCE in Assyria. Sumerians, Egyptians, Minoans and all the ancient civilizations treasured what is still the most expensive spice in the world, and in the Hebrew Song of Solomon we read: '*Your lips drop sweetness like a honeycomb, my bride, syrup and milk are under thy tongue, and your dress has the scent of Lebanon. Your cheeks are an orchard of pomegranates, and orchard full of rare fruits, spikenard* [lavender] *and saffron, sweet cane and cinnamon.*' Nero,

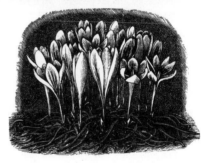

knowing its rarity, ordered the streets of Rome to be strewn with saffron for his triumphal entry. Medicinally, saffron was used in ancient times to treat a wide range of ailments, including stomach upsets, bubonic plague and smallpox. By medieval times, it was grown in Europe, with England's production being centred on Saffron Walden in Essex, and was mainly used for dyeing purposes. Clinical trials have revealed saffron's potential as an anticancer drug and an antiageing agent as it is an antioxidant. *Safranal*, a chemical in the spice, increases levels of the 'feel good' hormone, serotonin, and can ease depression.

SAGE

SALVIA OFFICINALIS
Family Lamiaceae/Labiatae, Mint

OTHER NAMES: Common sage, garden sage, red sage. There are over 500 varieties of sage, and most are medicinally useful, but only a handful are used in cooking.

DESCRIPTION: Hardy evergreen shrub, with a height and spread of 24 inches (60 cm), small mauve flowers and highly aromatic, grey-green, velvet-textured leaves.

PROPERTIES AND USES:
Culpeper relates: '*Jupiter claims this, and bids me tell you, it is good for the liver, and to breed blood. A decoction of the leaves and branches of Sage made and drank, says Dioscorides, provokes urine, brings down women's courses, helps to expel the dead child, and causes the hair to become black. It stays the bleeding of wounds, and cleanses foul ulcers. Three spoonfuls of the juice of Sage taken fasting, with a little honey, doth presently stay the spitting or casting of blood of them that are in a consumption... Matthiolus says, it is very profitable for all manner of pains in the head coming of cold and rheumatic humours: as also for all pains of the joints, whether inwardly or outwardly, and therefore helps the falling-sickness, the lethargy such as are dull and heavy of spirit, the palsy; and is of much use in all defluxions of rheum from the head, and for the diseases of the chest or breast... Pliny says, it procures women's courses, and stays them coming down too fast; helps the*

stinging and biting of serpents, and kills the worms that breed in the ear, and in sores. Sage is of excellent use to help the memory, warming and quickening the senses... The juice of Sage drank with vinegar, hath been of good use in time of the plague at all times. Gargles likewise are made with Sage, rosemary, honey-suckles, and plantain, boiled in wine or water, with some honey or alum put thereto, to wash sore mouths and throats, cankers, or the secret parts of man or woman, as need requires. And with other hot and comfortable herbs,

---

Improving the Memory

Sage was believed to increase mental capacity in Roman times and was associated with immortality. To be 'sage' means to be wise, from the belief that sage was thought to impart wisdom and improve memory. Gerard wrote, '*Sage is singularly good for the head and brain, it quickeneth the senses and memory, strengtheneth the sinews, restoreth health to those that have the palsy, and taketh away shakey trembling of the members.*' Sage indeed seems to slow the ageing process and is being used in research into Alzheimer's disease.

Sage is boiled to bathe the body and the legs in the Summer time, especially to warm cold joints, or sinews, troubled with the palsy and cramp, and to comfort and strengthen the parts. It is much commended against the stitch, or pains in the side coming of wind, if the place be fomented warm with the decoction thereof in wine, and the herb also after boiling be laid warm thereunto.'
An infusion of the leaves makes an excellent tonic with antiseptic, digestive and cleansing action, and acts as a gargle for sore throats and mouth ulcers. Rub the leaves on the gums and teeth to maintain oral health. Sage is helpful with menopausal symptoms and as a hair rinse. Sage adds a special flavour to biscuits, scones and bread and is renowned for sage-and-onion stuffing to accompany chicken, turkey and especially roast pork. 'Sage Derby' cheese is excellent. Sage was used as a method to darken greying hair by gypsies and people living in Turkey. Sage can only be picked by hand as no machine can adequately gather the delicate styles. It takes 20,000 flowers to produce 3.5 ounces (100 g) of spice.

> ## From *Love's Martyr*, 1601
>
> *Sage is an herb for health preservative,*
> *It doth expel from women barrenness:*
> *Ætius saith, it makes the child to live,*
> *Whose new-knit joints are full of feebleness,*
> *And comforteth the mothers weariness:*
> *Adding a lively spirit, that doth good*
> *Unto the painful labouring wives' sick blood.*
>
> *In Egypt when a great mortality,*
> *And killing Pestilence did infect the Land,*
> *Making the people die innumerable,*
> *The plague being ceased, the women out of hand*
> *Did drink of juice of Sage continually,*
> *That made them to increase and multiply,*
> *And bring forth store of children presently.*
>
> Robert Chester

HISTORY: The genus name *Salvia* derives from the Latin *salvare*, to heal. Sage has been prized in many cultures for its healing and medicinal properties, which include antiseptic, digestive and antibacterial uses. Theophrastus classified sage as a coronary herb, because it flushed disease from the body, easing any undue strain on the heart. The Romans considered sage to be a sacred herb and held highly elaborate ceremonies for its

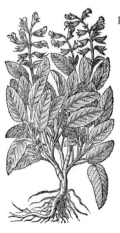

planting and harvesting. A sage gatherer would have a ceremonial bath to ensure that his feet were clean and pure before walking on the earth where the sage grew. In the Middle Ages, people drank sage tea to treat colds, fevers, liver trouble, epilepsy, memory loss and many other common ailments. Early Greeks drank, applied or bathed in sage tea. Charlemagne had it grown in his royal gardens.

CLARY SAGE

SALVIA SCLAREA
Family Lamiaceae/Labiatae, Mint

OTHER NAMES: Clear-Eye according to Culpeper. Clarysage, clarry, toute-bonne, see bright, eyebright (also another herb), muscatel sage.

DESCRIPTION: With large, strong-smelling, hairy leaves, clary sage grows 2–3 feet (60–90 cm) high, and bears cream and lilac flowers.

PROPERTIES AND USES:
'It is under the dominion of the Moon. The seed put into the eyes clears them from motes, and such like things gotten within the lids to offend them, as also clears them from white and red spots on them. The mucilage of the seed made with water, and applied to tumours, or swellings, disperses and takes them away; as also draws forth splinters, thorns, or other things gotten into the flesh. The leaves used with vinegar, either by itself, or with a little honey, doth help boils, felons, and the hot inflammations that are gathered by their pains, if applied before it be grown too great. The powder of the dried root put into the nose, provokes sneezing, and thereby purges the head and brain of much rheum and corruption. The seed or leaves taken in wine, provokes to venery. It is of much use both for men and women that have weak backs, and helps to strengthen the reins: used either by itself, or with other herbs conducing to the same effect, and in tansies often. The fresh leaves dipped in a batter of flour, eggs, and a little milk, and fried in butter, and served to the table, is not unpleasant to any, but exceedingly profitable for those that are troubled with weak backs, and the effects thereof. The juice of the herb put into ale or beer, and drank, brings down women's courses, and expels the after-birth. It is an usual course with many men, when they have gotten the running of the reins, or women the whites, they run to the bush of clary; maid, bring hither the frying-pan, fetch me some butter quickly, then for eating fried clary, just as hogs eat acorns; and this they think will cure their disease forsooth; whereas when they have devoured as much clary as will grow upon an acre of ground, their backs are as much the better as though they had pissed in their shoes; nay, perhaps much worse. We will grant that clary strengthens the back; but this we*

Love Potion

In one herbal, *Dream Pillows and Love Potions* by Jim Long (1997), we find this recipe for a love potion to attract a man: Mix equal parts of dried lavender, bachelor's buttons and clary sage, with a pinch of valerian and a sassafras leaf. Place in a small sachet and wear inside the clothing.

deny, that the cause of the running of the reins [kidneys] in men, or the whites in women, lies in the back, (though the back may sometimes be weakened by them) and therefore the medicine is as proper, as for me when my toe is sore, to lay a plaster on my nose.' Clary sage is used as a relaxant and tonic, and helps with stress-related problems such as headaches, insomnia and indigestion. Clary sage is strengthening and is good to take after childbirth, being said to have a special affinity with the female system, being recommended also for women who are experiencing hot flushes, pain and tension associated with menopause, menstrual problems and PMS. Clary sage also has a reputation for creating a sense of euphoria, and was formerly used in beer and wine to heighten the effects of the alcohol. Clary oil is used as a fixer in perfumery. The young tops of clary were used in soups and as pot herbs, to 'lift' omelettes, and flavour jellies. The leaves were chopped into salads.

HISTORY: The Romans called it *sclarea*, from *clarus* (clear) because they used it as an eyewash. German merchants added clary and elder flowers to Rhine wine to make it imitate a good muscatel. The practice was so common that Germans still call the herb *Muskateller Salbei* and the English knew it as *muscatel sage*. In some parts of Britain a wine has been made from the herb in flower, boiled with sugar, which had a sweet muscat flavour like a good Frontignac. It was considered an aphrodisiac in medieval times. It was employed in

Relaxing Treatment

The essential oil is clear, and has a sweet, nutty scent, almost a floral quality, being a good remedy for nervous stress. Clary contains a hormone-like compound similar to oestrogen that regulates hormonal balance, and a clary sage bath is warm and very relaxing. A sage lotion can be made to treat oily hair and skin, dandruff and wrinkles.

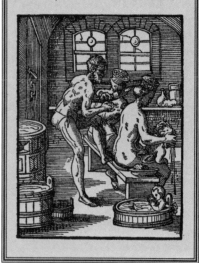

England as a substitute for hops, but the extra intoxication it induced gave severe headaches. Matthias de Lobel, a 17th-century Flemish physician and botanist, wrote: '*Some brewers of Ale and Beere doe put it into their drinke to make it more heady, fit to please drunkards, who thereby, according to their several dispositions, become either dead drunke, or foolish drunke, or made drunke.*'

287

ST JOHN'S WORT

HYPERICUM PERFORATUM
Family Hypericaceae, Hypericum

OTHER NAMES: Amber, scare-devil, goat weed, sol terrestris, Tipton weed, balm of the warrior's wound, rose of Sharon, Aaron's beard. *'Nature's Prozac'* is a fairly recent nickname.

DESCRIPTION: Hardy semi-evergreen perennial, growing from 1–3 feet (30–90 cm) tall with a 12-inch (30-cm) spread. Its pretty yellow flowers contain hypericin, and tiny resin glands on the leaves give off an unpleasant foxy scent. The stems exude a reddish-purple juice, *'the blood of St John'.*

PROPERTIES AND USES: It is used as an antidepressant, and for pain and inflammation caused by nerve damage. Oil infused with the flowers can help tissue repair in wounds, burns and shingles. Culpeper writes: *'It is under the celestial sign Leo, and the dominion of the Sun. It may be, if you meet a Papist, he will tell you, especially if he be a lawyer, that St. John made it over to him by a letter of attorney. It is a singular wound herb; boiled in wine and drank, it heals inward hurts or bruises; made into an ointment, it open obstructions, dissolves swellings, and closes up the lips of wounds. The decoction of the herb and flowers, especially of the seed, being drank in wine, with the juice of knot-grass, helps all manner of vomiting and spitting of blood, is good for those that are bitten or stung by any venomous creature, and for those that cannot make water. Two drams of the seed of St. John's Wort made into powder, and drank in a little broth, doth gently expel choler or congealed blood in the stomach. The decoction of the leaves and seeds drank somewhat warm before the fits of agues, whether they be tertians or quartains, alters the fits, and, by often using, doth take them quite away. The seed is much commended, being drank for forty days together, to help the sciatica, the falling sickness, and the palsy.'* An infusion of the flowers and olive oil offers a strong astringent, antibiotic, healing treatment for wounds, inflammations and aching joints. The tea is good for coughs and

---

St John the Baptist

The plant is named after St John the Baptist, whose feast day, 24 June, occurs close to Midsummer Day when daylight in Europe is longest and the plant is in full bloom. Its five yellow petals resemble a halo, and its red sap symbolizes the blood of the martyred saint.

---

insomnia. St John's wort is prescribed for depression and migraine but not in conjunction with other antidepressants or other drugs taken for migraine. The herb affects the levels of serotonin in the body, this being a chemical that affects anxiety, depression and migraine. There can be several unpleasant side-effects for those who are light-sensitive, suffering from the skin condition rosacea etc. The stems and flowers produce red and yellow dyes.

HISTORY : In medieval times, St John's wort was used for 'driving out the inner devil'. The philosopher Paracelcus (*c.*1525) recommended it for hallucinations and 'dragons', as well as for healing wounds. St John's wort is very effective as a compress for dressing wounds, and in the Middle Ages was commonly used to heal deep sword cuts. When held up to the light, the leaves appear to be peppered with what look like tiny translucent glands, perforations interpreted as punctures or 'wounds'. This led to the plant being identified as a wound-healer through the Doctrine of Signatures. St John's wort is a proven antidepressant used to treat both humans and animals. However, this versatile herb also contains dozens of chemical compounds that disinfect and heal wounds as well as boosting the entire nervous system. It gets its common name from the superstition that on St John's Day, 24 June, the dew which fell on the plant the evening before was efficacious in preserving the eyes from disease. The plant was collected, dipped

> ### Helping to Conceive
>
> If a childless wife walked naked to pick St John's wort in the woodlands, she would conceive within a year. (Whether the offspring was that of her husband could, no doubt, be the matter of some conjecture.)

in oil, and became transformed into a balm for every wound. Some say that its name *Hypericum* is derived from the Greek *hyper* (above) and *eikon* (icon), referring to the belief that the herb was so obnoxious to evil spirits that its smell would cause them to fly away. Others believe that the word comes from *hyper* and *ereike* (heath), possibly meaning the best heath of all. The plant was hung over a religious icon on St John's Day. Until comparatively recent times, it was gathered and hung in doorways and windows to ward off evil spirits. In Germany, the herb is commonly given to children and teenagers, and a 2008 study there compared the effects of *Hypericum perforatum* with placebos or a wide range of old and new antidepressants, including those from the new generation of SSRI drugs, such as Prozac and Seroxat. The herb was found to be as effective as the modern drugs, and causing fewer side effects than many standard drugs used to help those battling depression.

SAMPHIRE

CRITHMUM MARITIMUM
Family Apiaceae/Umbelliferae, Umbellifers

OTHER NAMES: Rock samphire, small samphire, marsh samphire, St Peter's herb, sampiere, sea asparagus, poor man's asparagus, sea pickle, crest marine.

DESCRIPTION: The leaves are narrow, sea-green, salty and succulent, and the flowers are borne in tiny greenish-white umbels. Samphire grows up to 12 inches (30 cm) in height and spread.

PROPERTIES AND USES:
'It is an herb of Jupiter, and was in former times wont to be used more than now it is; the more is the pity. It is well known almost to every body, that ill digestions and obstructions are the cause of most of the diseases which the frail nature of man is subject to; both which might be remedied by a more frequent use of this herb. If people would have sauce to their meat, they may take some for profit as well as for pleasure. It is a safe herb, very pleasant both to taste and stomach, helps digestion, and in some sort opening obstructions of the liver and spleen: provokes urine, and helps thereby to wash away the gravel and stone engendered in the kidneys or bladder.' – Culpeper. A diuretic, samphire can relieve flatulence and indigestion. The leaves can be eaten in salads, cooked in butter or steamed like asparagus or make an aromatic sauce.

HISTORY: It was originally *'sampiere'*, a corruption from *'herbe de St-Pierre'* named for the patron saint of fishermen because it grows in rocky regions and coastal marshes along the sea coast of northern Europe. The dangers involved in collecting rock samphire on sea cliffs are mentioned in Shakespeare's *King Lear: 'Half-way down / Hangs one that gathers samphire; dreadful trade!'* John Gerard wrote in 1597: *'The leaves kept in pickle and eaten in salads with oil and vinegar is a pleasant sauce for meat, wholesome for the stoppings of the liver, milt and kidneys. It is the pleasantest sauce, most familiar and best agreeing with man's body.'* Rock samphire used to be cried by the vendors in London streets as 'crest marine' and in the 19th century it was shipped in casks of seawater from the Isle of Wight to markets in London. By the 1960s, it had long fallen out fashion, and was known as *'poor man's asparagus'*. However, in 1981 it was served at the royal wedding breakfast of Charles and Diana, having been gathered from Sandringham marshes. It has regained favour as a garnish for restaurant fish, and sometimes as a lightly vinegared relish.

The Lone Species

It is the sole species of the genus *Crithmum*, and research is ongoing into its use as a treatment for obesity, samphire being rich in vitamin C, pectin, sulphates and iodine.

SANICLE

SANICULA EUROPAEA
Family Apiaceae/Umbelliferae, Umbellifers

OTHER NAMES: Wood sanicle, European sanicle, pool-root, self-heal (as is *Prunella vulgaris*) snakeroot (USA). It is the only representative in Britain of the *Sanicula* genus.

DESCRIPTION: A little like cow parsley, but with small, white to reddish flowers growing in small hemispherical umbels, from which appear bristly fruit with hooked prickles which attach to animal fur.

PROPERTIES AND USES:
Culpeper: '*This is one of Venus's herbs, to cure the wounds or mischiefs Mars inflicts upon the body of man. It heals green wounds speedily, or any ulcers, imposthumes, or bleedings inward, also tumours in any part of the body; for the decoction or powder in drink taken, and the juice used outwardly, dissipates the humours: and there is not found any herb that can give such present help either to man or beast, when the disease falls upon the lungs or throat, and to heal up putrid malignant ulcers in the mouth, throat, and private parts, by gargling or washing with the decoction of the leaves and roots made in water, and a little honey put thereto. It helps to stay women's courses, and all other fluxes of blood, either by the mouth, urine, or stool, and lasks* [diarrhoea] *of the belly; the ulcerations of the kidneys also, and the pains in the bowels, and gonorrhoea, being boiled in wine or water, and drank. The same also is no less powerful to help any ruptures or burstings, used both inwardly and outwardly. And briefly, it is as effectual in binding, restraining, consolidating, heating, drying and healing, as comfrey, bugle, self-heal, or any other of the vulnerary herbs whatsoever.*' European sanicle tea relieves mucous congestion in the chest, stomach, and intestines. As a gargle and mouthwash, it is used for mouth and throat inflammations and sores. It has been used externally to treat skin eruptions, scrofula and suppurating wounds. Its mildly styptic action made it helpful for internal haemorrhages.

HISTORY: In the Middle Ages it was believed that taking sanicle would make surgeons redundant. The plant gained its medical reputation as a vulnerary (wound healer), with the herbalist Henry Lyte writing that it will '*make whole and sound all wounds and hurts, both inward and outward*'. A decoction was used for scald-head (scalp disease characterised by pustules), bleeding piles and rashes.

Healing Herb

The whole herb is to be collected in June, only on the morning of a fine day, when the sun has dried the dew. The origin of the genus name is the Latin *sano* (I heal or cure), in reference to its medicinal virtues.

SARSAPARILLA

SMILAX REGELII (formerly *OFFICINALIS*)
Family Smilacaceae, Greenbriar

OTHER NAMES: Honduran sarsaparilla, Jamaican sarsaparilla, red-bearded sarsaparilla.

DESCRIPTION: A large perennial vine with a long, tuberous rootstock.

PROPERTIES AND USES: Culpeper observes: '*This is reckoned amongst the sorts of prickly Bindweeds, of which there are three sorts; one with red berries, another with black berries, and the third which was brought into Europe by the Spaniards about the year 1563…These are all plants of Mars; of an healing quality howsoever used. Dioscorides says, that both leaves and berries, drank before or after any deadly poison, are an excellent antidote. It is also said, that if some of the juice of the berries be given to a new-born child, it shall never be hurt by poison. It is good against all sorts of venomous things. Twelve or sixteen of the berries, beaten to powder, and given in wine, procure urine when it is stopped. The distilled waters, when drank, have the same effect, cleanses the reins and assuages inward inflammations. If the eyes be washed therewith, it heals them thoroughly. The true Sarsaparilla is held generally not to heat, but rather to dry the humours; yet it is easily perceived, that it does not only dry them but wastes them away by a secret property, chiefly that of sweating, which it greatly promotes. It is used in many kinds of diseases, particularly in cold fluxes from the head* and brain, rheums, and catarrhs, and cold griefs of the stomach, as it expels winds very powerfully. It helps not only the French disease but all manner of aches in the sinews or joints, all running sores in the legs, all phlegmatic swellings, tetters or ring-worms, and all manner of spots and foulness of the skin. It is reckoned a great sweetener of the blood, and has been found of considerable service in venereal cases. Infants who have received infection from their nurses, though covered with pustules and ulcers, may be cured by the use of this root without the help of mercurials; and the best way of administering it to them is to mix the powdered root with their food.'*

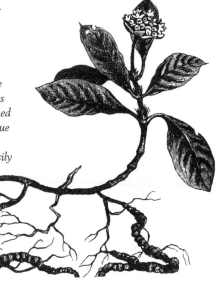

Sarsaparilla can act as an anti-inflammatory and cleansing agent, giving relief for skin diseases such as eczema, itching and psoriasis, and to treat rheumatic complaints and gout. Some believe the plant can treat impotence, as it has a testosterogenic action and can increase muscle bulk. The herb has been used to bring relief to women suffering from menopausal and menstrual problems, and to relieve depression and debility. As well as a liquid being used as a tonic pick-me-up, the smoke of sarsaparilla was inhaled by asthma sufferers.

HISTORY: The Aztecs used sarsaparilla in the treatment of syphilis, chronic skin ailments, especially those that cause putrid ulcerations, and in cases of bone disease. The plant was exported to Europe before 1530 from Mexico, often through Jamaica, and is named after Spanish *zarza* (bramble) and *parrilla* (little vine). Sarsaparilla was then used from the 16th century as a treatment for syphilis and rheumatism. Its products were also promoted as blood purifiers, tonics, diuretics, sweat inducers, and it was often used in patent medicines. The herb

Sugarfoot

In the US, before it was replaced by artificial agents, sarsaparilla root was the original flavouring for *root beer*. A few people may remember an old black and white TV cowboy series, *Sugarfoot* (1957–61). The unarmed hero, a fledgling lawyer in the lawless West, always ordered an alcohol-free sarsaparilla when he walked into a bar full of rowdy villains. The theme tune began: '*Sugarfoot, Sugarfoot, easy lopin', cattle ropin' Sugarfoot, / Carefree as the tumbleweeds, a joggin' along with a heart full of song / And a rifle and a volume of the law.*' For unfathomable reasons the show was aired as *Tenderfoot* in the UK.

contains a mixture of saponins, which have strong diuretic properties, as well as some laxative (as they act as gastric irritants), diaphoretic (sweat-causing), and expectorant uses. The 16th-century physician Nicolás Monardes devoted two chapters of his *Joyfulle Newes Out of the Newe Founde Worlde* to this 'new' herb.

Unreliable Treatment

Sarsaparilla was still being listed in the 1850s as a treatment for syphilis in the *U. S. Pharmacopoeia*. A tea made of sarsaparilla was used to treat venereal diseases such as syphilis and gonorrhoea. If any sufferers today would like to try it: bring two pints of water to the boil. Add 2 tablespoons each of yellow dock roots and sarsaparilla herb. Reduce the heat and simmer, covered, for five minutes, remove the cover and add 3½ teaspoonfuls of dried thyme herb. Then everything must be covered again and steeped an extra hour. However, it must be noted that neither the whole medication nor its saponins are actually effective in bringing in relief for syphilis and for purifying blood. Preferably, see a doctor.

SAVORY - SUMMER and WINTER

SATUREJA HORTENSIS and *SATUREJA MONTANA*
Family Lamiaceae/Labiatae, Mint

OTHER NAMES: Garden savory (summer savory), bean herb (both).

DESCRIPTION: Summer savory is a half-hardy annual growing to 12–18 inches (30–45 cm) high with a 10-inch (25-cm) spread, with aromatic oval leaves and small white to mauve flowers. Its smell is a cross between mint and thyme, with a peppery aftertaste. Winter savory is a hardy perennial with a height of around 12–15 inches (30–38 cm) and a spread of 8 inches (20 cm), with small aromatic pointed glossy leaves and small white to pink flowers.

PROPERTIES AND USES: Culpeper says: *'Mercury claims dominion over this herb. Keep it dry by you all the year, if you love yourself and your ease, and it is a hundred pounds to a penny if you do not.'* He considered summer savory better than winter savory for drying to make conserves and syrups: *'Keep it dry, make conserves and syrups of it for your use; for which purpose the Summer kind is best. This kind is both hotter and drier than the Winter kind...It expels tough phlegm from the chest and lungs, quickens the dull spirits in the lethargy, if the juice be snuffed up the nose; dropped into the eyes it clears them of thin cold humours proceeding from the brain...outwardly applied with wheat flour as a poultice, it eases sciatica and palsied members.'* Culpeper adds: *'The juice dropped into the eyes removes dimness of sight if it proceeds from thin humours distilled from the brain. The juice heated with oil of Roses and dropped in the ears removes noise and singing and deafness: outwardly applied with wheat flour, it gives ease to them.'*

Both are known mainly as culinary herbs, but also possess medicinal properties. Antiseptic, antifungal and antibacterial, both types of savory have therapeutic properties similar to those of oregano, thyme and rosemary. Savory is a carminative herb used for colic, diarrhoea and indigestion. Its antiseptic and astringent properties make it a good treatment for

Preventing Flatulence

Culpeper recommends savory as a *'good remedy for the colic'*. When used with bean dishes, it not only adds flavour but helps prevent flatulence, hence 'bean herb'. It is no coincidence that the German word for the herb is *Bohnenkraut*, meaning bean herb, as one of the components of the herb naturally aids their digestion.

Satyrs and Savory

The derivation of the genus name *Satureja* is not clear but it may refer (via Pliny) to the satyrs, the Greek demigods of the forest who where known for their half-man/half-goat shape and insatiable sexual appetites. In legend the satyrs lived in meadows of savory and wore crowns of the herb, so the herb was once thought to be an aphrodisiac as a result of this association. The French herbalist and healer Maurice Mességué (1921–) claims that savory is an essential ingredient in love potions he makes for couples. As a boy his father told him it was '*the herb of happiness*'.

sore throats, and a poultice of the leaves gives quick relief to wasp stings and insect bites. Winter savory has a stronger, more resinous flavour than summer savory, but both impart a peppery taste to foods and blend well with thyme, marjoram and basil. Both are used to marinate meats, and to add flavour to beans (especially in Italy) and vegetables. The leaves and tender tops are used, with marjoram and thyme, to season dressings for turkey, veal or fish. Its distinctive taste resembles that of marjoram, so it is not only added to stuffing, pork pies and sausages as a seasoning, but fresh sprigs of it may be boiled with broad beans and green peas, in the same manner as mint. It is also boiled with dried peas in making pea-soup. For garnishing it has been used as a substitute for parsley and chervil, and fresh leaves can replace pepper in cooking. In Bulgarian cookery, instead of salt and pepper being on the dinner table, there is salt, paprika and savory. It is a characteristic ingredient of *herbes de Provence*. Winter savory oil is used in preparations to prevent incipient

baldness. Cooks prefer to use summer savory. Use summer savory, with its more delicate flavour, for tender baby green beans, and winter savory to enhance dried beans and lentils.

HISTORY : Savory was known to the Greeks and Romans, and later imported to northern Europe. Both species were noticed by Virgil as being among the most fragrant of herbs, and on this account recommended to be grown near bee-hives to attract bees and so flavour the honey. Vinegar, flavoured with savory and other aromatic herbs, was used by the Romans in the same manner as mint sauce is used today. In Shakespeare's time, savory was a popular herb, and is mentioned, together with different mints, marjoram and lavender, in *The Winter's Tale*. Winter savory is the coarser and hardier, beloved by bees, and was extensively used as edging in Elizabethan knot gardens. The American colonists brought both winter and summer savory to North America, both being mentioned by the 17th-century American botanist John Josselyn.

(FIELD) SCABIOUS

KNAUTIA ARVENSIS
Family Dipsacaceae, Teasel

OTHER NAMES: Gypsy rose, pins and needles, blue bonnets, mournful widow, lady's pincushion, lady's hatpins, poor widow, blackamoor's beauty, Egyptian rose, blue buttons, bachelor's buttons, clafrllys (itch plant, Welsh).

DESCRIPTION: When first in flower, the stamens of this 12–24 inch (30–60 cm) perennial resemble pins sticking out of a pin cushion. The attractive flower heads range in colour from light blue to pale lilac.

PROPERTIES AND USES: Gerard tells us: *'The plant genders scabs, if the decoction thereof be drunk certain days and the juice used in ointments.'* The juice *'being drunk, procures sweat, especially with Treacle, and attenuates and makes thin, freeing the heart from any infection or pestilence.'* Culpeper relates that it is *'very effectual for coughs, shortness of breath and other diseases of the lungs,'* and says that the *'decoction of the herb, dry or green, made into wine and drunk for some time together,'* is good for pleurisy. The green herb, bruised and applied to any carbuncle, was stated by Culpeper to dissolve the same *'in three hours' space'*, and the same decoction removed pains and stitches in the side. The decoction of the root was considered a cure for all sores and eruptions, the juice being made into an ointment for the same purpose. Also, *'the decoction of the herb and roots outwardly applied in any part of the body, is effectual for shrunk sinews or veins and heals green wounds, old sores and ulcers.'* An attractive garden plant, the leaves are the food plants of the rare marsh fritillary butterfly and also the small skipper, Essex skipper, marbled white, red admiral and small tortoiseshell butterflies. It is also the food of the rare narrow bordered bee hawk moth and well as being popular with burnet, lime speck pug and shaded pug moths, so is environmentally valuable. Sheep and goats will eat the plant, but cattle dislike it.

HISTORY: It has been used as a blood purifier and as a treatment for eczema and other skin disorders for centuries. The juice of scabious, mixed with powder of borax and samphire, was recommended for removing freckles, pimples and leprosy, and also as a warm decoction to remove dandruff and scurf.

Scratchy and Itchy

The botanical name of corn scabious, *Scabiosa columbaria*, comes from the Latin word for itch, *scabiosa* (from *scabere*, to scratch). Herbalists used scabious, dried and added to juice, as a remedy for scabies, sores left by the plague and other skin complaints.

(DEVIL'S BIT) SCABIOUS

SUCCISA PRATENSIS
Family Dipsacaceae, Teasel

OTHER NAMES: Wild devil's bit, premorse.

DESCRIPTION: A slender plant with conspicuous stamens making a lilac 'pincushion' like those of other scabious species. Botanically, devil's bit has four-lobed flowers, whereas field scabious has five lobes, so they have been put in different genuses (*Knautia* and *Succisa*) within the family Dipsacaceae (Teasel).

PROPERTIES AND USES: Culpeper recommended it for many uses, saying that the root boiled in wine and drunk was very powerful against the plague and all pestilential diseases, and fevers and poison and bites of venomous creatures, and that '*it helpeth also all that are inwardly bruised or outwardly by falls or blows, dissolving the clotted blood.*' The root bruised and outwardly applied, took away black and blue marks on the skin. He considered '*the decoction of the herb very effectual as a gargle for swollen throat and tonsils, and that the root powdered and taken in drink expels worms.*' The juice or distilled water of the herb was a remedy for green wounds or old sores, cleansing the body inwardly and freeing the skin from sores, scurf, pimples, freckles, etc. The dried root was given in powder, promoting sweat, so making it beneficial in fevers. It made a tea for coughs, fevers and internal inflammation. It purified the blood, taken inwardly, and was used as a wash externally for cutaneous eruptions (hardenings and tumours of the skin). As with field scabious, the warm decoction has also been used as a wash to free the head from scurf, sores and dandruff. Also, as with field scabious, it is an excellent food source for butterflies, moths and bees.

HISTORY: The plant was used for its diaphoretic (sweat-inducing), soothing and fever-reducing properties, the whole herb being collected in September and dried.

Bitten by the Devil

John Gerard tells how '*The greater part of the root seems to be bitten away; old fantastic charmers report that the devil did bite it for envy, because it is an herb that hath so many good virtues and it is so beneficial to mankind.*' The devil reputedly found this herb in Paradise but, envying the good it might do to the human race, bit away a part of the root to destroy the plant. However, it still flourishes, with a strangely stumped root. The legend seems to have been very widely spread, for the plant bears this name across Europe.

SCENTED HERB GARDENS

The earliest scented gardens were built in the courtyards of the houses of Persian nobles more than 2500 years ago. These gardens were generally square or rectangular in form, often being divided into four sections by streams flowing from a central fountain. The name for these enclosed gardens was *pairi-daeza* (see The Origin of Paradise, page 254). The Persians, who honoured their gardeners, required three main qualities in their earthly paradises: running water, shade and scent. Through their adoption by the Byzantine church, such gardens eventually found their way into Western Europe, in the form of monastic cloister gardens. The idea of a walled, perfumed garden resonated with the medieval Christian tradition, which viewed the whole of creation in symbolic terms. Biblical references to flowers and plants, from the Song of Solomon to the Garden of Eden could be reinforced by such gardens appearing as images of Paradise itself. The Moors in Spain filled the caliph's gardens outside Cordoba with roses in 711 CE. During the centuries preceding the First Crusade in 1095, there are mentions of rose gardens being cultivated in Germany, France, and in many of the monasteries throughout Europe. Returning Crusaders introduced varieties that had been cultivated in Asia (damask roses, i.e. the Castilian rose) to Europe, and the English took plants of the *gallica* and *alba* varieties. The rose and

the lily were the first two flowers that Charlemagne ordered to be planted across his empire. In 1260 the Dominican monk Albertus Magnus specified the ingredients of a perfect paradise, or pleasure garden. There should be a fountain and a lawn of *'every sweet-smelling herb such as rue, and sage and basil, and likewise all sorts of flowers, as the violet, columbine, lily, rose, iris and the like'*. Albertus also recommended that *'Behind the lawn there may be great diversity of medicinal and scented herbs, not only to delight the sense of smell by their perfume but to refresh the sight with their flowers'*.

Along with the rose, the other major sacred flower of the early Christian church was the highly scented white Madonna lily, *Lilium candidum*. In monastery gardens, roses and lilies were grown together with especially aromatic herbs such as lavender and rosemary. The medieval romance garden and the Renaissance love garden were primarily rose and herb gardens, as esteemed for their aesthetic qualities as for their usefulness. The apogee of the scented garden came in the reign of Elizabeth I, when the upper classes demanded sweetly scented food, rooms and clothes. Elizabethan manor houses cultivated fragrant flowers and aromatic plants in a secluded formal garden, usually hedged with rose briars and fruit trees not only for the pleasure of walking and sitting there, but also to provide the ingredients for the stillroom. Here were prepared 'sweet waters' from rose petals and rosemary flowers, and healing lotions from the stems of the Madonna lily and spikes of lavender. Aromatic herbs, like hyssop and rue, were grown for strewing over the floors of rooms to purify the air, and their dried flowers were stuffed into pillows to encourage sleep. However, by the 18th century, scented gardens almost disappeared from sight, as aromatic flowers gave way to far grander designs.

Rose Garden

The original meaning of the word *rosary* is a round rose garden dedicated to the Virgin Mary (*rosarium* is Latin for rose garden). The earliest rosaries were built on holy ground, but 16th-century paintings show that the style was also adopted in private gardens, where rose gardens and arbours were built by royalty and the nobility.

Scented Gardens

Many herbs release their aroma when brushed against or touched. Suggested herbs for a **scented herb garden** include anise hyssop, basil, catmint, feverfew, lavender, lemon balm, lemon thyme, various mints, southernwood, wormwood, verbena, scented geraniums, lily-of-the-valley, sweet marjoram, sweet violets, rosemary and thyme. Roses, jasmine, nicotiana, stocks, wallflowers and lilacs can complement the garden. *Rosa gallica officinalis*, the apothecary's rose, would be a wonderful addition. On a small scale, one can establish a **scented lemon garden** with lemon balm, catmint, verbena, lemon grass, lemon thyme and lemon basil. For a **herbal tea garden**, try lemon basil, chamomile, lemon verbena, lemon balm, peppermint, orange mint, rose hips, bergamot, rosemary, pineapple sage, fennel and lavender.

Rosary Gardens

Rosary Gardens are designed to create a peaceful environment ideal for quiet reflection. They can also be designed to incorporate designated flowers to honour the Virgin Mary. Stepping stones can take the place of rosary beads. Five large stones and 50 small stones make the decades of Christ's birth, life and death (a sequence of prayers made during worship with a rosary is called a decade). The medallion with Mary's likeness is the central part of the rosary, so a statue of Mary can stand in the heart of the rosary garden. The flowers used can be the visual symbols of the Mysteries: glorious (yellow/gold), joyful (white), luminous (purple) and sorrowful (red).

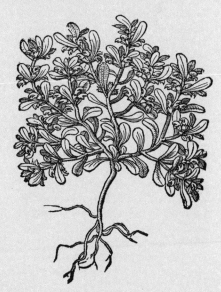

SELF HEAL

PRUNELLA VULGARIS
Family Lamiaceae/Labiatae, Mint

OTHER NAMES: Self-heal, heal-all, all-heal (shared with other plants), blue curls (USA), heart-of-the-earth (USA), prunella, brunella, carpenter-weed, hook heal, slough heal, carpenter weed, carpenter's herb.

DESCRIPTION: It has purple and violet flowers in dense spikes, often with white lower lips, and can grow from 1 to 2 feet (30–60 cm) high on a weak stem that is often supported by grass. Culpeper notes that the flowers are *'thick set together like an ear or spiky knap'* making it easy to recognize. Nectar lies at the bottom of the corolla tube, protected from tiny insects by a thick hedge of hairs placed just above it. The flower is adapted by this formation, like the rest of the Labiatae family, for fertilization by bees, which alight on the lower lip. They then thrust their proboscises down the corolla tube for nectar. In doing so their heads are dusted with pollen from the anthers, and on visiting the next flower, this pollen is smeared on the end of the curving style that runs up the arch of the upper lip, thus effecting fertilization.

PROPERTIES AND USES: Culpeper tells us: *'It is under the dominion of Mars, hot, biting, and choleric; and remedies what evils Mars afflicts the body of man with, by sympathy, as viper's flesh attracts poison, and the loadstone iron. It kills the worms, helps the gout, cramp, and convulsions, provokes urine, and helps all joint-aches.'* He explains its name as: *'Self-Heal whereby*

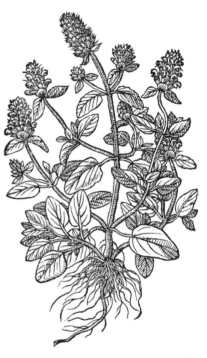

when you are hurt, you may heal yourself… it is an especial herb for inward or outward wounds. Take it inwardly in syrups for inward wounds, outwardly in unguents and plasters for outward. As Self-Heal is like Bugle in form, so also in the qualities and virtues, serving for all purposes, whereunto Bugle is applied with good success either inwardly or outwardly, for inward wounds or ulcers in the body, for bruises or falls and hurts. If it be combined with Bugle, Sanicle and other like wound herbs, it will be more effectual to wash and inject into ulcers in the parts outwardly…It is an especial remedy for all green wounds to close the lips of them and to keep the place from further inconveniences. The juice used with oil of roses to anoint the temples and forehead is very effectual to remove the headache, and the same mixed with honey of roses cleans and heals ulcers in the mouth and throat.' Self heal is still in use in modern herbal treatment as an astringent for inward or outward use on injuries and wounds with bleeding. Drops are made with milk for conjunctivitis, and an ointment made for bleeding piles. The plant is also useful for treating haemorrhage and excessive bleeding during menstruation. The whole plant was said to have antibacterial, antipyretic, antiseptic, antispasmodic, antiviral, astringent, carminative, diuretic, febrifuge, hypotensive, stomachic, styptic, tonic, vermifuge and vulnerary properties.

HISTORY: William Coles, in *Adam in Eden* (1657), explains its name: '*It is called by modern writers (for neither the ancient Greek nor Latin writers knew it) Brunella, from Brunellen, which is a name given unto it by the Germans, because it cureth that inflammation of the mouth which they call "die Breuen," yet the general name of it in Latin nowadays is Prunella, as being a word of a more gentile pronunciation.*' He also notes that '*die Breuen*' '*is common to soldiers when they lie in camp, but especially in garrisons, coming with an extraordinary inflammation or swelling, as well in the mouth as throat, the very signature of the Throat which the form of the Flowers so represent signifying as much*'. Thus the Doctrine of Signatures told apothecaries to prescribe prunella. Gerard wrote that: '*There is not a better Wound herb in the world than that of SelfHeale is, the very name importing it to be very admirable

upon this account and indeed the Virtues do make it good, for this very herb without the mixture of any other ingredient, being only bruised and wrought with the point of a knife upon a trencher or the like, will be brought into the form of a salve, which will heal any green wound even in the first intention, after a very wonderful manner, The decoction of Prunell made with wine and water doth join together and make whole and sound all wounds, both inward and outward, even as Bugle doth. To be short, it serves for the same that the Bugle serves and in the world there are not two better wound herbs as hath been often proved.*' Self heal was one of many plants that found their way to North America with the early settlers.

Carpenter's Herb

Although self heal is not as immediately effective as comfrey, yarrow or bugle, it is a useful herb because of its almost universal availability. Its name '*carpenters herb*' indicates that it was traditionally used for bruised or cut fingers.

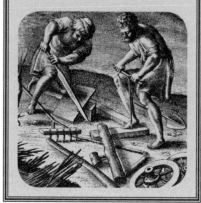

SHEPHERD'S PURSE

CAPSELLA BURSA-PASTORIS
Family Brassicaceae/Cruciferae, Cabbage

OTHER NAMES: Pickpurse, casewort, shepherd's bag, shepherd's scrip, shepherd's sprout, lady's purse, witches' pouches, rattle pouches, caseweed, pick-pocket, pick-purse, blindweed, pepper-and-salt, poor man's parmacettie, sanguinary, mother's heart.

DESCRIPTION: Its small white flowers are followed by triangular, notched seedpods. It is 6–18 inches (15–45 cm) high, growing from a rosette at its base.

PROPERTIES AND USES: Culpeper states: '*It is under the dominion of Saturn, and of a cold, dry, and binding nature, like to him. It helps all fluxes of blood, either caused by inward or outward wounds; as also flux of the belly, and bloody flux, spitting blood, and bloody urine, stops the terms in women; being bound to the wrists of the hands, and the soles of the feet, it helps the yellow jaundice.*' It is an important herb to stop bleeding, due to the tyramine and other amines it contains, and so it is used to prevent heavy menstrual bleeding, nosebleeds and as a post-partum herb. The herb acts as a vasoconstrictor, hastens coagulation and constricts blood vessels. The herb contains a protein that constricts the smooth muscles that support and surround blood vessels, especially those in the uterus. Other chemicals in the herb may accelerate clotting. Yet other compounds in the herb help the uterus contract, explaining the long-time use of the herb to help the womb return to normal size after childbirth. When the seeds are ripe, they have a fiery bite and have been ground as a pepper substitute.

HISTORY: Its flavonoids have a haemostatic action (stopping blood flow), so it has been used for most of recorded history to treat cuts, nose bleeds and uterine haemorrhages. Strangely, it used to be gathered and fed to chickens to make the yolks of their eggs much darker and more strongly flavoured. Shepherd's purse is also used in traditional Chinese medicine formulas for blurred vision, and spots before the eyes. During the First World War, as other styptics became unavailable, shepherd's purse was used as a replacement. In magical lore, eating the seeds of the first three plants you see will prevent illness for a whole year.

Seedpod Purses

The 'purses' are its small, delicate, heart-shaped seedpods, shaped like the leather purses which used to be carried by shepherds and herders. It is similarly called in France *bourse de pasteur*, and in Germany *Hirtentasche*. Each plant releases as many as 40,000 seeds.

SOAPWORT

SAPONARIA OFFICINALIS
Family Caryophyllaceae, Pink/Carnation

OTHER NAMES: Common soapwort, bouncing Bet, tumbling Ted, fuller's herb, fuller's grass bruisewort, old maids pink, sebonllys (soapflower, Welsh), sweet Betty, wild sweet William, dog cloves, soap root, latherwort, foam dock, gill-run-by-the-street, saponary, lady-by-the-gate, crow soap, hedge pink, farewell summer.

DESCRIPTION: Straggly perennial growing 2–4 feet (60–120 cm) high and with a 1–2-feet (30–60-cm) spread, with compact clusters of pink, fragrant flowers and smooth pointed leaves.

PROPERTIES AND USES: *'Venus owns this plant. The whole plant is bitter. Bruised and agitated with water it raises a lather like soap, which easily washes greasy spots out of cloths: a decoction of it, applied externally, cures the itch. The Germans make use of it, instead of sarsaparilla, for the cure of venereal disorders. In fact it cures virulent gonorrhœas, by giving the inspissated* [thickened] *juice of it to the amount of half an ounce daily. It is accounted opening and attenuating, and somewhat sudorific, and by some commended against hard tumours and whitlows, but it is seldom used.'* – Culpeper. When the rhizome and roots are boiled in water, their hormone-like saponins produce a lather, releasing a substance that can lift dirt and grease off clothes. Anti-inflammatory, it has been used for jaundice, dry and irritating skin conditions and for hair care. The flowers can be used in pot-pourris, and the plant is still used in shampoos, make-up removers and cleansers. Restorers and conservers still value its gentle qualities to lift dirt from fragile paintings, textiles, upholstery and silk. In the Middle East soapwort is still grown to use when washing woollen items.

HISTORY: Soapwort has an ancient reputation for treating skin conditions such as psoriasis, eczema, boils and acne. It was taken to the American colonies by early settlers. Soapwort used to be used for cleaning new wool, taking out the lanolin grease, and colonies of the plant have spread from their original positions growing near old wool mills. Thus the plant was known as *fuller's herb*, or *fuller's grass*. A fuller was the person in a mill who used the 'fulling' process in cleansing (usually woollen) cloth by first 'scouring' it, and then 'milling' it, making it thicker. Shepherds in the Alps washed their sheep with soapwort solution before shearing them. Soapwort was used to produce a head upon beer, and was also known as *bruisewort* as gipsies used it for black eyes and bruises. Maud Grieve's *Herbal* recommended soapwort for venereal diseases when mercury failed to clear them up.

SOLOMON'S SEAL

POLYGONATUM MULTIFLORUM
Family Ruscaceae, Ruscus

OTHER NAMES: King Solomon's seal, common Solomon's seal, lady's seals, St Mary's seal, dagrau Job (Welsh for Job's daggers), Jacob's ladder, David's harp, ladder-to-heaven, jade bamboo (in China, as its leaves resemble those of bamboo).

DESCRIPTION: This attractive perennial grows 12–30 inches (30–76 cm) high with a spread of 10 inches (25 cm), with white, waxy, fragrant tubular flowers hanging off arching stems.

PROPERTIES AND USES: Culpeper: '*Saturn owns the plant, for he loves his bones well. The root of Solomon's Seal is found by experience to be available in wounds, hurts, and outward sores, to heal and close up the lips of those that are green, and to dry up and restrain the flux of humours to those that are old. It is singularly good to stay vomitings and bleeding wheresoever, as also all fluxes in man or woman; also, to knit any joint, which by weakness uses to be often out of place, or will not stay in long when it is set; also to knit and join broken bones in any part of the body, the roots being bruised and applied to the places; yea, it hath been found by experience, and the decoction of the root in wine, or the bruised root put into wine or other drink, and after a night's infusion, strained forth hard and drank, hath helped both man and beast, whose bones hath been broken by any occasion, which is the most assured refuge of help to people of divers counties of the land that they can have. It is no less effectual to help ruptures and burstings, the decoction in wine, or the powder in broth or drink, being inwardly taken, and outwardly applied to the place. The same is also available for inward or outward bruises, falls or blows, both to dispel the congealed blood, and to take away both the pains and the black and blue marks that abide after the hurt. The same also, or the distilled water of the whole plant, used to the face, or other parts of the skin, cleanses it from morphew, freckles, spots, or marks whatsoever, leaving the place fresh, fair, and lovely; for which purpose it is much used by the Italian Dames.*'

It is astringent, demulcent and was used as a mucilaginous tonic, good in inflammations of the stomach and bowels, piles, and chronic dysentery. A strong decoction given every two or three hours was used to cure erysipelas (a skin infection), and the powdered roots made a poultice for bruises, piles,

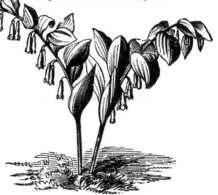

inflammations and tumours. The bruised roots were a popular cure for black eyes, mixed with cream. A decoction of the root in wine was recommended for people with broken bones, as Gerard wrote: *'As touching the knitting of bones and that truly which might be written, there is not another herb to be found comparable to it for the purposes aforesaid; and therefore in brief, if it be for bruises inward, the roots must be stamped, some ale or wine put thereto and strained and given to drink…as well unto themselves as to their cattle.'* According to traditional Chinese medical principles, *Polygonatum* has sweet and neutral properties, and is associated with the lung, heart, kidney and spleen meridians. Its main uses are to strengthen the spleen and stomach, thus improving appetite and reducing fatigue; to moisten the lungs by reducing coughs and expelling phlegm; and to strengthen the kidneys, helping reduce pain and weakness in the lower back. It is also used as a tonic herb, and has been used for respiratory and lung disorders, and to reduce inflammation. *Polygonatum* is also, in Chinese medicine, applied topically to treat bruises, skin ulcers and boils, haemorrhoids and oedema. The young shoots are an excellent vegetable when boiled and were commonly eaten like asparagus in Turkey.

HISTORY: In Galen's time, the distilled water was used as a cosmetic, to which Culpeper refers. Gerard rather more ungraciously notes: *'The roots of Solomon's Seal, stamped while it is fresh and green and applied, takes away in one night or two at the most, any bruise, black or blue spots*

gotten by falls or women's wilfulness in stumbling upon their hasty husband's fists, or such like.' The flowers and roots were used as snuff, and also had a wide vogue as aphrodisiacs, for love philtres and potions. Native North Americans made tea from the roots of *Polygonatum biflorum* (the New World close relative of *Polygonatum multiflorum*) for women's complaints and general internal pains. They also used the tea to counteract the pain caused by contact with poison ivy.

Approved by Solomon

The flat, round scars on the rootstocks are said to resemble a six-pointed seal, like the Star of David or Solomon's Biblical Seal. Another explanation is that these round depressions, or the marks which appear when the root is cut transversely, resemble Hebrew characters, and Solomon was said to have approved the plant's use as a poultice to help heal ('seal') broken limbs.

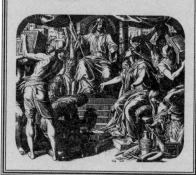

SORREL
RUMEX ACETOSA
Family Polygonaceae, Knotweed

OTHER NAMES: Narrow leaved dock, spinach dock, broad leafed sorrel, common sorrel, garden sorrel, meadow sorrel, green sauce, sour sabs, sour grabs, sour suds, sour sauce, cuckoo sorrow, cuckoo's meat. Although often called French sorrel, that is a close relative, buckler leaf sorrel, *Rumex scutatus.* Culpeper also mentions Wild Sorrel, which is sheep's sorrel, *Rumex acetosella.*

DESCRIPTION: This hardy perennial grows to 24 inches (60 cm) with a 24-inch (60-cm) spread, and has shield-shaped leaves up to 6 inches (15 cm) in length and whorled spikes of reddish-green flowers which turn purple. Its sourness is sharpest at the height of its growing season – before that it is almost tasteless.

PROPERTIES AND USES:
Culpeper tells us: '*Sorrel is prevalent in all hot diseases, to cool any inflammation and heat of blood in agues pestilential or choleric, or sickness or fainting, arising from heat, and to refresh the overspent spirits with the violence of furious or fiery fits of agues: to quench thirst, and procure an appetite in fainting or decaying stomachs: For it resists the putrefaction of the blood, kills worms, and is a cordial to the heart, which the seed doth more effectually, being more drying and binding, and thereby stays the humors of the bloody flux, or flux of the stomach…Both roots and seeds, as well as the herb, are held powerful to resist the poison of the scorpion…The leaves, wrapt in a colewort leaf and roasted in the embers, and applied to a large imposthume, botch boil, or plague-sore, doth both ripen and break it. The distilled water of the herb is of much good use for all the purposes aforesaid.'* When used as a dried herb, the leaves of the antioxidant plant have been used to treat itchy skin, fever, scurvy and ringworm. Sorrel can be cut thinly and sprinkled over soups and salads to help relieve these ailments. Sorrel is thought to cleanse the blood, and the leaves can be used as a poultice for acne or boils. Medicinally the tea has been used to treat kidney and liver ailments, and to help mouth ulcers. Sorrel tea is a popular and refreshing summer tea in Jamaica, but has to be sweetened to be palatable. When taken as tea, the herb can be helpful

---

Thirst Quencher
Sorrel is named from the French *surelle,* sour. Roman legionaries were said to suck on sorrel leaves when marching to prevent thirst.

in treating jaundice, kidney stones and rashes. When the leaves are consumed dry and fresh, it acts as a diuretic and can clear out the body's system, being said to 'cleanse' the prostate gland. The sorrel plant contains nutraceuticals, which can help prevent and treat several diseases including diabetes, hypertension, heart disease and cancer. The body's immune system is also enhanced due to its flavonoids, and sorrel contains high amounts of vitamin C, vitamin A, magnesium, calcium and potassium.

Maud Grieve in 1932 wrote that '… *in this country, the leaves are now rarely eaten, unless by children and rustics, to allay thirst, though in Ireland they are still largely consumed by the peasantry with fish and milk. Our country people used to beat the herb to a mash and take it mixed with vinegar and sugar, as a green sauce with cold meat, hence one of its popular names: Greensauce.*' However, sorrel is now a popular item of diet once more, the young leaves giving not just a slight acidity but also a hint of fresh apple or lemon flavour to salads. Because of their acidity, the leaves can be treated as spinach, and sorrel can be quickly heated by itself, without water, as an accompaniment to roast goose or pork, instead of apple sauce. The related *Rumex scutatus* is used by the French in their excellent sorrel soup.

HISTORY: Greeks, Egyptians and Romans ate sorrel as an appetite and digestion stimulant, and to counteract rich or fatty foods. In the Middle Ages, it was considered one of the finest vegetables but after

> ## Stain Remover
>
> The juice from crushed leaves can remove rust marks, mould and ink stains from furniture and clothes, wicker and silver. In the past, when lemons were very expensive, the lemon flavour of sorrel was a good substitute for lemon juice.

the introduction of French sorrel, with its large succulent leaves, it gradually lost its position as a salad and a potherb. John Evelyn (1620–1706), the English diarist and cultivator of gardens, wrote in 1720: '*Sorrel sharpens the appetite, assuages heat, cools the liver and strengthens the heart; is an antiscorbutic, resisting putrefaction and in the making of sallets [salads] imparts a grateful quickness to the rest as supplying the want of oranges and lemons. Together with salt, it gives both the name and the relish to sallets from the sapidity, which renders not plants and herbs only, but men themselves pleasant and agreeable.*' The plant is also called *cuckoo's meat* from an old belief that the bird cleared its voice by eating sorrel.

SOUTHERNWOOD

ARTEMISIA ABROTANUM
Family Asteraceae/Compositae, Aster/Daisy

OTHER NAMES: Garden Southernwood, Old Man Tree (Culpeper). Old man, boy's love, lad's love, lover's plant, miss-in-my-corner, apple ringie, appleringie, garderobe, our lord's wood, maid's ruin, maiden's ruin, garden sagebrush, European sage, lad's love, southern wormwood, lemon plant, sitherwood.

DESCRIPTION: Hardy evergreen bushy shrub with a spread up to 3 feet (90 cm). Tiny yellow flowers form dense panicles and the feathery grey-green leaves are camphor/lemon scented.

PROPERTIES AND USES:
'*Government and virtues. It is a gallant mercurial plant, worthy of more esteem than it hath. Dioscorides says that the seed bruised, heated in warm water, and drank, helps those that are bursting, or troubled with cramps or convulsions of the sinews, the sciatica, or difficulty in making water, and bringing down women's courses. The same taken in wine is an antidote, or counter-poison against all deadly poison, and drives away serpents and other venomous creatures; as also the smell of the herb, being burnt, doth the same. The oil thereof anointed on the back-bone before the fits of agues come, takes them away. It takes away inflammations in the eyes, if it be put with some part of a roasted quince, and boiled with a few crumbs of bread, and applied. Boiled with barley-meal it takes away pimples, pushes or wheals that arise in the face, or other parts of the body.*

The seed as well as the dried herb, is often given to kill the worms in children. The herb bruised and laid to, helps to draw forth splinters and thorns out of the flesh. The ashes thereof dries up and heals old ulcers, that are without inflammation, although by the sharpness thereof it bites sore, and puts them to sore pains; as also the sores in the privy parts of man or woman. The ashes mingled with old salad oil, helps those that have hair fallen, and are bald, causing the hair to grow again either on the head or beard. It is a powerful diuretic, and good in hysteric complaints; for this purpose, the best way of taking it is in a conserve, made with the young tops, and twice their weight of sugar. A strong decoction of the leaves is a good worm medicine, but it is a very disagreeable and nauseous one. The leaves are likewise a good ingredient in fomentations for easing pain, dispersing swellings, or stopping the progress

---

Quick Love

According to the starchild.co.uk website: '*Southernwood was said to attract "quick love" and a sprig placed beneath the pillow could counteract any evil spells intended to hinder successful cohabitation. A man could win a girl's affection if he managed to secretly place a sprig of Southernwood beneath her apron. However, the affections would not last long and would turn to hatred in a few years.*'

of gangrene.' – Culpeper. It was used as a bitter digestive tonic, emmenagogue (to stimulate menstrusation), anthelmintic (antiworm treatment), antiseptic and uterine stimulant, according to Maud Grieve. Southernwood was used to treat liver, spleen and stomach problems and encourage menstruation. The leaves can be mixed with other herbs in aromatic baths and are said to counter drowsiness. An infusion of the leaves can act as a natural insect repellent when applied to the skin, and as a hair rinse is said to combat dandruff. Burned as incense, in magical lore, southernwood guards against trouble of all kinds. It has been used as a culinary herb with greasy meats. The foliage is used in aromatic vinegars, floral waters and pot-pourris. A yellow dye can be extracted from the branches of the plant, for use with wool.

HISTORY: The genus *Artemisia* was named for the Greek goddess Artemis. Historically southernwood was used as an air freshener or strewing herb, and the Greeks and Romans used the leaves in love potions, and placed the leaves in their bedding to rouse lust. Later users also thought it protected against impotence,

Moth Repellent

The leaves are an excellent mosquito repellent when rubbed on the skin, and are also one of the best natural moth and insect repellents. The French call it *garderobe* (to guard, or preserve, clothes) because when it is laid among clothes, it repels moths. It became customary to lay sprays of the dried herb amongst clothes in drawers, or hang them in closets and wardrobes.

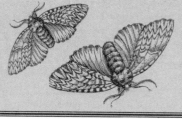

hence the later name of *lovers' plant*. Such was its reputation for increasing virility that teenage boys rubbed an ointment on their cheeks to speed up the growth of facial hair. The common nicknames of *lad's love* and *maiden's ruin* refer to the habit of including a spray of the plant in country bouquets presented by young men to their fancied ladies in order to seduce them. Southernwood was traditionally believed to ward off infection and, up until the early 18th century, a bunch of southernwood and rue was placed at the side of a prisoner in the dock to prevent the contagion of jail fever. Women carried sprigs of the herb for its pungent fragrance, which they hoped might keep them awake during church services. It has been used as a wash for wounds and ulcers.

(FIELD) SOUTHERNWOOD

ARTEMISIA CAMPESTRIS
Family Asteraceae, Aster/Daisy

OTHER NAMES: Field wormwood, tall wormwood, sand wormwood, beach wormwood, northern wormwood, Pacific wormwood, boreal wormwood, field sagewort, field mugwort, wild sage (USA).

DESCRIPTION: A non-aromatic perennial with a branched creeping woody stock, rare in the UK and consequently a protected plant. The greyish-green leaves are oblong, and the small brown flowers stand in thick spikes at the tops of the branches.

PROPERTIES AND USES: Culpeper notes: '*Government and virtues. It is a powerful diuretic, and is good in hysteric cases. The best way of using it is in conserve made of the fresh tops, beaten up with twice their weight of sugar. It is a Mercurial plant, and worthy of more esteem that it has. It wants but to be more known to be very highly prized, having a fine, pleasant, warm, aromatic taste, with a little bitterness, but not enough to be disagreeable: it is best given in the form of conserve, and with a great deal of success in weaknesses of the stomach. The manner is thus:- Clip four ounces of the leaves fine, and beat them in a mortar, with six ounces of loaf sugar, till the whole is like a paste; three times a day take the bigness of a nutmeg of this; it is pleasant, and very effectual; and one thing in its favour is particular, it is a composer, and always disposes to sleep. Opiates weaken the stomach, and must not be given often where their assistance is wished for; this possesses the soothing quality without the mischief. This quality is not singular to this plant; the columba is a bitter and an opiate, and thus nature mixes powers which to us appear contradictory.*'
This species of *Artemisia* has the same qualities, to a lesser degree, as the garden southernwood, and Linnaeus recommended an infusion of it to alleviate pleurisy.

HISTORY: Dr John Hill in *The British Herbal* of 1756 says that it has a '*warm, fine, pleasant, aromatic taste, with a little bitterness, not enough to be disagreeable. It wants but to be more common and more known to be very highly valued…*' The leaves were chewed in order to treat stomach problems.

Tribal Treatments

The plant was used by some Native North American tribes as an abortifacient to terminate difficult pregnancies. The Lakota people pulverized the roots for use as perfume and also put crushed roots on the face of a sleeping man so he would not wake up while his horses were stolen. A tea from the roots was used for the treatment of those who cannot urinate.

(GERMANDER) SPEEDWELL

VERONICA CHAMAEDRYS
Family Plantaginaceae, Plantain

OTHER NAMES: Bird's eye speedwell, veronica, Paul's betony, eye of Christ, angels' eyes, cat's eye, bird's eye, farewell, goodbye, fluellin, fluellin the male, fluellen (all from the Welsh, llysiau Llewelyn), rhwyddlwyn (Welsh), groundhele, common gypsyweed. There is a similar speedwell, common speedwell, *Veronica officinalis*, but which is not as common as germander speedwell, despite its name.

DESCRIPTION: Small plant forming clumps with pale blue flowers with four petals and a white eye.

PROPERTIES AND USES: Culpeper: '*Venus governs this plant and it is also reckoned among the vulnerary plants, both used inwardly and outwardly: it is likewise pectoral, and good for coughs and consumptions; and is helpful against the stone and strangury, as also against pestilential fevers. An infusion of the leaves, drank constantly in the manner of tea, is greatly recommended as a provocative to venery, and a strengthener; it has been called a cure for barrenness, taken a long time in this manner.*' Speedwell can be used in herbal tea cough remedies as an expectorant, and according to Maud Grieve in 1931 has diaphoretic (sweat-producing), diuretic and tonic properties. Germander speedwell is rich in tannins and its glycoside content has anti-inflammatory, diuretic and liver protective actions. Speedwell extracts are added to skin ointments to treat eczema and help heal skin irritations and wounds.

HISTORY: Ancient writers regard highly the virtues of the speedwell as a vulnerary (wound healer), a blood purifier and a remedy in various skin diseases, its outward application being considered efficacious for the 'itch'. It was also believed to cure smallpox and measles, and to be a panacea for many ills. Gerard recommended it for cancer, '*given in good broth of a hen*', and advocated the use of the root as a specific against pestilential fevers. Its blossoms wilt very quickly after picking, so in Germany it is known ironically as '*Maennertreu*' (men's faithfulness). A common medieval benediction to a friend was either 'forget me not' or 'speedwell'/'farewell' (or 'speed thee well'/'fare thee well'), equivalent to today's 'goodbye' or 'see you soon'. Sometimes such language was accompanied with parting gifts of small blue flowers. It was actually the germander speedwell that in literature and botany was most commonly known as the 'forget-me-not' for hundreds of years, until around 1880. When the *Mayflower* and her sister ships were launched, '*Speedwell*' was considered the 'luckiest' name for a vessel.

SPIGNEL

MEUM ATHAMANTICUM
Family Apiaceae, Umbellifers

OTHER NAMES: Wood spignel, spicknel, spikenel, baldmoney, mew, meu, bearwort (USA).

DESCRIPTION: This aromatic northern plant has cloud-like flowerheads arranged in rayed umbels of white or pinkish florets. The unusual feathery, dark green leaves give off a strong aroma similar to curry when crushed. As with most plants, Culpeper describes it in great detail.

PROPERTIES AND USES:
Culpeper writes: '*It grows wild in Lancashire, Yorkshire, and other northern counties, and is also planted in gardens. Government and virtues. It is an herb of Venus. Galen says, the roots of Spignel are available to provoke urine, and women's courses; but if too much thereof be taken, it causes head-ache. The roots boiled in wine or water, and drank, helps the stranguary and stoppings of the urine, the wind, swellings and pains in the stomach, pains of the mother, and all joint-aches. If the powder of the root be mixed with honey, and the same taken as a licking medicine, it breaks tough phlegm, and dries up the rheum that falls on the lungs. The roots are accounted very effectual against the stinging or biting of any venomous creature, and is one of the ingredients in Mithridate and other antidotes of the same.*'

HISTORY: The name *baldmoney* is said to be a corruption of Balder, the god of the old Norse and German religions, to whom the plant was dedicated. *Spicknel* is derived from spike nail, a large, long nail, an allusion to the shape of the plant's capillary leaves. The roots have sometimes been eaten in the Scottish Highlands as a vegetable. The seeds have been used as substitutes for pepper, or other pungent aromatics.

Spignel produces grooved fruits which taste strongly of curry, so it was an unpopular plant with dairy farmers as it flavoured the milk.

Bärwurz

Many of the herbs in this book are used in local alcoholic specialities. Bärwurz is an excellent distilled spirit made in Lower Bavaria from the root of the baldmoney or spignel plant. It is colourless, clear and its typical aroma is marketed as '*reminiscent of forests and moss*'. Bärwurz is mainly bottled in slim, brown, earthenware bottles and said to have a beneficial effect on the stomach. Its makers claim that Bärwurz relieves the bloated sensation following a large meal, which is why it is popular as a digestive schnapps.

SPINACH

SPINACIA OLERACEAE
Family Amaranthaceae, Amaranth

OTHER NAMES: Culpeper calls this plant Spinage.

DESCRIPTION: An edible flowering plant growing to a height of around 1 foot (30 cm), with triangular leaves.

PROPERTIES AND USES: Culpeper writes: '*It is more used for food than medicine, being a good boiled salad, and much eaten in the spring, being useful to temper the heat and sharpness of the humours; it is cooling and moistening, diuretic, and renders the body soluble.*' It is more nourishing than other green vegetables, being valuable for anaemia sufferers because of its high iron and chlorophyll content. Chlorophyll is known to have a chemical formula remarkably similar to that of haemoglobin, and it is stated that the ingestion of chlorophyll will raise the haemoglobin of the blood without increasing the formed elements. The plant contains from 10 to 20 parts per 1000 by weight of chlorophyll. It is rich in vitamin A, and is thought to speed recovery after a heart attack. Spinach was the first vegetable to be frozen and sold commercially, by American inventor Clarence Birdseye in 1930.

HISTORY: The word spinach is derived from the Farsi (Persian) *aspanakh*, meaning 'green hand'. It was introduced into China from Persia via Nepal around 647 CE, and was known as 'the Persian vegetable.' Cultivated for over 2000 years and probably of Persian origin, spinach was not introduced into Europe until the ninth century, when the Saracens invaded Sicily. During the First World War, wine fortified with spinach juice was given to French soldiers weakened by haemorrhage. The plant is mentioned in 1390 in the first known English cookbook, *The Forme of Cury*, where it is called *spinnedge* or *spynoches*. Catherine de' Medici was queen of France from 1547 to 1559 and asked for spinach to be served at every meal. This is why culinary dishes containing spinach are known as '*Florentine*', reflecting the place of her birth. The cartoon character *Popeye the Sailor Man* dates from 1929 and is represented as having superhuman powers whenever he eats spinach, because of its high iron content. However, it appears that a German scientist named von Wolf misplaced a decimal point when measuring the iron content in 1870, an error which multiplied its iron content tenfold. His error was not discovered and rectified until the 1930s by which time Popeye was already well established as a popular character.

STOCK GILLIFLOWER

MATTHIOLA INCANA
Family Brassicaceae, Cabbage

OTHER NAMES: Culpeper also calls it the Castle Gilliflower and the Great Castle Gilliflower. Brompton stock, cluster-leaved stock, common stock, hoary stock, hopes, queen's stock, wallflower stock, tenweeks stock.

DESCRIPTION:
A bushy annual or short-lived perennial, 2 feet (60 cm) tall, with grey-green, lance-shaped leaves. The oldest variety bears spikes of fragrant four-petalled, light purple flowers; Culpeper mentions white, pink and scarlet flowers, but there are now even more colours available. The name '*hoary stock*' refers to the grey tinge on the leaves.

PROPERTIES AND USES: Culpeper referred to them as being garden flowers: '*They are of temperature hot and dry, of a similar nature with the yellow or wall gilliflowers, and are plants of Mercury. The flowers of the stock gillyflower, boiled in water and drunk, are good to remedy all difficulty of breathing, and help the cough, They also promote the menses and urine, and, by bathing or sitting over the decoction, it causes perspiration.*'

HISTORY: In addition Culpeper mentions an annual 'Small Stock Gilliflower' – '*...leucoion or "white violets", because the leaves are white; the leaves of the flowers are of various colours, and called by some writers dames matronales,*

or dames violets.' It grows about 1 foot (30 cm) high, and is *Hesperis matronalis (alba)*, known as dames rocket, sweet rocket, white sweet rocket (in white form), mother of the evening, damask violet, dames-wort, dame's gilliflower, night-scented gilliflower, winter gillflower, summer lilac or queen's gilliflower, the latter as it was the favourite flower of Marie Antoinette. The genus name *Hesperis* is Greek for evening, as the flower's clove scent becomes more noticeable then, and *matronalis* refers to mother. In *The Great Herball, or Generall Historie of Plantes* by John Gerard (1597) it is listed under the name *Dames Violets* or *Queens Gillofloures*. Gerard remarked that it was grown in gardens '*for the beauty of their floures...The distilled water of the floures hereof is counted to be a most effectuall thing to procure a sweat*', implying that it was used to help break a fever. Dames rocket was taken to America in the 1700s and has naturalized, being a prolific seed producer.

Gilliflower Names

Culpeper describes several 'gilliflowers'. His 'Clove Gilliflower' is the carnation, *Dianthus caryophyllus*, and his 'Wall, or Yellow Gilliflower' is the wallflower, *Erysimum cheiri*.

(COMMON) STONECROP

SEDUM ACRE
Family Crassulaceae, Orpine

OTHER NAMES: Biting stonecrop, golden moss, wall ginger, wallpepper, gold chain, creeping Tom, mousetail, Jack-of-the-buttery, bird bread (the French also call it pain d'oiseau).

DESCRIPTION: It is the commonest of the stonecrops, forming tufts or cushions, 3–10 inches (8–25 cm) across, which in June and July are a mass of golden star-like flowers.

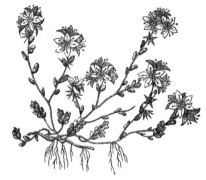

PROPERTIES AND USES: Some writers considered biting stonecrop to possess considerable virtues, but others, because of the long-lasting effects of its acridity (biting quality), thought it unsafe to be administered. Culpeper noted: '*Its qualities are directly opposite to the other Sedums, and more apt to raise inflammations than to cure them; it ought not to be put into any ointment, nor any other medicine.*' However, he considered it good for scurvy both inwardly in decoction and outwardly, and also commended it for king's evil (scrofula).

Other herbalists recommended it for some scorbutic diseases, when properly and carefully used, recommending it in the form of a gargle for scurvy of the gums, and as a lotion for scrofulous ulcers. It has been used to treat intermittent fevers and dropsy. In large doses it is emetic and cathartic, and applied externally will sometimes produce blisters. The herb has been used as an astringent, hypotensive (to lower blood pressure), laxative, rubefacient (increasing blood flow to the skin), vermifuge and vulnerary (wound healing). A homeopathic remedy is made from the plant, used in the treatment of piles and anal irritations.

HISTORY: Pliny recommended common stonecrop to help one sleep, for which purpose it must be wrapped in a black cloth and placed under the pillow of the patient, without his knowing it, otherwise it will not be effective. The pungency of the leaves has given its specific name of *acre*, and the popular English names of *wallpepper* and *wall ginger*. Gerard tells us it was called *mousetail*, or *Jack of the butterie*. Dr Fernie wrote: '...*this and the Sedums album and reflexum were ingredients in a famous worm-expelling medicine or "theriac" (treacle), and "Jack of the Buttery" is a corruption of Bot. theriaque.*' Matthias de Lobel called it *vermicularis*, partly because of the grub-like shape of the leaves, and partly from its medical efficacy as a vermifuge (to expel intestinal worms).

(ORPINE) STONECROP

SEDUM (or HYLOTELEPHIUM) TELEPHIUM
Family Crassulaceae, Orpine

OTHER NAMES: Culpeper calls it Orpine. Live long, life everlasting, frog's stomach, harping Johnny, live forever, midsummer men, orphan John, witch's moneybags, herbe aux charpentiers.

DESCRIPTION: A succulent groundcover, and the largest British species of *Sedum*, it is readily distinguished from most allied plants by its large, broad, flattened leaves. It has pinkish red flowers, and can grow from 1–3 feet (30–90 cm) in height.

PROPERTIES AND USES: Culpeper: '*Orpine is seldom used in inward medicines with us, although Tragus saith from experience in Germany, that the distilled water thereof is profitable for gnawings or excoriations in the stomach or bowels, or for ulcers in the lungs, liver, or other inward parts, as also in the matrix, and helps all those diseases, being drank for certain days together. It stays the sharpness of humours in the bloody-flux, and other fluxes in the body, or in wounds. The root thereof also performs the like effect. It is used outwardly to cool any heat or inflammation upon any hurt or wound, and eases the pains of them; as, also, to heal scaldings or burnings, the juice thereof being beaten with some green salad oil, and anointed. The leaf bruised, and laid to any green wound in the hand or legs, doth heal them quickly; and being bound to the throat much helps the quinsy; it helps also* ruptures and burstenness. If you please to make the juice thereof into a syrup with honey or sugar, you may safely take a spoonful or two at a time, (let my author say what he will) for a quinsy, and you shall find the medicine pleasant, and the cure speedy.' The leaves have sometimes been used as a salad, like the other sedums, and sheep and goats eat it, but horses will refuse it.

HISTORY: Its hold on life has earned it the names of *live long* and *life everlasting*, as it stays fresh for a long time after being gathered, living on the store of nourishment in its fleshy leaves and swollen roots. It was as a popular remedy for diarrhoea, kidney problems, piles and haemorrhages.

Colour Confusion

Its name is derived from Telephus, the son of the Greek mythological hero Heracles, who is said to have discovered its virtues. Its most familiar English name, *orpine*, is derived from *auripigmentum*, the gold-coloured pigment called *orpiment*, or *orpin*, a yellow sulphur compound of the metal arsenic. The name might have been appropriate for the brilliant yellow flowers of other sedums, but is out of place applied to the crimson blossoms of orpine stonecrop.

(WHITE) STONECROP

SEDUM ALBUM
Family Crassulaceae, Orpine

OTHER NAMES: Culpeper calls it the Small Houseleek, Prick-Madam and Wall Pepper.

DESCRIPTION: It has prostrate bulbous cylindrical leaves, and 6–10 inch (15–25 cm) stems with small white star-like flowers. There is also an earlier flowering white stonecrop, *Sedum anglicum*.

PROPERTIES AND USES:
Culpeper observes: *'It is under the dominion of the Moon, cold in quality, and something binding, and therefore very good to stay defluxions, especially such as fall upon the eyes. It stops bleeding, both inward and outward, helps cankers, and all fretting sores and ulcers; it abates the heat of choler, thereby preventing diseases arising from choleric humours. It expels poison much, resists pestilential fevers, being exceeding good also for tertian agues. You may drink the decoction of it, if you please, for all the foregoing infirmities. It is so harmless an herb, you can scarce use it amiss. Being bruised and applied to the place, it helps the king's evil* [scrofula], *and any other knots or kernels in the flesh; as also the piles, but it should be used with caution. It is also so very acid that it will raise blisters, if applied externally to the skin. The juice taken inwardly excites vomiting. In scorbutic cases, and quartan agues, it is a most excellent medicine, under proper management. A decoction of it is good for sore mouths, arising from a scorbutic taint in the constitution. The leaves bruised and applied to the skin, are excellent in paralytic contractions of the limbs'.*

HISTORY: The older herbalists considered the white stonecrop to possess all the virtues of the houseleek. The leaves and stalks were recommended for all kinds of inflammation, being applied as a cooling plaster to painful haemorrhoids. It was also custom to prepare and eat it as a pickle, in the same way as samphire.

Getting Acclimatized

This plant can acclimatize according to the environment in which it grows. If one compares a plant growing on top of a wall, with less water and fewer nutrients, to one growing in the earth at the bottom of the wall with more water and nutrients, the ground-based stonecrop will be faster-growing and larger. The plant on top of the wall may be red in colour because of lack of water, which causes it to synthesize carotenoids to protect itself from the effects of photoinhibition (a reduction in the process of photosynthesis).

STRAWBERRY

FRAGARIA VESCA
Family Rosaceae, Rose

OTHER NAMES: Woodland strawberry, wild (European) strawberry, European strawberry, alpine strawberry. What we know as the cultivated garden strawberry, much larger, did not become common until the 18th century.

DESCRIPTION: Height up to 12 inches (30 cm) in grassy hedges, with trifoliate leaves and small white flowers with yellow centres followed by the fruits, which have their seeds on the outside.

PROPERTIES AND USES: Culpeper: '*Venus owns the herb. Strawberries, when they are green, are cool and dry; but when they are ripe, they are cool and moist. The berries are excellently good to cool the liver, the blood, and the spleen, or an hot choleric stomach; to refresh and comfort the fainting spirits, and quench thirst. They are good also for other inflammations; yet it is not amiss to refrain from them in a fever, lest by their putrefying in the stomach they increase the fits. The leaves and roots boiled in wine and water, and drank, do likewise cool the liver and blood, and assuage all inflammations in the reins and bladder, provoke urine, and allay the heat and sharpness thereof. The same also being drank stays the bloody flux and women's courses, and helps the swelling of the spleen. The water of the Berries carefully distilled, is a sovereign remedy and cordial in the panting and beating of the heart, and is good for the yellow jaundice. The juice dropped into foul ulcers, or they washed therewith, or the decoction of the herb and root, doth wonderfully cleanse and help to cure them. Lotions and gargles for sore mouths, or ulcers therein, or in the privy parts or elsewhere, are made with the leaves and roots thereof; which is also good to fasten loose teeth, and to heal spongy foul gums. It helps also to stay catarrhs, or defluxions of rheum in the mouth, throat, teeth, or eyes. The juice or water is singularly good for hot and red inflamed eyes, if dropped into them, or they bathed*

A Tangle of Strawberries

Some people believe that the name strawberry is derived from the habit of placing straw under the cultivated plants when the berries are ripening, to keep garden pests away. The name in fact comes from the past historic tense '*straw*' of the verb '*strew*'. It refers to the tangle of vines with which the strawberry strews or stretches over the ground.

therewith. It is also of excellent property for all pushes, wheals and other breakings forth of hot and sharp humours in the face and hands, and other parts of the body, to bathe them therewith, and to take away any redness in the face, or spots, or other deformities in the skin, and to make it clear and smooth. Some use this medicine: Take so many Strawberries as you shall think fitting, and put them into a distillatory, or body of glass fit for them, which being well closed, set it in a bed of horse dung for your use. It is an excellent water for hot inflamed eyes, and to take away a film or skin that begins to grow over them.' The trifoliate leaves can be used in salad or make a tea, which can be also used as a gargle for sore throats. The fruit is a diuretic, laxative and astringent and was used by those suffering with rheumatic gout. The root is astringent and used in diarrhoea. There is a common allergy to strawberries.

HISTORY: The earliest mention of the strawberry in England is in a tenth-century Saxon plant list, and in 1265 the 'straberie' is mentioned in the household roll of the Countess of Leicester. 'Strawberry ripe' was a favourite cry of street vendors in the 15th century as they offered the fresh fruit for sale. Ben Jonson, in his unfinished play *The Sad Shepherd* writes: *'My Son hath sent you / A pot of Strawberries, gathered i' the wood / (His Hogs would else have rooted up, or trod) / With a choice dish of wildings* [crab apples] *here, to scald / And mingle with your Cream.'* Linnaeus is said to have discovered and proved the efficacy of strawberries as a cure for rheumatic gout.

Whiten Your Teeth with Strawberries

The fruit helps to stop teeth discoloration as it contains malic acid. Mash a strawberry to a pulp, mix with half a teaspoon of baking soda, and use a toothbrush to spread the paste over your teeth, especially any stained areas. Leave this mixture on for five minutes, then remove with a fresh toothbrush to clean the stains off the teeth. Repeat once a week, and in four to five weeks there should be a noticeable difference. Cost – virtually nothing – as opposed to hundreds of pounds at a dental clinic. Also a cut strawberry rubbed over the face immediately after washing will whiten the skin and remove slight sunburn.

For a badly sunburnt face, however, it is recommended that you should rub the juice well into the skin, leave it on for half an hour, and then wash off with warm, soap-less water.

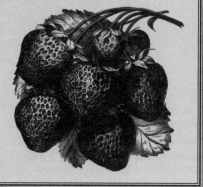

SUNDEW

DROSERA ROTUNDIFOLIA
Family Droseraceae, Sundew

OTHER NAMES: Common sundew, round-leaved sundew, dew plant, red rot, herba rosellae.

DESCRIPTION: A small insectivorous plant 2–6 inches (5–15 cm) high, found around ponds, bogs and rivers, where the soil is peaty. Its leaves have a covering of sticky red glandular hairs, and its white flowers only open in sunshine. In winter, sundew produces a *hibernaculum* (a protective bud of tightly curled leaves at ground level) to survive the cold.

PROPERTIES AND USES: Culpeper tells us: *'The Sun rules it, and it is under the sign Cancer. Some authors gravely tell us that a water distilled from this plant is highly cordial and restorative; but it is more than probable that it never deserved the character given of it in that respect. The leaves, bruised and applied to the skin, erode it, and bring on such inflammations as are not easily removed. The ladies in some parts mix the juice with milk, as to make an innocent and safe application for the removal of freckles, sun-burn, and other discolourings of the skin. The juice, unmixed, will destroy warts and corns, if a little of it be frequently put upon them. These are effects which pronounce its internal use to be dangerous; and if it is not productive of bad consequences, when distilled with other ingredients, for cordial waters, &c, it is because its pernicious qualities are not of a nature to rise in distillation.'* It relaxes the muscles of the respiratory tract, easing breathing and relieving wheezing and so is of great value in the treatment of various chest complaints. Sundew has been used for whooping cough, incipient phthisis (early tuberculosis), chronic bronchitis and asthma. Sundew juice, mixed with thyme in a syrup, is a remedy for children's coughs. The juice is said to take away corns and warts, and in America it has been advocated as a cure for old age. The flowering plant is said to be antibacterial, antibiotic, antispasmodic, antitussive (cough suppressant), demulcent, expectorant and hypoglycaemic (raising blood sugar levels), as well as having aphrodisiac properties. It has also been used to treat sunburn, toothache and prevent freckles.

HISTORY: In the 12th century, Italian herbalists were using sundew as a herbal remedy for coughs, naming it *herba sole* (sun herb), and for the following centuries it was used in cough preparations across Europe. At the same time, alchemists and scholars of the Medical School of Salerno had identified the sundew flower as beneficial in the cure of whooping cough and also effective as an aphrodisiac. It is now known that the sundew contains carotenoids that enhance the function of

Coming to a Sticky End

The moment a small insect alights upon a leaf of sundew, it is hopelessly trapped. At the base of the plant's long flowering stems are dish-shaped leaves covered with hairs that exude a mucilage at their tips. In sunshine this sap sparkles and attracts insects. Upon an insect's touch, the hairs bend in and down upon the creature. According to Charles Darwin, the mere contact of the legs of a small gnat with a single tentacle is enough to induce this response. All species of sundew are able to move their tentacles in response to contact with digestible prey. The tentacles are extremely sensitive and will bend towards the centre of the leaf in order to bring the insect into contact with as many stalked glands as possible. Eventually, the prey either succumbs to death through exhaustion or through asphyxiation as the mucilage envelops them and clogs their spiracles. Death usually occurs within a quarter of an hour and additional amounts of sap, which contains digestive enzymes, then convert the insect's protein into a nutrient soup to sustain the plant. The nutrients are absorbed through the leaf surface and used to help fuel plant growth.

the immune and reproductive systems, its flavonoids have beneficial antioxidant effects and its vitamins are helpful for coughs, lung infections, asthma and other

Dew of the Sun

Each leaf hair has a small gland at the top containing a sticky fluid which looks like a glistening dewdrop, hence its name, sundew, derived from Latin *ros solis*, meaning dew of the sun. Sundews are adapted to living on wet boggy soil, which does not contain the nutrients needed for their survival, so they are carnivorous, feeding on small insects that are attracted by their bright colour and sugary secretions.

conditions. When the infusion of Ros Solis (sundew) was prepared in Salerno, because of its therapeutic attributes and pleasant taste, '*Rosolio*' became sought-after in all European courts. As early as the 13th century, alchemists also noted positive results from the use of sundew's sap in the treatment of consumption, or tuberculosis. In the 16th century John Gerard observed in his *Herball* that '*physicians have thought this herb to be a rare and singular remedy for all those that be in a consumption of the lungs*'. Sundew tea was recommended for bronchitis, whooping cough, asthma and dry coughs, and recent studies have confirmed its efficacy as a cough suppressant. It is also used today in treatments for lung infections and stomach ulcers, and is a listed ingredient in around 250 registered medications. A purple or yellow dye was prepared in the Scottish Highlands from sundew plants.

SWEET CICELY

MYRRHIS ODORATA
Family Apiaceae/Umbelliferae, Parsley/Umbellifers

OTHER NAMES: Sweet chervil, anise cicely, English cicely, Spanish chervil, anise chervil, garden myrrh, sweet-scented myrrh, British myrrh, great chervil, smooth cicely, sweet bracken, sweet-fern, sweet-humlock, sweets, the Roman plant, shepherd's needle, smoother cicely, cow chervil.

DESCRIPTION: A hardy perennial, it grows 3–5 feet (90–150 cm) tall and spreads 2 feet (60 cm). It has large, flat umbels of sweetly scented, frothy cream flowers. The leaves are finely divided and feathery. There is a strong fragrance, reminiscent of liquorice, anise or myrrh.

PROPERTIES AND USES: Culpeper: *'This whole plant, besides its pleasantness in salads, hath its physical virtue. The root boiled and eaten with oil and vinegar, (or without oil) do much please and warm old and cold stomachs oppressed with wind or phlegm, or those that have the phthisic* [tuberculosis] *or consumption of the lungs. The same drank with wine is a preservation from the plague. It provokes women's courses, and expels the after-birth, procures an appetite to meat, and expels wind. The juice is good to heal the ulcers of the head and face; the candied roots hereof are held as effectual as angelica, to preserve from infection in the time of a plague, and to warm and comfort a cold weak stomach.*

It is so harmless, you cannot use it amiss.' Its leaves taste strongly of a cross between aniseed and parsley. The boiled roots were chewed to freshen the breath, and the flowers can be made into a cordial, like those of elderflower. The plant has been used as a herbal tonic, for coughs and for digestive problems and all parts can be eaten.

HISTORY: Cicely derives from the obscure Greek plant name *seselis*, which was seemingly used as a collective term for a number of umbelliferous herbs. The botanical genus name *Myrrhis* is Greek and denotes both an unidentified plant and an aromatic oil from western Asia. The scientific species name *odoratus* is Latin, meaning scented. *'Sweet Chervil or Sweet Cis is so like in taste unto Anis seede that it much delighteth the taste among other herbs in a sallet* [salad]' – John Parkinson, *Paradisus* (1629). A decoction was used to treat the bites of snakes and mad dogs.

Many Uses

It is the sole species in the genus *Myrrhis*. Like its relatives anise, fennel, and caraway, sweet cicely can also be used to flavour aquavit. The roots can make a wine, and the crushed seeds were used as a furniture polish, especially for oak.

SWEET FLAG

ACORUS CALAMUS
Family Acoraceae (formerly Araceae), Palm

OTHER NAMES: Calamus (from the Greek for reed), sweet sedge, sweet myrtle, sweet flag, sweet rush, sweet grass, sweet root, sweet calomel, sweet cane, myrtle grass, myrtle sedge, cinnamon sedge, gladdon, flagroot, beewort. Culpeper calls it Sweet-Smelling Reed, Aromatical Reed, True Acorus and Calamus Aromaticus.

DESCRIPTION: It is a vigorous, reed-like, aquatic plant with sword-shaped leaves and small yellow and green flowers on a fleshy, cane-like stalk. It can reach to 5 feet (1.5 m), and although it resembles 'yellow flag' iris, a member of the lily family and the reason calamus is called *sweet flag*, it is actually a member of the palm family.

PROPERTIES AND USES: Culpeper recommended calamus as a '*strengthener of the stomach and head.*' It has been used since ancient times for its effects on the digestive system and the lungs. It is said that the herb eliminates phlegm and tranquillizes the mind, and sweet flag has been used to treat amnesia, heart palpitations, insomnia, tinnitus,

chronic bronchitis and bronchial asthma. In Europe it is used as a digestive aid, helping to counter acidity and ease heartburn and dyspepsia. The sweet-scented roots and leaves are used in perfumes, and its pungent, cinnamon-spicy qualities add flavour to sweets, medicines, beers, gins and schnapps.

HISTORY: Sweet flag was brought to Europe by the Tartars in the 13th century, and it is one of the herbs mentioned in the book of Exodus. Dioscorides prescribed it for eye problems, and '*Acorus*' is derived from the Greek word '*acoron*', the adjectival form of '*coreon*' (pupil), because it was used as a treatment for inflammation of the eye. *Acorus calamus* was used as a popular '*strewing herb*' to ward off disease and to add a pleasing fragrance to churches and houses. Native North Americans had so many medicinal uses for calamus that it was actually considered a commodity and medium of exchange. Some Native Americans used the herb to increase strength and endurance, while others used it as a digestive aid and to help improve mental clarity and sharpness (echoing Culpeper's beliefs). Calamus is thought to be a parasiticide, so has been used to destroy and expel parasites from the intestines. An insecticide is also made from the essential oil. Calamus has also been used to stimulate and regulate menstrual flow, and externally applied to relieve burns, skin problems, eruptions and neuralgia.

No Smoking

The powdered root of calamus was formerly smoked or chewed. It was thought to destroy the taste for tobacco, and thus discourage and break the smoking habit.

SWEET WOODRUFF

GALIUM ODORATUM (formerly ASPERULA ODORATA)
Family Rubiaceae, Madder/Bedstraw/Coffee

OTHER NAMES: Wild baby's breath, master of the woods new mowed hay, woodrove, ladies in the hay, Waldmeister (German for master of the woods), woodward, kiss me quick.

DESCRIPTION: With white star-shaped flowers and a trailing stem, it only grows to 6 inches (15 cm) tall but spreads to 12 inches (30 cm) or more. It often forms carpets in beech woods, and is excellent ground cover under trees and shrubs in gardens.

PROPERTIES AND USES: Culpeper related that sweet woodruff was a restorative herb, good for people suffering from consumption. He wrote that it was also good for opening obstructions in the liver and spleen and as a provocative to venery, i.e. an aphrodisiac. Sweet woodruff contains medicinally active compounds such as coumarin, tannins, anthraquinones and iridoids. Some properties are anticoagulant, so woodruff has been used to counteract blood clotting and for varicose vein sufferers. It has also been used as a tonic tea for anxiety or insomnia but has diuretic properties. Topically it has been used as a compress for boils, ulcers, varicose veins and phlebitis (an inflammation of the veins, usually in the legs). It is said to have anti-inflammatory and antispasmodic properties, soothes intestinal discomfort, especially abdominal cramps, and can be used to treat headaches and migraine. Sweet woodruff has also been given to children and adults to help with insomnia, and is also a good source of flavonoids, which are useful for their antioxidant properties and for their effectiveness in keeping small blood vessels efficient and healthy. It has also been recommended as a treatment for liver disease and kidney stones and as a strengthener for the heart. The flowers can be added to salads and

Squinancywort

In some descriptions of sweet woodruff, the writers claim that it went by the names *woodrowel* and *woodrow*. In fact those were the folk names of another of the woodruff family, *squinancy woodruff (Asperula cynanchica)* which was also known as *quinsywort* and *squinancywort*. These names indicate that squinancywort was formerly used for treating quinsy, a disease similar to tonsillitis. Squinancywort is no longer used by herbalists because it became harder to source and is now a rare plant in most of the British Isles.

summer drinks. Another use for sweet woodruff is as a natural plant dye. The leaves produce a light brown dye and the roots a light red one when used with alum as a mordant or fixative.

HISTORY : Woodruff tastes like a mixture of cinnamon and chamomile. At the beginning of May fresh sprigs were crushed and added to white wine in Europe, to make wine cups for celebrating May Day or other ancient May festivals such as Beltane. In Germany one of the favourite hock cups is still made by steeping the fresh sprigs in Rhine wine to make *Maibowle*, which is drunk on the first of May. The name of the plant appears in the 13th century as '*wuderove*',

and later as '*wood-rove*'. Rove is probably derived from the French *rovelle*, a wheel, an allusion to the spoke-like arrangement of the leaves in whorls. In the Middle Ages the fresh leaves were bruised and applied to cuts and wounds to aid healing, and a strong decoction of the fresh herb was often used as a cordial and to tone the stomach. Medieval soldiers believed sweet woodruff promoted success in battle, and carried it tucked into their helmets when they engaged the enemy. In the Middle Ages sweet woodruff was woven into wreaths and swags and hung on the walls and strewn on the floors of churches. The herb was said to represent humility. It is now grown commercially to produce anticoagulant drugs such as Warfarin.

Refreshing Scent

The plant when newly gathered has little fragrance but, when dried, has a most refreshing scent of new-mown hay or vanilla, which is retained for years. Gerard tells us: '*The flowers are of a very sweet smell as is the rest of the herb, which, being made up into garlands or bundles, and hanged up in houses in the heat of summer, doth very well temper the air, cool and make fresh the place, to the delight and comfort of such as are therein. It is reported to be put into wine, to make a man merry, and to be good for the heart and liver, it prevails in wounds, as Cruciata and other vulnerary herbs do.*' In Old French works it is known as *muge-de-bois*, musk of the woods. The powdered leaves were mixed with fancy snuffs, because

of their enduring fragrance, and also put into pot-pourri. To help bring restful sleep, make a pillow stuffed with sweet woodruff. In the Middle Ages sweet woodruff was used as a strewing herb and as a stuffing for mattresses to sweeten the room. It was also popular in Elizabethan England for use in nosegays, wreaths, garlands and sachets. For a sweet-smelling insect repellent, make sachets of sweet woodruff to place with stored linen. Woodruff can also add fragrance to your bath. On St Barnabas' Day and on St Peter's Day, bunches of box, sweet woodruff, lavender and roses were strewn in churches.

TANSY

TANACETUM VULGARE
Family Asteraceae, Aster/Daisy

OTHER NAMES: Common tansy, bitter buttons, cow bitter, golden buttons.

DESCRIPTION: A strong hardy perennial up to 3 feet (90 cm) high, with yellow button flowers that can be dried for decoration.

PROPERTIES AND USES:
Culpeper: '*The decoction of the common Tansy, or the juice drank in wine, is a singular remedy for all the griefs that come by stopping of the urine, helps the strangury* [painful urination in small volumes, often related to prostate problems or cystitis] *and those that have weak reins* [loins, or kidney region] *and kidneys. It is also very profitable to dissolve and expel wind in the stomach, belly, or bowels, to procure women's courses, and expel windiness in the matrix, if it be bruised and often smelled unto, as also applied to the lower part of the belly. It is also very profitable for such women as are given to miscarry. It is used also against the stone in the reins, especially to men. The herb fried with eggs (as it is the custom in the Spring-time) which is called a Tansy, helps to digest and carry downward those bad humours that trouble the stomach. The seed is very profitably given to children for the worms, and the juice in drink is as effectual. Being boiled in oil, it is good for the sinews shrunk by cramps, or pained with colds, if thereto applied...It is an agreeable bitter, a carminative, and a destroyer of worms...outwardly it is used as a cosmetic, to take off freckles, sun-burn, and morphew* [an eruption of scurf]; *as also in restringent gargarisms* [gargles]...*It cleanses and heals ulcers in the mouth or secret parts, and is very good for inward wounds, and to close the tips of green wounds, and to heal old, moist, and corrupt running sores in the legs or elsewhere. Being bruised and applied to the soles of the feet and hands and wrists, it wonderfully culls the hot fits of agues, be they never so violent. The distilled water cleanses the skin of all discolourings therein, as morphew, sun-burnings, &c. as also pimples, freckles, and the like; and dropped into the eyes, or cloths wet therein and applied, takes away the heat and inflammations in them.*' The most well known medicinal use was to bring on menstruation by drinking a strong tea made of tansy leaves and flowers. However, it could cause miscarriage and there have been reports of deaths in women attempting to use the tea as an abortifacient. It is useful as a vermifuge (treatment to expel worms), and as a poultice to treat skin infections, but can be toxic. The plant produces a yellow dye.

HISTORY: The name tansy is probably derived from the Greek *athanasia* (immortality), either, says the Flemish botanist Rembert Dodoens, because it lasts so long in flower or, as Ambrosius wrote, because it is excellent for preserving dead bodies from corruption. The first president of Harvard was buried in 1668 wearing a tansy wreath in a coffin packed with tansy. When his body was exhumed in 1846, the tansy had maintained its shape and fragrance. Tansy was said to have been given to Ganymede to make him immortal. Tansy was hung on the house by Germanic peoples as a protection against monsters, was burned as incense and was one of the many herbs taken to America by the early colonists. At Easter, even archbishops and bishops played handball with men of their congregation, and a tansy cake was the reward of the victors. The cakes were made from the young leaves of the plant, mixed with eggs, to purify the humours of the body after the limited diet of Lent. William Coles (1656) wrote that '*tansies*' (tansy cakes) were eaten in the spring because tansy is very wholesome after

A Strewing Herb

Tansy was one of the strewing herbs mentioned by Thomas Tusser in 1577, and was one of the native plants dedicated to the Virgin Mary. The fresh leaves smell of camphor and were rubbed into pets' coats to repel fleas, and also used to deter blowflies from meat and corpses. Dried bunches make an effective fly, ant, insect and mice repellent. Plant tansy outside the kitchen door, on window sills and around the edges of the vegetable garden to discourage flies and predatory insects, and as a companion plant for roses, cucumbers and squashes. It is known to repel the colorado beetle from potato crops.

the salt fish consumed during Lent, and counteracts the ill-effects which the '*moist and cold constitution of winter has made on people…though many understand it not, and some simple people take it for a matter of superstition to do so.*'

From *The Cross Roads; or, The Haymaker's Story,* 1821

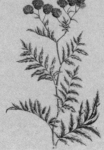

And where the marjoram
      once, and sage, and rue,
And balm, and mint, with
      curl'd-leaf parsley grew,
And double marigolds, and
      silver thyme,
And pumpkins 'neath the
      window climb;
And where I often, when a
      child, for hours

Tried through the pales to get
      the tempting flowers,
As lady's laces, everlasting peas,
True-love-lies-bleeding, with the
      hearts-at-ease,
And golden rods, and tansy
      running high,
That o'er the pale-tops smiled
      on passers-by.

John Clare

TAMARISK

TAMARIX GALLICA
Family Tamaricaceae, Tamarisk

OTHER NAMES: French tamarisk, manna tree, salt cedar (along with other tamarisk species). It is assumed that this is the tamarisk species to which Culpeper refers, having been taken by the Moors to the Iberian Peninsula. Culpeper believed that its place of origin was Spain, although it was grown throughout Europe.

DESCRIPTION: A small ornamental tree, indigenous to the Sinai Peninsula and Saudi Arabia, which grows all around the Mediterranean, with attractive pink flowers on narrow, feather-like spikes.

PROPERTIES AND USES: Culpeper: *'The root, leaves, young branches, or bark boiled in wine, and drank, stays the bleeding of the haemorrhoid veins, the spitting of blood, the too abounding of women's courses, the jaundice, the colic, and the biting of all venomous serpents, except the asp; and outwardly applied, is very powerful against the hardness of the spleen, and the toothache, pains in the ears, red and watering eyes. The decoction, with some honey put thereto, is good to stay gangrenes and fretting ulcers, and to wash those that are subject to nits and lice…give it also to those who have the leprosy, scabs, ulcers, or the like. Its ashes doth quickly heal blisters raised by burnings or scaldings. It helps the dropsy, arising from the hardness of the spleen, and therefore to drink out of cups made of the wood is good for splenetic persons. It is also helpful for melancholy, and the black jaundice that arise thereof… The bark is sometimes used for the rickets in children.'* A sweet and mucilaginous manna is produced in response to insect damage to the stems. There is some confusion over whether the manna is produced by the plant, or whether it is an exudation from the insects. The insects in question live in the deserts around Israel, and it is not known if the manna can be produced in Britain.

HISTORY: The generic name possibly comes from the Tambre River in Galicia, Spain, known to the Romans as the River Tamaris. In North Africa it has been used medicinally for rheumatism and diarrhoea.

Fire and Salt

All the tamarix species are adapted to survive fires, having long taproots that allow them to access deep water tables. They also limit competition from other plants, as they take up salt from deep ground water, accumulating it in their foliage. The trees then deposit the salt in the surface soil where it builds up concentrations, temporarily detrimental to some plants. The salt is washed away during heavy rains.

TARRAGON

ARTEMISIA DRACUNCULUS
Family Asteraceae/Compositae, Aster/Sunflower

OTHER NAMES: French tarragon, dragon's wort, little dragon, dragons.

DESCRIPTION: It is closely related to wormwood and mugwort, and has thin, blade-like and highly aromatic leaves smelling of anise. Its small, pale yellow flowers are rarely fully open.

PROPERTIES AND USES: *'The leaves, which are chiefly used, are heating and drying, and good for those who have the flux, or any preternatural discharge. It is a mild martial plant. An infusion of the young tops increases the urinary discharge, and gently promotes the menses.'* – Nicholas Culpeper. Tarragon was formerly used in the treatment of toothache, and by the 13th century was a popular seasoning for vegetables, a sleep-inducing drug and a breath sweetener. It makes an excellent vinegar, and gives a spicy, sweet flavour to fish, eggs, cheese and sauces. John Evelyn, in *Kalendarium Hortense* (1666) wrote *'… the tops and shoots like those of Rocket must never be excluded from salads. 'Tis highly cordial and friendly to the head, heart, and liver.'* Tarragon tea can relieve insomnia, constipation and aid digestion.

HISTORY: Tarragon is native to the southern Russia/western Asia area of Siberia, so was seemingly unknown in the ancient world. Through the trade routes, it found its way to Europe and into Italian and French cuisine during medieval times, but is a relative newcomer to the herb garden. By the 15th century, tarragon was imported to England, but was grown only in the Royal Gardens. By the 16th century it began to find common use as a culinary herb, but not until the 18th century was it introduced to America, with Thomas Jefferson being an early distributor. The name tarragon derives from the French *estragon* (little dragon), which is derived from the Arabic *tarkhun*. Because of the serpentine nature of its roots, according to the Doctrine of Signatures the herb was understood to have the ability to cure the bites of venomous reptiles, insects and mad dogs.

Full of Flavour

Tarragon is famous as being used in the French classic dish *escalopes de veau a l'estragon* (veal escalops with tarragon), as well as *fines herbes*, *herbes de Provence* and Dijon mustard, and also is the defining herb in sauce béarnaise and remoulade. French tarragon complements fish, shellfish, pork, beef, lamb, game, poultry and most vegetables and makes a delicious vinegar, alone or in combination with chives, lemon balm, shallots and garlic.

TEASEL - COMMON, FULLER'S and SMALL

DIPSACUS SYLVESTRIS, DIPSACUS FULLONUM (or *SATIVUS*),
DIPSACUS PILOSUS
Family Dipsacaceae, Teasel

OTHER NAMES: (Common teasel) wild teasel, Venus' basin, water thistle. (Fuller's teasel) fuller's thistle, teazel, tame teasel, manured teasel, card thistle, barber's brush, brushes and combs, church broom, brush and comb, Johnny-prick-the-finger. (Small teasel) shepherd's rod, small wild teazle.

DESCRIPTION:

Some botanists believe *fuller's teasel* to be a variety of the *common wild teasel*, in which the spines of the flower heads have strongly developed into a hooked form, a feature preserved by cultivation and apt to disappear by neglect, or on poor soil, causing it to relapse into the ordinary wild variety. Thus Culpeper calls the *fuller's teasel* the *manured teasel*. The inflorescence is a cylindrical array of lavender flowers which dries to a cone of spine-tipped hard bracts. The plant grows to a height of 5 feet (1.5 m). The whole plant is very harsh and prickly to the touch. The *small teasel* known as *shepherd's rod* grows with a fleshy, thick, and somewhat hairy stem with golden yellow flowerheads, followed by seedheads of a green and purple colour,

stuck round with tenacious prickles. It is sometimes found with white flowers, and looks more like the related scabious than a teasel.

PROPERTIES AND USES: Culpeper tells us about the medicinal uses of both the common and fuller's teasel: '*The virtues of both these Teasels are much the same: the roots, which are the only part used, being reckoned to have a cleansing faculty; the ancients commend a decoction of them in wine, boiled to a consistence, and kept in a brazen vessel, to be applied to the rhagades, or clefts of the fundament, and for a fistula therein; and to take away warts. The water found standing in the hollow of the leaves is commended as a collyrium to cool inflammations of the eyes and as a cosmetic to render the face fair. They are under the dominion of Venus.*' He tells us, on the authority of Dioscorides, that an ointment made from the bruised roots is good, not only for warts and wens, but also against cankers and fistulas. Other writers have recommended an infusion of the root for strengthening the stomach, creating an appetite, removing obstructions of the liver, and as a remedy for jaundice. As regards the small teasel,

Culpeper relates: '*It is a plant of Mars, and like the Teazle, is cultivated in many places for the use of clothiers, who employ the heads to raise the knap on wollen cloths. The flowers appear in June, and the heads ripen in autumn. The root is bitter, and given in a strong infusion, strengthens the stomach, and creates an appetite: it is also good against obstructions of the liver, and the jaundice. Many people have an opinion, that the water contained in the bason formed by the leaves, is a good cosmetic, but there is no real foundation for such a conjecture.*'

HISTORY: Dioscorides recommended the teasel root for its cleansing properties and the use of a decoction for effective treatment of fistulas and warts. The prickly leaves of both common and fuller's teasels are joined together at the base, forming a natural water reservoir for dew and rain in which insects can drown, whereby the plant can extract nutrients. This conspicuous feature has earned the plant its name of *Venus' basin*, and it was held that the water which collects there acquired curative properties. It was regarded as a remedy for warts, and was also used as a cosmetic and an eyewash. The generic name of the plant, *Dipsacus*, also refers to this structure, derived from the Greek verb, to be thirsty. Henry Lyte, in his 1586 translation of Rembert Dodoens's *Cruydeboeck*, says that the small worms found often within the heads '*do cure and heal the quartaine ague, to be worn or carried about the neck or arm*'.

Fleecing Wool

The English name, *teazle* or *teasel*, is from the Anglo-Saxon *taesan*, signifying to tease cloth, and refers to the use of the flowerheads by clothworkers. These heads are a mass of semi-stiff spines, the spines longest at the top of the head, each head being enclosed by curving, narrow, green bracts, set with small prickles. The principal use of the teasel from Roman times has been for 'fleecing' or 'fulling', i.e. raising the nap on woollen cloth. Gerard called the cultivated variety '*Tame Teasell*', which is used because its spines are crooked, not straight. Teasel heads are fixed on the rim of a wheel, or on a cylinder, which is made to revolve against the surface of the cloth to be 'fulled', thus raising the nap. They were gradually replaced by steel combs during the Industrial Revolution. However, until the mid-20th century, no machine was invented which could compete with the plant in its combined rigidity and elasticity. Its great utility is that while raising the nap, it would break at any serious obstruction in the production process, whereas all metallic substances (prior to plastics being used) in such a case would cause the cloth to yield first and tear the material.

(BLESSED) THISTLE

CNICUS BENEDICTUS
Family Asteracea/Compositae, Aster/Sunflower

OTHER NAMES: Culpeper also calls it Carduus Benedictus and Holy Thistle. Spotted thistle, St Benedict's thistle. Do not confuse blessed thistle with milk thistle, *Silybum marianum*. Both thistles share the common name holy thistle, but they are two entirely different plants from different families. Cotton thistle and melancholy thistle are given similar attributes and properties.

DESCRIPTION:
A handsome annual plant, the thistle grows about 2 feet (60 cm) high, is reddish, slender, with pale yellow flowers.

PROPERTIES AND USES: Culpeper: *'It is an herb of Mars, and under the sign of Aries. Now, in handling this herb, I shall give you a rational pattern of all the rest; and if you please to view them throughout the book, you shall, to your content, find it true. It helps swimming and giddiness in the head, or the disease called vertigo, because Aries is in the house of Mars. It is an excellent remedy against the yellow jaundice and other infirmities of the gall, because Mars governs choler. It strengthens the attractive faculty in man, and clarifies the blood, because the one is ruled by Mars. The continually drinking the decoction of it, helps red faces, tetters, ring-worms, because*

Mars causes them. It helps the plague, sores, boils, and itch, the biting of mad dogs and venomous beasts, all which infirmities are under Mars; thus you see what it doth by sympathy. By antipathy to other planets it cures the French-pox, by antipathy to Venus who governs it. It strengthens the memory, and cures deafness by antipathy to Saturn, who hath his fall in Aries, which rules the head. It cures quartain agues, and other diseases of melancholy, and adjusts choler, by sympathy to Saturn, Mars being exalted in Capricorn. Also it provokes urine, the stopping of which is usually caused by Mars or the Moon.' Blessed thistle is a bitter tonic, used for both the liver

Pestilence

It is said to have been named 'blessed' because of its high reputation as a heal-all. It is mentioned in many treatises on the Plague, especially by Thomas Brasbridge, who in 1578 published his *Poore Man's Jewell*, that is to say, *a Treatise of the Pestilence*, unto which is annexed a declaration of the vertues of the Hearbes Carduus Benedictus and Angelica.

Bitter Vegetable Drug

Because of its bitter properties, blessed thistle increases the flow of gastric juices, relieving dyspepsia, indigestion and headaches associated with liver congestion. British and German pharmacopoeias both recommended the consumption of *'bitters'*, including blessed thistle, to stimulate bile flow and cleanse the liver. In Europe, blessed thistle, classified as a 'bitter vegetable drug', was used as a medicinal agent to stimulate appetite, aid digestion and promote health. Recent studies tell us that bitters increase gastric juice and bile acid secretions, by increasing the flow of saliva through stimulation of specific receptors on the mucous membrane lining of the mouth. Alcoholic *digestifs* contain such bitters or carminative herbs to aid digestion, are usually around 45 per cent proof and drunk neat, with the exception of Angosturas bitters which is usually added to gin.

and digestion. The herb is a diuretic and induces perspiration, helping to purify the system and rid the body of toxins. It was also applied as a poultice herb to treat chilblains. The green leaf may be eaten, with bread and butter, like watercress, and was recommended for breakfast. The remains of old thistle mills can be found across Wales and Scotland. When beaten up or crushed in a mill to destroy the prickles, the leaves of all thistles are excellent food for cattle and horses. This kind of fodder was formerly used to a great extent before the introduction of hardy green crops for the purpose.

HISTORY: Medieval monks and apothecaries esteemed this plant as a cure for everything from smallpox to headaches, and it was supposed to even cure the plague. It is described in William Turner's *Herball* of 1568: '*It is very good for the headache and the migraine, for the use of the juice or powder of the leaves, preserves and keeps a man from the headache, and heals it being present. It is good for any ache in the body and strengthens the members of the whole body, and fastens loose sinews and weak. It is also good for the dropsy. It helps the memory and amends thick hearing. The leaves provoke sweat. There is nothing better for the canker and old rotten and festering sores than the leaves, juice, broth, powder and water of Carduus benedictus.*' Shakespeare in *Much Ado about Nothing* writes: '*Get you some of this distilled Carduus Benedictus and lay it to your heart; it is the only thing for a qualm…I mean plain Holy Thistle.*' Blessed thistle was a traditional tonic for women, and was used as a *galactaloge* to stimulate a mother's milk. Recent research suggests that blessed thistle has anti-inflammatory, antitumour and anticancer properties.

(MILK) THISTLE

SILYBUM MARIANUM
Family Asteraceae/Compositae, Aster/Sunflower

OTHER NAMES: Our Lady's thistle, Marian thistle, ysgall Mair (Mary's thistle, Welsh), blessed milk thistle, Mary thistle, Saint Mary's thistle, Mediterranean milk thistle, variegated thistle, sow thistle, wild artichoke.

DESCRIPTION: The name milk thistle derives from two features of the glossy green leaves: they are mottled with splashes of white and they contain a milky sap. It grows from 1–6 feet (30 cm to 1.8 m) tall and is very prickly, with white to purple, disc-shaped flowers.

PROPERTIES AND USES: Culpeper thought the milk thistle to be as efficient as *Carduus benedictus* for agues, preventing and curing the infection of the plague, and also for removal of obstructions of the liver and spleen. He recommended the infusion of the fresh root and seeds, not only as good against jaundice, also for breaking and expelling stone and being good for dropsy when taken internally. Culpeper also recommends the young, tender plant (after removing the prickles) to be boiled and eaten in the spring as a blood cleanser. An excellent liver remedy, milk thistle increases the flow of bile and helps prevent travel sickness. It was formerly cultivated in gardens for its attractiveness,

and the stalks may be eaten. The young leaves may be eaten as a salad. Charles Bryant, in *Flora Dietetica*, writes: *'The young shoots in the spring, cut close to the root with part of the stalk on, is one of the best boiling salads that is eaten, and surpasses the finest cabbage. They were sometimes baked in pies. The roots may be eaten like those of Salsify.'* In some districts the leaves are called 'pig leaves', presumably because pigs like them, and the seeds are a favourite food of goldfinches.

HISTORY: Pliny the Elder (23–79 CE) reported that the juice of the plant mixed with honey is indicated for 'carrying off bile'. There is an old Saxon remedy which states: *'this wort if hung upon a man's neck it setteth snakes to flight.'* It has been grown as a medicinal plant in

---

Our Lady's Thistle

Traditionally the milk-white veins of the leaves were believed to have been caused by the milk of the Virgin Mary which once fell upon a thistle plant, and so it was called *Our Lady's thistle*. The Latin name of the species has the same derivation.

Liver Protector

Scientists in Germany noticed that milk thistle seemed to protect the livers of animals from poisoning with highly toxic carbon tetrachloride. A previously unknown flavonol was isolated and given the name *silymarin*. Further studies showed that it is effective in the treatment of a number of disorders affecting the liver. Cirrhosis, deathcap mushroom poisoning, all types of hepatitis, gallstones, occupational toxic chemical exposure and skin disease all showed positive results under tests. Milk thistle has been used for liver ailments for two millennia, but until recently was little known. Silymarin, a constituent of milk thistle, is now listed medicinally as a liver protector.

It is an antioxidant, i.e. a free radical-scavenging agent, thus stabilizing and protecting the membrane lipids of the hepatocytes (liver cells). *Silybin*, a constituent chemical of silymarin, also alters the membrane structure of the liver cell, blocking the absorption of penetrating toxins into the cell. Additionally, it stimulates the production of new liver cells to replace damaged cells. An injection of silybin is an antidote for death cap mushroom poisoning. Recently Kate Moss, Orlando Bloom and Tracey Emin have been reported as being devotees of Pincer vodka, which combines the apple-flavoured milk thistle and vodka, to help protect the liver from toxins and ease any potential hangovers.

monastic gardens since the early medieval period. John Evelyn wrote: '*Disarmed of its prickles and boiled, it is worthy of esteem, and thought to be a great breeder of milk and proper diet for women who are nurses* [i.e. women who feed other women's babies, milk-nurses].' It was popular in Germany for curing jaundice and other bile-related illnesses. It was used as a demulcent to treat catarrh and pleurisy. Gerard wrote: '*...the root if borne about one doth expel melancholy and remove all diseases connected therewith... My opinion is that this is the best remedy that grows against all melancholy diseases...*

Dioscorides affirmed that the seeds being drunk are a remedy for infants that have their sinews drawn together, and for those that be bitten of serpents.' William Westmacott, writing in 1694, says of this thistle: '*It is a Friend to the Liver and Blood: the prickles cut off, they were formerly used to be boiled in the Spring and eaten with other herbs; but as the World decays, so doth the Use of good old things and others more delicate and less virtuous brought in.*' The seeds were thought to cure hydrophobia. The heads of this thistle formerly were eaten, boiled and treated like those of the globe artichoke.

THYME

THYMUS VULGARIS
Family Lamiaceae/Labiatae, Mint

OTHER NAMES: Garden thyme, common thyme, summer thyme, English thyme, French thyme, winter thyme.

DESCRIPTION: A small perennial, usually from 4 to 8 inches (10–20 cm) high, with small leaves and bearing flowers which bees love. The plant has an agreeable aromatic smell and a warm pungent taste. Thyme is a member of the mint family, and includes lemon, orange, woolly and broad-leafed varieties and more than 400 others including caraway, coconut, basil, lavender, camphor and nutmeg thyme.

PROPERTIES AND USES: *'It is a noble strengthener of the lungs, as notable a one as grows; neither is there scarce a better remedy growing for that disease in children which they commonly call the chin-cough, than it is. It purges the body of phlegm, and is an excellent remedy for shortness of breath. It kills worms in the belly, and being a notable herb of Venus, provokes the terms, gives safe and speedy delivery to women in travail, and brings away the after birth. It is so harmless you need not fear the use of it. An ointment made of it takes away hot swellings and warts, helps the sciatica and dullness of sight, and takes away pains and hardness of the spleen. It is excellent for those that are troubled with the gout. It eases pains in the loins and hips. The herb taken any way inwardly, comforts the stomach much, and expels wind.'* – Nicholas Culpeper. The medicinal virtues of thyme are due to its volatile oil constituents, such as *thymol*, which is the main active ingredient of *Listerine* mouthwash. Thyme has primarily been used in respiratory ailments because it fights infections and suppresses coughs. Thyme is also used as a digestive aid and its oil is recommended for those suffering from mental stress, PMT, fatigue and depression. Thymol also acts as a expectorant. Thyme tea is an excellent cold and hangover remedy, especially when sweetened with thyme honey. You can also wash and disinfect a wound with thyme tea. An

Stuffings and Marinades

It is best fresh or bought freeze-dried, and complements other robust herbs such as rosemary and sage. Use it chopped in stuffings for poultry or lamb, or in a marinade for olives, and add sprigs to marinades for meat, fish or vegetables. Tuck a few sprigs, with half a lemon and an onion, inside a chicken before roasting.

infusion of thyme leaves can be used to mop the kitchen floor. The fragrant dried leaves can be added to pot-pourris, and put into scented sachets for cupboards and drawers to repel insects. It is one of the herbs used in bouquet garni, along with parsley and bay. Thyme is excellent in dishes that require long, slow cooking, as it is one of the few herbs that won't lose its flavour when cooked for a long time. Fresh leaves and flowers can be used in salads and as garnishes, and you can use the leaves, fresh or dried, for making thyme butter, oil and vinegar. Fresh leaves are much more pungent than dried, when using in recipes. Thyme honey is one of the finest available, recommended by herbalists and gourmets alike.

HISTORY: Thyme was known as an antiseptic by the Sumerians *c.*3000 BCE, and Ancient Egyptians used it as part of the mummification process – it was known to preserve meat. Greeks and Romans used it in massage oil, bath oil and incense, as well as for medicinal purposes. The Greeks burned thyme in their temples for consecration and purification, and also as an offering to the gods. It was especially sacred to Adephaghia, the Greek goddess of food and gluttony. It was used to cure headaches, enhance moods, relieve poor digestion, and for respiratory problems. It was strewn, or worn on clothes to ward off plague as well as fleas and lice. In 1725 a German apothecary discovered that the plant's essential oil was effective against bacteria and fungi. In the 19th century, thyme was used to disinfectant hospital and to promote the recovery of patients. Across Europe, thyme has traditionally been used to repel insects, prevent nightmares, kill intestinal worms, disinfect wounds and alleviate diarrhoea in children. A pillow stuffed with thyme dispels nightmares and assists with peaceful sleep. Before the advent of modern antibiotics, thyme was used to medicate bandages. The oil is known as an excellent antiseptic for fungal infections such as athlete's foot.

Seeing Fairies

Traditionally, any place where thyme grows wild is reputedly blessed by the fairies. The following recipe dating from 1600 can be found in Oxford's Ashmolean Museum:

TO ENABLE ONE TO SEE THE FAIRIES: A pint of sallet oyle and put in into a vial glasse; and first wash it with rose-water and marygolde water; the flowers to be gathered towards the east. Wash it till the oyle becomes white, then put into the glasse, and then put thereto the budds of hollyhocke, the flowers of marygolde, the flowers or toppes of wild thyme, the budds of young hazle, and the thyme must be gathered near the side of a hill where fairies use to be; and take the grasse of a fairy throne; then all these put into the oyle in the glasse and sette it to dissolve three dayes in the sunne and then keep it for thy use.

(INDIAN) TOBACCO

NICOTIANA TABACUM
Family Solanaceae, Nightshade

OTHER NAMES: Indian tobacco, tabac. Culpeper also mentions *English Tobacco*.

DESCRIPTION: A New World annual, 3–6 feet (90 cm to 1.8 m) high with long flat leaves.

PROPERTIES AND USES:
Culpeper: '*It is a hot martial plant. A slight infusion of the fresh-gathered leaves causes vomiting, and that very roughly; but for constitutions that can bear it, it is a good medicine for rheumatic pains; an ointment made of them, with hog's-lard, is good for the piles when they get painful and are inflamed. The distilled oil is sometimes dropped on cotton, and applied to aching teeth, and it seldom fails to give temporary relief. The powdered leaves, or a decoction of them, kill lice, and other vermin. The smoke of tobacco injected in the manner of a glister [syringe], is of a singular efficacy in obstinate stoppages of the bowels, for destroying those small worms called ascarides [roundworm], and for the recovery of persons apparently drowned. A constant chewing, or smoking of tobacco, hurts the appetite, by depriving the constitution of too much saliva; but though it is improper for lean dry, hectic people, it may be useful to the more gross, and to such as are subject to cold diseases. Snuff is seldom productive of any bad effects, unless it be swallowed, but it should not be used by such as are inclined to an apoplexy. Tobacco is a great expeller of phlegm when smoked in a pipe, in which vast quantities are consumed, the greatest part by way of amusement, though some commend it as a helper of digestion; many extol it as a preservative from the plague; but Rivinus says, that is the plague of Leipzig several died, who were great smokers of tobacco. The distilled oil is of a poisonous nature: a drop of it taken inwardly, will destroy a cat.*' Maud Grieve tells us in 1931: '*A wet Tobacco leaf applied to piles is a certain cure…A pipe smoked after breakfast assists the action of the bowels…The smoke injected into the rectum or the leaf rolled into a suppository has been beneficial in strangulated hernia, also for obstinate constipation, due to spasm of the bowels, also for retention of urine, spasmodic urethral stricture, hysterical convulsions, worms, and in spasms caused*

No Smoking

In 2006 Bhutan was rated by *Business Week* magazine as the happiest country in Asia, and the 8th happiest of more than 200 in the world, based on global survey campaigns. Bhutan is the only country in the world where tobacco sales are illegal.

Stupefying Drug

From A.F.M. Willich's *Domestic Encyclopedia Or A Dictionary Of Facts, And Useful Knowledge*, 1802: '*Various properties have been attributed to this stupefying drug, since it was first introduced into Europe, about the middle of the 16th century. Its smoke, when properly blown against noxious insects, effectually destroys them; but the chief consumption of this plant, is in the manufactures of Snuff and Tobacco, or the cut leaves for Smoking. It is likewise (though we think, without foundation), believed to prevent the return of hunger; and is therefore chewed in considerable quantities by mariners, as well as the labouring classes of people; a disgusting practice, which cannot be too severely censured. For, though in some cases, this method of using tobacco, may afford relief in the rheumatic tooth-ach, yet, as the constant mastication of it induces an uncommon discharge of saliva, its narcotic qualities operate more powerfully, and thus eventually impair the digestive organs...It is remarkable, that the daily smoking of tobacco, is a practice which has only within the last century become general throughout Europe, especially in Holland and Germany; where it constitutes one of the greatest luxuries with which the industrious, poor peasants, as well as the more indolent and Wealthy classes, regale themselves and their friends. In Britain, however, the lower and middle ranks, only, appear to be attached to such fumigations; which, though occasionally useful in damp and mephitic situations, are always hurtful to persons of dry and rigid fibres, weak digestion, or delicate habits; but particularly to the young, plethoric, asthmatic, and those whose ancestors have been consumptive; or who are themselves threatened with pulmonary diseases. In proof of this assertion, we shall only remark, that a few drops of the oil distilled from the leaves of this powerful plant, taken internally, have operated as fatal poison: and, a considerable portion of such oil being disengaged within the tuba of tobacco-pipes, during combustion, the noxious effects of inhaling and absorbing it by the mouth, may be easily inferred.*'

by lead, for croup, and inflammation of the peritoneum, to produce evacuation of the bowels, moderating reaction and dispelling tympanitis [inflammation of the middle ear], and also in tetanus.'

HISTORY: The *Nicotiania* genus derives its name from the French diplomat Jean Nicot (1530–1600), who introduced the plant to Europe in the mid-16th century, and *tabaco* probably comes from the Arawak word for the pipe in which it is smoked. Over a billion people are regular smokers, and in 2005 the World Health Organization attributed 5.4 million of 58.8 million deaths in that year to tobacco. Around 100 million deaths were caused by tobacco in the 20th century, and the WHO predicts, on current trends, up to 1 billion deaths in the 21st century.

TOMATO

SOLANUM LYCOPERSICUM
Family Solanaceae, Nightshade

OTHER NAMES: Love apple (Culpeper), golden apple, wolf apple, wolf peach, apple of love. *Lycopersicum* means *'wolf peach'*, which derived from German legends that deadly nightshade was used to summon werewolves. Thus the tomato, which bears similar flowers but much larger fruit, was called the 'wolf peach' when it arrived in Europe. The Aztecs called the fruit *xitomatl*, meaning 'chubby object with a navel'. Other Mesoamerican peoples took the name as *tomatl*, from we derived the name tomato.

DESCRIPTION: A climbing fruit (see box) probably only known as a small yellow variety to Culpeper. Various 17th-century illustrations show the fruit being only as large as the flowers.

PROPERTIES AND USES: Culpeper said that a salve of the juice cured inflammations and burning, and that the *'leaves boiled with olive oil, till crisped, then strained and afterwards boiled with wax, rosin and a little turpentine, to a salve, are an infallible remedy for old sores and ulcers of the private parts, or for wounds and ulcers in other parts of the body, coming of heat, or viscous humours of the blood.'* One medium tomato provides half the recommended daily dose of vitamin C. Lycopene is a carotenoid that is responsible for the red colour of tomatoes, watermelon and pink grapefruit.

It is regarded as a 'wonder chemical', an antioxidant which, when absorbed into the body, helps to prevent and repair damaged cells by inactivating free radicals in the body. It has thus been credited with reducing wrinkles, which are also caused by free radicals ageing the skin. People with high lycopene levels are at lower risk of developing prostate, cervical, bladder and pancreatic cancers, and lycopene protects against Age-Related Macular Degeneration (AMD) the most common

Superior Superfood

There seems to be a new 'super' superfood. The gac *(Momordica cochinchinensis)* is a Southeast Asian fruit variously known as *Baby Jackfruit, Spiny Bitter Gourd* and *Sweet Gourd*. Relative to mass, it contains up to 70 times the amount of lycopene found in tomatoes, and up to ten times the amount of good beta-carotene of carrots or sweet potatoes. Its carotenoids are bound to long-chain fatty acids, making them more easily absorbed by the body, and gac also contains a protein that may inhibit the proliferation of cancer cells. Gac provides high levels of antioxidants and of vitamin A that is good for the skin and eyes.

form of blindness for elderly people in the Western world. Lycopene is more easily absorbed by the body after processing, for example into tomato ketchup or purée, and when tomatoes are cooked with certain oils, such as olive oil.

HISTORY: Some believe that the Spanish explorer Hernán Cortés was the first to send the small yellow tomato to Europe after he captured the Aztec city of Tenochtítlan, now Mexico City, in 1521. Others think Columbus brought the tomato back in 1493. It appears appeared in a 1544 herbal written the Italian Pietro Andrea Mattioli, who named it *pomo d'oro* (apple of gold). The French misheard the name as *pomo d'amore*, or *love apple*, and the term passed into English towards the end of the 16th century. When first introduced from the Americas, the tomato was treated as a novelty. If children ate its berries, they were 'purged' by a physician. However, Italian dandies came to believe that eating the berries was an aphrodisiac and it gradually became a salad ingredient. It is assumed by some to be the true 'apple', the forbidden fruit that Eve offered to Adam in the Garden of Eden. They were not grown in England until the 1590s, and Gerard grew them, but believed that it was poisonous, a view held in England and America until the early 18th century. By the mid-18th century, tomatoes were widely eaten, and cultivated upon an almost industrial scale in glass-houses. *La Tomatina* is a week-long food fight festival, held each year in the town of Buñol in the Valencia region of Spain. This event is attended by tens of thousands of people from all over the world, during which some 90,000 pounds (over 40,000 kg) of tomatoes are thrown in an enormous food fight.

Fruit and Vegetable

Botanically, a tomato is a fruit: it comprises the ovary together with its seeds, of a flowering plant. Typically served as part of a salad or main course of a meal, rather than at dessert, it is considered a vegetable for most culinary purposes. In 1887, US tariff laws that imposed a duty on vegetables, but not on fruits, caused the tomato's status to become defined legally. The U.S. Supreme Court in 1893 declared that the tomato is a vegetable, based on a definition that classifies vegetables by use, i.e. that they are generally served with dinner and not as a dessert. However, in 2001 the Council of the European Union directed that tomatoes should be considered fruits. Tomatoes have been designated the state vegetable of New Jersey, but Arkansas took both sides in declaring the 'South Arkansas Vine Ripe Pink Tomato' to be both the state fruit and the state vegetable in the same law, citing both its culinary and botanical classifications. In 2009, the state of Ohio passed a law making the tomato the state's official fruit.

TORMENTIL

POTENTILLA ERECTA (formerly *POTENTILLA TORMENTILLA*)
Family Rosaceae, Rose

OTHER NAMES: Common tormentil, septfoil, seven leaves, thormantle, Thor's mantle, biscuits, bloodroot, earthbank, ewe daisy, five fingers, flesh and blood, shepherd's knapperty, shepherd's knot, English sarsaparilla.

DESCRIPTION: A low, clump-forming plant, growing up to 6–12 inches (15–30 cm) tall and with non-rooting runners. There are usually four notched petals on the yellow flowers. From the rootstock come leaves on long stalks, divided into three or five oval leaflets (occasionally, but rarely, seven, hence unusually the names *septfoil* and *seven leaves*) toothed towards their tips.

PROPERTIES AND USES: Culpeper writes: '*This is a gallant herb of the Sun. Tormentil is most excellent to stay all kind of fluxes of blood or humours in man or woman, whether at nose, mouth, or belly. The juice of the herb of the root, or the decoction thereof, taken with some Venice treacle, and the person laid to sweat, expels any venom or poison, or the plague, fever, or other contagious diseases, as pox, measles, &c. for it is an ingredient in all antidotes or counter poisons. Andreas Urlesius is of opinion that the decoction of this root is no less effectual to cure the French pox than Guiacum or China; and it is not unlikely, because it so mightily resists putrefaction.*

The root taken inwardly is most effectual to help any flux of the belly, stomach, spleen, or blood; and the juice wonderfully opens obstructions of the liver and lungs, and thereby helps the yellow jaundice. The powder or decoction drank, or to sit thereon as a bath, is an assured remedy against abortion, if it proceed from the over flexibility or weakness of the inward retentive faculty; as also a plaster made therewith, and vinegar applied to the reins of the back, doth much help not only this, but also those that cannot hold their water, the powder being taken in the juice of Plaintain, and is also commended against the worms in children.' It is considered one of the safest and most powerful aromatic astringents, and for its tonic properties was called '*English sarsaparilla.*'

HISTORY: A lotion prepared from the dried root has been used both as medicine to treat a number of ailments, e.g. to stop bleeding or diarrhoea, and to dye leather red. Maud Grieve in 1931 also recommended it '*…as a gargle in sore, relaxed and ulcerated throat and also as an injection in leucorrhoea* [vaginal discharge]*…If a piece of lint be soaked in the decoction and kept applied to warts, they will disappear. It was much given for cholera, and also sometimes in intermittent fevers, and used in a lotion for ulcers and long-standing sores.*'

TURNSOLE

HELIOTROPUM EUROPAEUM
Family Boraginaceae, Borage

OTHER NAMES: European turnsole, European heliotrope, great turnsole, turnsol, caterpillar weed.

DESCRIPTION: It reaches 12–18 inches (30–45 cm) in height with curled sprays of small white flowers; the stem and leaves are covered with soft downy hairs. Because of its curly shape and hairy stem it gets the name of caterpillar weed. The scent resembles that of jasmine.

PROPERTIES AND USES: Culpeper relates: '*It grows in gardens, and flowers and seeds with us, notwithstanding it is not natural to this land, but to Italy, Spain, and France, where it grows plentifully. Government and virtues. It is an herb of the Sun, and a good one too. Dioscorides says that a good handful of this, which is called the Great Turnsole, boiled in water, and drank, purges both choler and phlegm; and boiled with cumin, helps the stone in the reins, kidneys, or bladder, provokes urine and women's courses, and causes an easy and speedy delivery in child-birth. The leaves bruised and applied to places pained with the gout, or that have been out of joint and newly set, and full of pain, do give much ease; the seed and juice of the leaves also being rubbed with a little salt upon warts and wens, and other kernels in the face, eye-lids, or any other part of the body, will, by often using, take them away.*' A tincture of the whole fresh plant was said to be used for a clergyman's sore throat. The plant is said to be poisonous to sheep and humans.

HISTORY: In Greek mythology, the nymph Clytie adored the Sun god Apollo. Clytie gazed at him longingly when he drove his chariot through the heavens from east to west every day. Apollo never glanced at her, so she began weeping and fell to the ground. For nine days and nights she did not eat or drink but just lay there, watching Apollo traverse the skies. Her limbs became rooted in the ground and green leaves enveloped her and tiny flowers covered her face. In this way she changed into a flower and evermore became known as heliotrope gazing upwards and following the course of the Sun. The sap of its flowers was used as a food colouring in the Middle Ages.

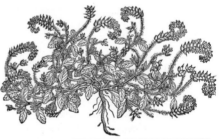

Facing the Sun

After opening, the flower gradually turns from the east to the west and during the night turns back again to the east to meet the rising Sun. *Helios* is Greek for Sun and *tropaios* means to turn back. Turnsole has the same origins, turning to face *Sol*, the sun.

THOMAS TUSSER
(1524-80)

This farmer wrote the instructional poem *Five Hundred Points of Good Husbandry* (1557) and is remembered for the popular proverb, '*A fool and his money are soon parted.*' In the long poem he lists the following:

SEEDS AND HERBS FOR THE KITCHEN

Avens (herb bennet); *betony;* *beets or bleets – white or yellow; bloodwort; bugloss; burnet; borage; cabbage – remove in June; clary sage; coleworts; cresses; endives; fennel; French mallows; French saffron, set in August; lang de beef* (oxtongue); *leeks – remove in June; lettuce – remove in May; longwort* (pellitory of Spain); *liverwort; marigolds – often cut; mercury; mints – at all times; nep* (catmint); *onions – from December to March; orach or arach – red and white; patience?; parsley; pennyroyal; primrose; poret* (porret, a young leek); *rosemary – in the springtime, to grow south or west; sage, red and white; English saffron – set in August; Summer savory; sorrel; spinach; succory* (chicory); *siethes* (a kind of chives); *tansy; thyme; violets – of all sorts.*

HERBS AND ROOTS FOR SALADS AND SAUCE

Alexanders – at all times; artichokes; blessed thistle – or Carduus benedictus; cucumbers – in April and May; cresses – sow with lettuce in the spring; endive; musk-million (muskmelon) – *in April and May; mustard-seed – sow in the spring, and at Michaelmas; mints; purslane; radish – and after remove them; rampions* (bellflower); *rocket – in April; sage; sorrel; spinach – for the summer; sea-holly; sparage* (asparagus) – *let grow for two years, and then remove; skirrets* (crummock) – *set these plants in June; succory* (chicory); *tarragon – set in slips in March; violets, of all colours. These buy with the penny, or look not for any: capers, lemons, olives, oranges, rice, samphire.*

HERBS AND ROOTS, TO BOIL OR TO BUTTER

Beans – set in winter; cabbages – sow in March, and afterwards remove; carrots; citrons – sow in May; gourds – in May; navews (rape, wild cabbage or wild turnips) – *sow in June; pompions* (pumpkin) – *in May; parsneps* (parsnips) – *in winter; runcival pease* (runcible, or large peas) – *set in winter; rapes – sow in June; turneps* (turnips) – *in March and April.*

STREWING HERBS OF ALL SORTS

Basil – fine and bushed, sow in May; baulm (lemon balm) – *set in March; camomile; costmary* (alecost); *cowslips and paggles* (primrose, *Primula officinalis*); *daisies of all sorts; sweet fennel; germander; hyssop –*

set in February; lavender; lavender spike; lavender cotton; knotted marjoram – sow or set, at the spring; maudeline; penny royal; roses of all sorts – in January and September; red mints; sage; tansy; violets; winter savory.

HERBS, BRANCHES AND FLOWERS, FOR WINDOWS AND POTS

Bays – sow or plant in January; bachelors' buttons; bottles – blue, red and tawny; columbines; campions; cowslips; daffodils, or daffadon-dillies; eglantine, or sweet-briar; fetherfew (feverfew); flower amour – sow in June; flower de luce; flower gentle – white and red; flower nice; gillyflowers – red, white, and carnations set in spring, and at harvest in pots, pails, or tubs, or for summer, in beds; holyoaks (hollyhocks) – red, white and carnations; Indian eye – sow in May, or set in slips in March; lavender of all sorts; lark's foot; laus tibi (white narcissus); lilium convallium (lilies of the valley); lilies – red and white, sow in March and September; marigolds double; nigella romana; pansies or heartsease; paggles – green and yellow; pinks of all sorts; queen's gilliflowers; rosemary; roses of all sorts; snap-dragon; sops in wine; sweet Williams; sweet Johns (pinks); star of Bethlehem; star of Jerusalem; stock gilliflowers of all sorts; tuft gilliflowers; velvet flowers, or French marigolds; violets – yellow and white; wall gilliflowers of all sorts.

Note: in the 1876 edition the editor commented, 'The delicate olfactory nerves of modern females would revolt at feverfew, and several other plants in this list, if placed in their windows; while many more which are here enumerated might be easily raised in the natural ground, without the trouble and expense of pots.' However, these herbs were used to repel insects, not for their sweet scent.

HERBS TO STILL (DISTILL) IN SUMMER

Blessed thistle; betony; dill; endive; eyebright; fennel; fumitory; hyssop; mints; plantain; roses – red and damask; respies (raspberries); saxifrage, strawberries; sorrel; succory; woodruff – for sweet waters and cakes.

NECESSARY HERBS TO GROW IN THE GARDEN FOR PHYSIC, NOT REHEARSED BEFORE

Anise; archangel; betony; chervil; cinquefoil; cumin; dragons; dittany, or garden ginger; gromwell seed, for the stone; hartstongue; horehound; lovage, for the stone; liquorice; mandrake; mugwort; peony; poppy; rue; rhubarb; smallage (wild celery), for the swellings; saxifrage, for the stone; savin (juniper), for the botts (worms); stitchwort; valerian; woodbine.

Thus ends the brief / Of herbs the chief. / To get more skill, / Read whom you will: / Such more to have, / Of field go crave.

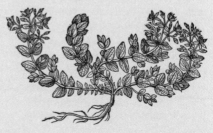

VALERIAN

VALERIANA OFFICINALIS
Family Valerianaceae, Valerian

OTHER NAMES: Culpeper calls it Garden Valerian. Common valerian, all heal, garden heliotrope, St George's herb, bloody butcher, capon's tail, capon's trailer, cat's valerian, vandal root, English valerian, fragrant valerian, sete wale (set well), red valerian.

DESCRIPTION: An attractive fern-like plant with fragrant pinkish flowers, and lance-shaped leaves that get progressively smaller at the top. It can reach 5 feet (1.5 m) in height.

PROPERTIES AND USES: Culpeper describes it: *'This is under the influence of Mercury. Dioscorides says, that the Garden Valerian has a warming faculty, and that being dried and given to drink it provokes urine, and helps the stranguary. The decoction thereof taken, doth the like also, and takes away pains of the sides, provokes women's courses, and is used in antidotes. Pliny says, that the powder of the root given in drink, or the decoction thereof taken, helps all stoppings and stranglings in any part of the body, whether they proceed of pains in the chest or sides, and takes them away. The root of Valerian boiled with liquorice, raisins, and aniseed, is singularly good for those that are short-winded, and for those that are troubled with the cough, and helps to open the passages, and to expectorate phlegm easily. It is given to those that are bitten or stung by any venomous creature,*

being boiled in wine. It is of a special virtue against the plague, the decoction thereof being drank, and the root being used to smell to. It helps to expel the wind in the belly. The green herb with the root taken fresh, being bruised and applied to the head, takes away the pains and prickings there, stays rheum and thin distillation, and being boiled in white wine, and a drop thereof put into the eyes, takes away the dimness of the sight, or any pin or web therein. It is of excellent property to heal any inward sores

---

Stimulating Sedative

Valerian is sedative to humans, but excites cats, rats and mice. The roots smell strongly of new leather and are sometimes dug up by cats, being a cat attractant like catnip. Valerian is also attractive to rats, and has been used to bait traps. In one version of the legend of the Pied Piper of Hamelin, he lured the rodents with valerian to drive them out of the city.

St Vitus's Dance

Valerian was a traditional remedy for St Vitus's dance, now known as Sydenham's chorea. It is a disorder associated with rheumatic fever, affecting children and characterized by jerky, uncontrollable movements, either of the face or of the arms and legs. There is no specific treatment, with sedatives and tranquillizers are helpful in suppressing the involuntary movements. Thus valerian would have been an effective choice of treatment. St Vitus (died *c.*303) is the patron saint of Prague, Bohemia, dogs, domestic animals, young people, dancers, coppersmiths, actors, comedians, epileptics, mummers and those who oversleep. The help of the saint is invoked to protect against epilepsy, lightning, poisoning by dog bite or snake bite, sleeplessness, animal attacks, storm, and St Vitus's dance. Vitus is one of the Fourteen Holy Helpers, a collective cult of saints that originated in the 14th-century Rhineland, who were believed to intercede effectively against various diseases. His nurse and her husband, St Crescentia and St Modestus, martyred with St Vitus, share his feast of 15 June.

Sydenham's chorea gets its name from the Graeco-Latin word implying the act of dancing, which we recognise in the word 'choreography'. The term *chorea* was first applied by Paracelsus to the frenzied movements of religious fanatics who in the Middle Ages journeyed to the healing shrine of St Vitus Cathedral in Prague.

---

or wounds, and also for outward hurts or wounds, and drawing away splinters or thorns out of the flesh.' Valerian is the most widely recognized herbal sedative, used for insomnia, nervous anxiety and to help the body relax in the presence of pain. Although potent, fortunately it is neither habit-forming nor addictive. Additionally, it helps one sleep, but does not cause a morning hangover or interact with alcohol. Research shows that root extracts help one to fall asleep faster and also improve sleep quality. The strange, pungent odour of the root is an indicator of the strength of its medicinal properties. Valerian root does not lose effectiveness over time, so dried roots were often placed in linen cupboards and drawers to deter insects.

HISTORY: Valerian is used in the 11th-century herbal recipes of the Anglo Saxon leeches, medical men who drew blood. In the Middle Ages it was known as amentilla or amantilla, and a 14th-century saying reads: *'Men who begin to fight and when you wish to stop them, give to them the juice of Amantilla id est Valeriana and peace will be made immediately.'* Thomas Hill in 1577 wrote: *'...it provoketh sweat and urine, amendeth stitches, helpeth the straightness of breath, the headache, fluxes and Shingles, procureth clearness of sight and healeth the piles.'* Valerian has traditionally been used as a nerve tonic, to cure anxiety, to relieve the symptoms of the falling sickness (epilepsy). The flowers were used in charm bags to encourage love, protection and sleep.

VERVAIN

VERBENA OFFICINALIS
Family Verbenaceae, Vervain

OTHER NAMES: Common vervain, common verbena, herb of grace (as is rue), herb of the cross, holy herb, holy wort, herba sacra, herb of enchantment, Britannica, enchanter's plant, enchanter's herb, Juno's tears, pigeon's grass, pigeonwood, simpler's joy, divine wood, wild hyssop, mosquito plant. It must be picked before flowering, and dried promptly. Do not confuse this with *Verbena boniarensis*, also known as blue vervain, the statuesque purple-topped plant we see in many gardens, which originated in the New World.

DESCRIPTION: A hardy perennial growing to 3 feet (90 cm), with small pale lilac flowers carried on slender spikes.

PROPERTIES AND USES: Culpeper notes: *'This is an herb of Venus, and excellent for the womb to strengthen and remedy all the cold griefs of it, as plantain does the hot. Vervain is hot and dry, opening obstructions, cleansing and healing. It helps the yellow jaundice, the dropsy and the gout; it kills and expels worms in the belly, and causes a good colour in the face and body, strengthens as well as corrects the diseases of the stomach, liver, and spleen; helps the cough, wheezings, and shortness of breath, and all the defects of the reins and bladder, expelling the gravel and stone. It is held to be good against the biting of serpents, and other venomous beasts, against the plague, and both tertian and quartian agues. It consolidates and heals also all wounds, both inward and outward, stays bleedings, and used with some honey, heals all old ulcers and fistulas in the legs or other parts of the body; as also those ulcers that happen in the mouth; or used with hog's grease, it helps the swellings and pains in the secret parts in man or woman, also for the piles or hæmorrhoids; applied with some oil of roses and vinegar unto the forehead and temples, it eases the inveterate pains and ache of the head, and is good for those that are frantic. The leaves bruised, or the juice of them mixed with some vinegar, does wonderfully cleanse the skin, and takes away morphew [facial scurf], freckles, fistulas, and other such like inflammations and deformities of the skin in any parts of the body. The distilled water of the herb when it is in full strength, dropped into the eyes, cleanses them from films, clouds, or mists, that darken the sight, and wonderfully strengthens the optic nerves. The said water is very powerful in all the diseases aforesaid, either inward or outward, whether they be old corroding sores, or green wounds.'* An infusion cured insomnia and stress, prevented stones

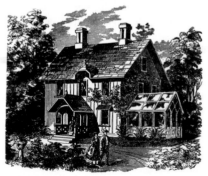

Found at Calvary

Its multiple virtues may be due to the legend of its discovery on the Mount of Calvary, where it staunched the wounds of the crucified Saviour. Hence, it was crossed and blessed with a commemorative verse when it is gathered.

and boosted the immune system, and its diuretic qualities aided lactation. Vervain is useful as a pain reliever and natural tranquillizer, an expectorant used to treat chronic bronchitis, and as an antirheumatic used to relieve joint pain. Herbalists consider vervain helpful when depression is related to chronic illness. As an added benefit, it can help to heal any damage that has occurred to the liver. It is a noted honey plant.

HISTORY: Vervain is said to be derived from the Welsh *ferfaen*, from *ferri* (to drive away or ferry) and *faen* (the soft mutation of *maen*, stone), as the plant was popularly used for afflictions of the bladder, especially calculus (stones). Another derivation is possibly from *herba veneris*, because of the aphrodisiac qualities attributed to it. Romans used it as an altar plant, as it was the 'sacred bough' used in their sacrifices, and Druids also revered it. Associated with the Passion of Christ, it was used in ointments to make demons fly away. Pliny the Elder relates that in Rome the bridal wreath was of verbena, gathered by the bride herself. Bruised, it was worn round the neck for general good luck, as a charm against headaches, and against snake and other venomous bites. Vervain was thought to

be good for the sight. According to Maud Grieve: '*It is recommended in upwards of thirty complaints, being astringent, diaphoretic, antispasmodic, etc. It is said to be useful in intermittent fevers, ulcers, ophthalmia, pleurisy, etc., and to be a good galactogogue* [promoting lactation]. *It is still used as a febrifuge in autumn fevers. As a poultice it is good in headache, ear neuralgia, rheumatism, etc. In this form it colours the skin a fine red, giving rise to the idea that it had the power of drawing the blood outside.*' Today vervain is used to treat stress-induced conditions and nervous exhaustion.

Iron Herb

Vervain was placed around fields to prevent bad weather and was sacred to the mighty Thor, the Norse thunder god. The ancient smiths used vervain in a procedure for hardening steel, so it comes as no surprise to learn that this herb was mixed into love potions to make love as hot as burning iron. In Holland, Germany, Denmark, Slovakia and Finland it is known as '*iron herb*'.

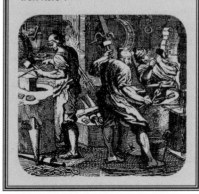

VIOLET

VIOLA ODORATA
Family Violaceae, Violet

OTHER NAMES: Scented violet, dog violet, English violet, common violet, garden violet. Culpeper also includes the common dog-violet or wood violet *(Viola riviniana)*, the early dog-violet *(Viola reichenbachiana)* and the yellow violet or field pansy *(Viola arvensis)*.

DESCRIPTION: The leaves are heart-shaped, slightly downy beneath and the wonderfully scented flowers are generally deep purple or violet like their name, but lilac, pale rose-coloured or white variations are also common.

PROPERTIES AND USES: Culpeper says: *'All the Violets are cold and moist, while they are fresh and green, and are used to cool any heat or distemperature of the body, either inwardly or outwardly, as the inflammation in the eyes, to drink the decoction of the leaves and flowers made with water or wine, or to apply them poultice wise to the grieved places; it likewise eases pains in the head caused through want of sleep, or any pains arising of heat if applied in the same manner or with oil of Roses. A dram weight of the dried leaves or flowers of Violets, but the leaves more strongly, doth purge the body of choleric humours and assuages the heat if taken in a draught of wine or other drink; the powder of the purple leaves of the flowers only picked and dried and drank in water helps the quinsy and the falling sickness in children, especially at the* beginning of the disease. It is also good for jaundice. The flowers of the Violets ripen and dissolve swellings. The herbs or flowers while they are fresh or the flowers that are dry are effectual in the pleurisy and all diseases of the lungs. The green leaves are used with other herbs to make plasters and poultices for inflammation and swellings and to ease all pains whatsoever arising of heat and for piles, being fried with yoke of egg and applied thereto.'

HISTORY: The violet was thought to have been present at the Crucifixion and, having been touched by the shadow of the Cross, now hangs its sweet head in mourning. To the Greeks, it was the flower of the goddess of love, Aphrodite and the symbol of Athens. Aristophanes called Athens the *'violet-crowned city'* because its king had the same name as the violet, *Ion*. Petals were strewn as air fresheners, and they are an old popular remedy for bruises.

Violet Remedies

'The common dark-blue violet makes a slimy tea, which is excellent for the canker. Leaves and blossoms are both good. Those who have families should take some pains to dry these flowers.'

American Frugal Housewife, 1833

WALLFLOWER

ERYSIMUM CHEIRI (CHEIRANTHUS CHEIRI)
Family Brassicaceae, Cabbage

OTHER NAMES: Culpeper calls them Wall-Flowers, or Winter Gilliflowers. Bloody warriors, Aegean wall gillifower, gillyflower, wallstock-gillofer, giroflier, handflower, beeflower, baton d'or, cherisaunce. Cruciferae was previously used as their family name, because the petals are well spaced and make a clearly visible cross.

DESCRIPTION: A small plant with dark green, pointed leaves and fragrant, deep yellow, four-petalled single flowers.

PROPERTIES AND USES: Culpeper: '*Government and virtues: The Moon rules them. Galen, in his seventh book of simple medicines, says, that the yellow Wall-flowers work more powerfully than any of the other kinds, and are therefore of more use in physic. It cleanses the blood, and fretteth the liver and reins from obstructions, provokes women's courses, expels the secundine, and the dead child; helps the hardness and pain of the mother, and of spleen also; stays inflammations and swellings, comforts and strengthens any weak part, or out of joint; helps to cleanse the eyes from mistiness or films upon them, and to cleanse the filthy ulcers in the mouth, or any other part, and is a singular remedy for the gout, and all aches and pains in the joints and sinews. A conserve made of the flowers, is used for a remedy both for the apoplexy and palsy.*' If the flowers are steeped in oil for some weeks, the oil is useful in massaging rheumatic or neuralgic limbs. Gerard suggests that the '*oyle of Wallflowers is good for use to annoint a paralyticke*'. An infusion of the flowers relieves headaches and nervous disorders.

HISTORY: It is one of the earliest garden flowers in Britain, being found growing around castles and old ruins. Gerard noted '*This Wallflower and the Stock Gilliflower are used by certain empiricks and quack salvers about love and lust, matters which for modesty I omit.*' In times past, this flower was carried in the hand at festivals, hence the name *handflower*. William Turner called it *Wallgelouer*, or *Hartisease*, and this is the plant to which the name heart's-ease was originally given.

From *Hesperides,* 1647

Why this flower is now called so
List, sweet maids, and you shall know:
Understand this firstling was
Once a bright and bonny lass
Kept as close as Danae was
Who a sprightly springal loved,
And to have it fully proved
Up she got upon a wall
Tempting down to slide withal:
But the silken twist untied,
So she fell, and bruised and died.
Love, in pity of the deed,
And her loving, luckless speed,
Turned her to this plant we call
Now, the 'Flower of the Wall.'

Robert Herrick

WALNUT

JUGLANS REGIA
Family Juglandaceae, Walnut

OTHER NAMES: Jupiter's nuts, common walnut, Persian walnut, English walnut, Carpathian walnut, royal walnut.

DESCRIPTION: A large, slow-growing, deciduous tree reaching 100 feet (30 m) with a trunk up to 7 feet (2.1 m) in diameter. It commonly has a short trunk and a broad crown.

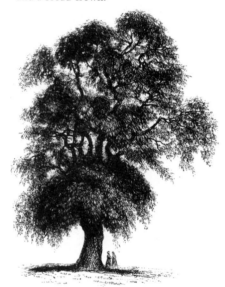

PROPERTIES AND USES: Culpeper found uses for the bark, leaves and nuts, and continued: '... *The juice of the other green husks boiled with honey is an excellent gargle for sore mouths, or the heat and inflammations in the throat and stomach. The kernels, when they grow old, are more oily, and therefore not fit to be eaten, but are* then used to heal the wounds of the sinews, gangrenes, and carbuncles. The said kernels being burned, are very astringent, and will stay lasks [diarrhoea] and women's courses, being taken in red wine, and stay the falling of the hair, and make it fair, being anointed with oil and wine. The green husks will do the like, being used in the same manner. The kernels beaten with rue and wine, being applied, help the quinsy; and bruised with some honey, and applied to the ears, ease the pains and inflammation of them. A piece of the green husks put into a hollow tooth, eases the pain. The catkins hereof, taken before they fall off, dried, and given a dram thereof in powder with white wine, wonderfully helps those that are troubled with the rising of the mother. The oil that is pressed out of the kernels, is very profitable,*

Walnuts for Health

Walnuts are unique among nuts because they contain large amounts of alpha-linoleic acid, one of the two major types of omega-3 fatty acids. Walnut oil is recommended in cooking as walnuts contain omega-3 essential fats and can reduce the inflammation and joint pain of rheumatoid arthritis. A handful of walnuts each day can cut the size of prostate tumours and inhibit their growth. Omega-3 fatty acids have also been shown to help stave off breast cancer and heart disease.

taken inwardly like oil of almonds, to help
the cholic, and to expel wind very effectually;
an ounce or two thereof may be taken at any
time. The young green nuts taken before they
be half ripe, and preserved with sugar, are of
good use for those that have weak stomachs,
or defluxions thereon. The distilled water
of the green husks, before they be half ripe,
is of excellent use to cool the heat of agues,
being drank an ounce or two at a time: as
also to resist the infection of the plague, if
some of the same be also applied to the sores
thereof. The same also cools the heat of green
wounds and old ulcers, and heals them,
being bathed therewith. The distilled water
of the green husks being ripe, when they are
shelled from the nuts, and drank with a little
vinegar, is good for the place, so as before
the taking thereof a vein be opened. The
said water is very good against the quinsy,
being gargled and bathed therewith, and
wonderfully helps deafness, the noise, and
other pains in the ears. The distilled water
of the young green leaves in the end of May,
performs a singular cure on foul running
ulcers and sores...' The green husks of the
fruit, boiled, make a good yellow dye.

Nutty Foreigners

The word walnut derives from Old
English *wealhhnutu*, literally foreign
nut, *wealh* or *wealsc* meaning foreign.
When the English invaded Britain,
they used this term for the native
Britons, calling them the Wealsch, or
Welsh, and pushing them westwards
into Wales, the West Country and
Cumbria. Thus the Welsh are called
'foreigners' in their own country. The
walnut was so called because it was
introduced from Gaul and Italy, the
Latin name for the walnut being *nux
Gallica*, Gallic nut.

HISTORY: The wood has been used for
making furniture, the wheels and bodies
of coaches, gun-stocks, and by cabinet-
makers for inlaying. The oil has been used
for frying, eaten as butter and employed
as lamp oil. Walnut oil was called
'*vegetable arsenic*', because of its curative
effect in eczema and other skin diseases
where arsenic was traditionally used.

Signature of the Skull

The English botanist William Coles
related walnuts to the Doctrine of
Signatures in *Adam in Eden*,
1657: '*Wall-nuts have the perfect
Signature of the Head: The outer
husk or green Covering, represent
the Pericranium, or outward skin
of the skull, whereon the hair
groweth, and therefore salt made of
those husks or barks, are exceeding good
for wounds in the head. The inner woody
shell hath the Signature of the Skull,*

*and the little yellow skin, or Peel, that
covereth the Kernel, of the hard Meninga
and Pia-mater, which are the thin
scarves that envelope the brain.
The Kernel hath the very figure
of the Brain, and therefore it is
very profitable for the Brain, and
resists poisons; For if the Kernel
be bruised, and moistened with the
quintessence of Wine, and laid upon the
Crown of the Head, it comforts the brain
and head mightily.*'

WATER AGRIMONY

BIDENS TRIPARTITA
Family Asteraceae/Compositae, Aster/Daisy

OTHER NAMES: Burr marigold, bur marigold, three-lobe beggarticks, three-part beggarticks, leafy-bracted beggarticks, triffid burr-marigold. Culpeper names it: Water-agrimony, Eupatorium, Hepatorium, Water Hemp, Bastard Hemp, Bastard Agrimony.

DESCRIPTION: It is worthwhile reading the full description of the plant given by Culpeper: '*The root continues a long time, having many long slender strings; the stalk grows up about two feet high, sometimes higher; they are of a dark purple colour; the branches are many, growing at distances the one from the other, the one from the one side of the stalk, the other from the opposite point; the leaves are winged, and much indented at the edges; the flowers grow at the tops of the branches, of a brown yellow colour, spotted with black spots, having a substance within the midst of them like that of a daisy; if you rub them between your fingers they smell like rosin, or cedar when it is burnt; the seeds are long, and easily stick to any woollen thing they touch.*'

PROPERTIES AND USES: Culpeper states that it was called hepatorium '*... because it strengthens the liver...It is a plant of Jupiter, as well as the other agrimony; only this belongs to the celestial sign Cancer. It healeth and dryeth, cutteth and cleanseth, thick and tough tumours of the breast; and for this I hold it inferior to but few herbs that grow. It helps the cachexia, or evil disposition of the body; also the dropsy and yellow jaundice. It opens obstructions of the liver, mollifies the hardness of the spleen; being applied outwardly, it breaks imposthumes; taken inwardly, it is an excellent remedy for the third-day ague; it provokes urine and the terms; it kills worms, and cleanseth the body of sharp humours, which are the cause of itch, scabs &e. The smoke of the herb, being burnt, drives away flies, wasps, &c. It strengthens the lungs exceedingly. Country people give it to their cattle when they are troubled with the cough, or brokenwinded.*' The plant produces a weak yellow dye.

HISTORY: The plant was valued for its diuretic and astringent properties, and used in fevers, gravel, stone, bladder and kidney troubles, consumption and excessive bleeding.

Gold Fish Killer

Most *Bidens* species share the trait of having seeds that stick to anything passing their way. In Latin, *bidens* refers to having two teeth, in this case the two teeth on the seed. According to Maud Grieve in 1931, its burrs '*... when the plant has been growing on the borders of a fish-pond, have been known to destroy gold fish by adhering to their gills.*'

WATER BETONY

SCROPHULARIA AURICULATA
Family Scrophulariaceae, Figwort

OTHER NAMES: Culpeper also calls the plant *'Broomwort, and in Yorkshire Bishop's Leaves'*. Brook or water betony, bishop-leaves, brownwort, bullwort, stinking Christopher, cressel, cressil, crowdy-kit, crowdy, fiddles, fiddler, fiddlewood, figwort, huntsman's cap, poor man's salve, stinking Roger, babes in a cradle, water figwort.

DESCRIPTION: A handsome semi-aquatic plant which can grow to 4 feet (1.2 m) high, with maroon and green two-lipped flowers. Its leaves resemble those of wood betony, hence its name.

PROPERTIES AND USES: Culpeper notes: *'Water betony is an herb of Jupiter in Cancer, and is appropriated more to wounds and hurts in the breast than wood-betony, which follows; it is an excellent remedy for sick hogs. It is of a cleansing quality: the leaves bruised and applied are effectual for all old and filthy ulcers: and especially if the juice of the leaves be boiled with a little honey, and dipped therein, and the sores dressed therewith; as also for bruises or hurts, whether inward or outward; the distilled water of the leaves is used for the same purpose; as also to bathe the face and hands spotted or blemished, or discoloured by sun burning. I confess I do not much fancy distilled waters, I mean such waters as are distilled cold; some virtues of the herb they may haply have (it were a strange thing else;) but this I am confident of, that being distilled in a pewter still, as the vulgar and apish fashion is, both chemical oil and salt is left behind, unless you burn them, and then all is spoiled, water and all, which was good for as little as can be, by such a distillation in my translation of the London dispensatory.'*

HISTORY: Maud Grieve tells us: *'This plant has vulnerary and detergent properties…In modern herbal medicine, the leaves are employed externally as a poultice, or boiled in lard as an ointment for ulcers, piles, scrofulous glands in the neck, sores and wounds. It is said to have been one of the ingredients in Count Matthei's noted remedy, "AntiScrofuloso". In former days this herb was relied on for the cure of toothache and for expelling nightmare.'*

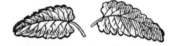

Fiddling Plant

Because the stalks are coloured it was called *brownwort*. It was called *fiddlewood* because the stems are stripped by children of their leaves and scraped across each other fiddle-fashion to produce a squeaking sound. Similarly, in the name *crowdy kit, kit* is a West Country word for fiddle. It is called figwort because of the form of the root in another member of the genus *Scrophularia*, the knotted figwort, *S. nodosa*.

WATERCRESS
NASTURTIUM OFFICINALE
Family Brassiceae/Cruciferae, Cabbage

OTHER NAMES: Two-rowed watercress, water pepper, winter cress, brooklime, pepper cress, true nasturtium, tall nasturtium.

DESCRIPTION: Watercress has shiny compound leaves on creeping or floating hollow stems, with fibrous roots. A fast-growing perennial, it is one of the oldest known leaf vegetables cultivated by humans, with mild pepper-flavoured leaves and stems. Watercress produces small white and green flowers in clusters. Watercress is so named because it naturally favours wet areas around springs and along riverbanks.

PROPERTIES AND USES:
A nutritional culinary food, it can also be considered a medicinal plant. The leaves have a high vitamin and mineral content and help digestion. It is a diuretic, antibiotic and lowers blood sugar. Watercress contains significant amounts of iron, calcium, iodine and folic acid, in addition to vitamins A and C, and is believed to have cancer-suppressing properties. Culpeper said: '*It is an herb under the dominion of the Moon. It is more powerful against the scurvy, and to cleanse the blood and humours, than brooklime, and serves in all the other uses in which brooklime is available; as to break the stone,*

and provoke urine and women's courses. It is also good for them when troubled with the green sickness, and it is a certain restorative of their lost colour if they use it in the following manner: chop and boil them in the broth of meat, and eat them for a month together, morning, noon, and night. The decoction thereof cleanses ulcers by washing therewith; the leaves bruised, or the juice, is good to be applied to the face or other parts troubled with freckles, pimples, spots, or the like, at night, and washed away in the morning. The juice mixed with vinegar, and the forepart of the head bathed therewith, is very good for those that are dull and drowsy, or have the lethargy. Watercress pottage is a good remedy to cleanse the blood in the spring, and help headaches, and consume the gross humours winter has left behind; those who would live in health, may

---

Wrinkled Nose

It is referred to as true nasturtium, but is not closely related to the nasturtium family, Tropaeolaceae. Loosely translated, nasturtium is derived from Latin words meaning 'wrinkled nose', alluding to its pungent odour. *Officinale* denotes that it is a plant used medicinally.

Liver Fluke Parasite

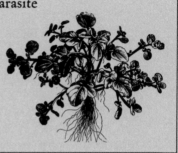

Care must be taken if harvesting from the wild. Any watercress growing in water that drains from fields where animals, particularly sheep, graze should not be used raw, as it may be infected with the liver fluke parasite. However, cooking the leaves will destroy any parasites. Like many plants in this family, the foliage of watercress becomes bitter when the plants begin producing flowers.

make use of this: if any fancy not pottage, they may eat the herb as a salad.'

Watercress was used to prevent scurvy and in the treatment of tuberculosis. Considered a cleansing herb, its high content of vitamin C makes it a herbal remedy that is valuable for chronic illnesses, and it has been used in the treatment of tuberculosis. The freshly pressed juice has been used internally and externally in the treatment of chest and kidney complaints. A medicinal poultice of the leaves was said to be an effective treatment for healing glandular tumours or lymphatic swellings and chronic irritations and inflammations of the skin. It was believed that a watercress lotion could reduce blemishes. Recently, watercress has been the focus of several scientific studies regarding its potential for fighting malignant disease, mainly due to its high antioxidant content. As a nutritional supplement, it contains a large quantity of vitamins A and C, beta-carotene, folic acid, iodine, iron, protein and especially calcium. Applied externally, it has a long-standing reputation as an effective hair tonic, helping to promote the growth of thick hair. It makes

wonderful salads, sandwiches and soups. The seed can be ground into a powder and used as a mustard.

HISTORY: First cultivated by the Persians, it spread to Greece and Rome. It has been used since the time of Hippocrates as a stimulant and expectorant in the treatment of coughs and bronchitis. The Ancient Greeks believed that watercress made one witty, healthy and had the potential to cure insanity. Watercress was a staple food for Greek and Persian soldiers, who noticed that it improved their health and conditioning. It is now used in salads and sandwiches but in the 18th century it was simmered with scurvy grass and oranges as a 'spring cleansing' soup and to cure headaches. It was a useful winter vegetable in the Middle Ages, and is today used in popular 'detox' diets. New Market, Alabama, was known in the 1940s as the *'Watercress Capital of the World'* in America. Alresford, near Winchester, is considered the *'Watercress Capital of Britain'* and a local steam railway route in Hampshire, which used to take watercress to London markets, is called the Watercress Line.

WILD GARLIC

ALLIUM URSINUM
Family Alliaceae, Onion

OTHER NAMES: Broad-leaved garlic, wood garlic, ramsons, badger's flower, bear's garlic, badger's garlic, devil's garlic, gipsy onion, stinking Jenny, buckrams.

DESCRIPTION: Culpeper: '*The root of this is round and whitish; the leaves are oblong, very broad, of a fine deep green. The stalk of a pale green, three square, and ten inches high, whereon grow small white flowers.*' Maud Grieve was rather more dismissive: '*…it grows in woods and has a very acrid taste and smell, but it also has very small bulbs, which would hardly render it of practical use.*' Its clusters of star-shaped white flowers spread across swathes of woodland in spring, and the plant can be smelt from yards away.

PROPERTIES AND USES: Culpeper observes: '*It is under Mars as well as the former* [garlic]. *The root is only known in physic; it is a powerful opener…It wonderfully opens the lungs, and gives relief in asthmas; nor is it without its merit in wind colic; and is a good diuretic, which appears by the smell it communicates to the urine. It is very useful in obstructions of the kidneys, and dropsies, especially in that which is called anasarca* [oedema, excess fluid in tissues and body cavities]. *It may be taken in a morning fasting, or else the conserve of Garlic which is kept in the shops may be used.*' The freshly pressed juice was used to treat sore throats, coughs and colds. If the leaves are boiled, the juice can be used as a disinfectant wipe.

HISTORY: The familiar term ramsons comes from the Old English *hramson* or *hramsa*. Many old English villages have the prefix '*Ram*' and were named after the abundance of wild garlic growing there. Its Latin species name comes from the European brown bear's (*Ursus arctos*) taste for the bulbs, and habit of digging them out of the ground, as do badgers and wild boar. Ramsons leaves have also been used as fodder. Cows that have fed on ramsons give milk that tastes slightly of garlic, and butter made from this milk was popular in 19th-century Switzerland.

Popular Ingredient

The stems are preserved by salting and eaten as a salad in Russia. The bulbs, leaves and flowers are also edible, and becoming increasingly popular once more, being featured by popular chefs such as Gordon Ramsay and Jamie Oliver to flavour salads, soups, sauces and egg dishes. The leaves can be used as salad, spice, boiled as a vegetable, in soup, or as an ingredient for pesto instead of basil. It is best to pick and use the leaves before the plant flowers.

WILD THYME

THYMUS SERPYLLUM
Family Lamiaceae/Labiatae, Mint

OTHER NAMES: Creeping thyme, running thyme, mother of thyme, breckland thyme, serpolet.

DESCRIPTION: It is shorter, with broader leaves and a weaker smell than garden thyme, from which it is probably derived, hence Culpeper's name of *Mother of Thyme*. It is the lowest-growing common variety of thyme, around 1 inch (2.5 cm) high, and is good for ground-cover; it smells of oregano or lemon.

PROPERTIES AND USES: Culpeper: *'Mother of Thyme is under Venus. It is excellent in nervous disorders. A strong infusion of it, drank in the manner of tea, is pleasant, and a very effectual remedy for head-aches, giddiness, and other disorders of that kind; and it is a certain remedy for that troublesome complaint, the night-mare. A gentleman afflicted for a long space of time with this complaint in a terrible manner, and having in vain sought for relief from the usual means employed for that purpose, was advised to make trial of the infusion of this plant, which soon removed it, and he continued free for several years, after which the disorder sometimes returned, but always gave way to the remedy.'* Drunk by itself or mixed with other plants such as rosemary, it was a remedy for headaches and other nervous affections.

HISTORY: An old tradition says that thyme was one of the herbs that formed the fragrant bed of the Virgin Mary. Since the Egyptians used thyme for embalming,

> ## From *A Midsummer Night's Dream*
> *I know a bank whereon the wild thyme blows*
> *Where oxlips and the nodding violet grows;*
> *Quite over-canopied with luscious woodbine,*
> *With sweet musk roses and with Eglantine.*
>
> William Shakespeare

the herb has also been associated with death. It was one of the fragrant flowers planted on graves, and the Order of Oddfellows (a benevolent fraternal organization) carry sprigs of thyme at funerals and throw them into the grave of a dead brother. In some areas it was a custom for girls to wear sprigs of thyme, with mint and lavender, to bring them sweethearts. According to Maud Grieve: *'In medicine, Wild Thyme or Serpolet has the same properties as Common Thyme, but to an inferior degree. It is aromatic, antiseptic, stimulant, antispasmodic, diuretic and emmenagogue* [stimulating blood flow in the pelvic area and uterus].' She tells us that the infusion was used *'for chest maladies and for weak digestion, being a good remedy for flatulence, and favourable results have been obtained in convulsive coughs, especially in whooping cough, catarrh and sore throat'.*

(WHITE) WILLOW

SALIX ALBA
Family Salicaceae, Willow

OTHER NAMES: European willow.

DESCRIPTION: A large tree up to 100 feet (30 m) high, with a rough greyish bark, its name derives from the white tone to the undersides of the leaves.

PROPERTIES AND USES: Culpeper: *'The Moon owns it. Both the leaves, bark, and the seed, are used to stanch bleeding of wounds, and at mouth and nose, spitting of blood, and other fluxes of blood in man or woman, and to stay vomiting, and provocation thereunto, if the decoction of them in wine be drank. It helps also to stay thin, hot, sharp, salt distillations from the head upon the lungs, causing a consumption. The leaves bruised with some pepper, and drank in wine, helps much the wind cholic. The leaves bruised and boiled in wine, and*

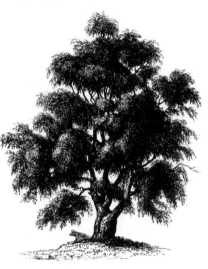

drank, stays the heat of lust in man or woman, and quite extinguishes it, if it be long used. The seed also is of the same effect. Water that is gathered from the Willow, when it flowers, the bark being slit, and a vessel fitting to receive it, is very good for redness and dimness of sight, or films that grow over the eyes, and stay the rheums that fall into them; to provoke urine, being stopped, if it be drank; to clear the face and skin from spots and discolourings. Galen says, the flowers have an admirable faculty in drying up humours, being a medicine without any sharpness or corrosion; you may boil them in white wine, and drink as much as you will, so you drink not yourself drunk. The bark works the same effect, if used in the same manner, and the tree hath always a bark upon it, though not always flowers; the burnt ashes of

---

Discovering Aspirin

The Reverend Edward Stone (1702–68) discovered the active ingredient of aspirin when he noted in 1763 that willow bark was effective in reducing a fever. He experimented by gathering and drying a pound of willow bark and creating a powder which he gave to about 50 persons. It was consistently found to be a *'powerful astringent and very efficacious in curing agues and intermitting disorders'*. He had discovered salicylic acid, the active ingredient in aspirin.

---

the bark being mixed with vinegar, takes away warts, corns, and superfluous flesh, being applied to the place. The decoction of the leaves or bark in wine, takes away scurff and dandrif by washing the place with it. It is a fine cool tree, the boughs of which are very convenient to be placed in the chamber of one sick of a fever. In the fifty-third volume of the Philosophical Transactions, page 195, we have an account given by Mr. Stone, of the great efficacy of the bark of this tree, in the cure of intermitting fevers. He gathered the bark in summer, when it was full of sap, and having dried it by a gentle heat, gave a drachm of it in powder every four hours between the fits. While the Peruvian bark remained at its usual moderate price, it was hardly worth while to seek for a substitute, but since the consumption of that article is become nearly as equal to the supply of it, from South America, we must expect to find it dearer, and very much adulterated every year, and consequently the white Willow bark is likely to become an object worthy the attention of the faculty; and should its success, upon a

more enlarged scale of practice, prove equal to Mr. Stone's experiments, the world will be much indebted to that gentleman for his communication.' The tree has been used in dyspepsia connected with debility of the digestive organs, in convalescence from acute diseases, in worms, in chronic diarrhoea and dysentery. The bark contains up to 13 per cent tannin as its chief constituent, and also a small quantity of salicin.

HISTORY: Hippocrates wrote in the fifth century BCE about a bitter powder which could be extracted from willow bark to ease aches and pains and reduce fevers (see box), a remedy also mentioned in Egyptian, Sumerian and Assyrian texts and by Dioscorides, Pliny and Galen. The tree has always been the willow most used for pollarding (cutting back) to make fences and stakes. It has also provided the brakes on railway wagons, the sides and bottoms of carts, the rims of pails, wood for charcoal, and in Russia the trunks were used for log cabins.

Making Cricket Bats

Salix alba 'Caerulea' (cricket bat willow) is grown as a specialist timber crop in Britain, mainly for the production of cricket bats, and for other uses where a tough, lightweight wood that does not splinter easily, is needed. It may be a hybrid between white willow and crack willow. *Salix fragilis*, crack willow, has brittle branches which can easily be broken (cracked) off. *Salix caprea*, also known as pussy willow, goat willow, sallow and sally is small and bushy with beautiful catkins. *Salix babylonica* is the familiar weeping willow. *Salix babylonica* 'Tortuosa', corkscrew willow, has elaborately twisted shoots and branches.

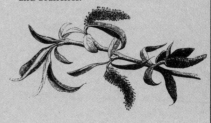

WINTER CHERRY

PHYSALIS ALKEKENGI
Family Solanaceae, Nightshade

OTHER NAMES: Chinese lantern, Japanese lantern, strawberry tomato, bladder cherry, jamberry.

DESCRIPTION: The plant and its varieties are grown for the decorative value of their brilliantly coloured, swollen orange calyces which surround the fruit – they are colloquially known as Chinese lanterns.

PROPERTIES AND USES: Culpeper: *'The leaves being cooling, may be used in inflammations, but not opening as the berries and fruit are: which by drawing down the urine, provoke it to be voided plentifully when it is stopped or grown hot, sharp, and painful in the passage; it is good also to expel the stone and gravel out of the reins, kidneys and bladder; helping to dissolve the stone, and voiding it by grit or gravel sent forth in the urine; it also helps much to cleanse inward imposthumes or ulcers in the reins of bladder, or in those that void a bloody or foul urine. The distilled water of the fruit, or the leaves together with them, or the berries, green or dry, distilled with a little milk and drank morning and evening with a little sugar, is effectual to all the purposes before specified, and especially against the heat and sharpness of the urine. I shall only mention one way, amongst many others, which might be used for ordering the berries, to be helpful for the urine and the stone, which is this; Take three or four good handfuls of the berries, either green or fresh, or dried, and having bruised them, put them into so many gallons of beer or ale when it is newly tunned up; This drink taken daily, hath been found to do much good to many, both to ease the pains, and expel urine and the stone, and to cause the stone not to engender.'*

HISTORY: Dioscorides prescribed its stem as a sedative and its berries as diuretics and a cure for epilepsy. The berries were said to be aperient and highly recommended in fevers and in gout. John Ray stated that a gout sufferer had prevented returns of the disorder by taking eight berries at each change of the moon. Mixed with honey, the berries were said to improve eyesight. With wine they supposedly cured toothache. The leaves and stems were used for the malaise that follows malaria and scarlet fever.

Japanese Contraceptive

In Japan, its seeds are used as part of the Bon Festival, given as offerings to guide the souls of the deceased. Its balloon-like qualities also caused it to be used as a contraceptive in early Japan, an example of the Doctrine of Signatures being employed elsewhere in the world.

WITCH HAZEL

HAMAMELIS VIRGINIANA
Family Hamamelidaceae, Witch Hazel

OTHER NAMES: Spotted alder, striped alder, winterbloom, snapping hazelnut, tobacco wood.

DESCRIPTION: Deciduous twisted shrub which can grow to 15 feet (4.5 m), with yellow thread-like blossoms; it grows best in moist light shade. It blooms from September to November, hence the name *winterbloom*, and some varieties have an intense fragrance.

PROPERTIES AND USES: Distilled and combined with alcohol, the aromatic oil extracted from the bark makes a soothing and mildly astringent lotion.

Witching a Well

Witch comes from '*wyche*' or '*wice*', the Anglo-Saxon for bend. The pliable branches of witch hazel became a favourite among the American colonists dowsing to dig wells for water, so it is thought that wyche became witch. While in Europe the native common hazel (*Corylus avellana*) was used for dowsing rods, in North America the early settlers used *Hamamelis virginiana*. They called this new tree a hazel. Finding a well was thought to be evidence of witchcraft, and locating a well through dowsing was called '*witching a well*', so this is a more likely explanation of the name of witch hazel.

It has become a general and proven treatment for abrasions, burns, scalds, insect bites and inflammatory conditions of the skin such as acne. It is also an excellent astringent, toning facial cleanser, used to decrease bags under eyes, skin puffiness, and to reduce pore size, having become a valued ingredient in natural skin care formulations and anti-ageing products. Frozen witch hazel is very soothing for insect bites, varicose veins and bruises, and a cotton ball dampened with witch hazel relieves painful haemorrhoids. Its ability to shrink swollen tissue makes witch hazel appropriate to treat laryngitis. '*Swimmer's ear*' is associated typically with pus and moisture in the outer ear canal, and generally it is annoying and difficult to cure. However, a cotton swab dipped in a witch hazel, goldenseal and calendula tea, and then applied to the outer ear, is useful in treating the infection.

HISTORY: The plant is not included in the earlier editions of Culpeper as it is a native of North America. When the seed-bearing capsules of witch hazel break open, they throw the seeds up to a distance of 20 feet (6 m), giving rise to the name of *snapping hazel*. It has long been used by the Native North Americans to make poultices for painful swellings and tumours. The distilled witch hazel widely sold commercially is not as astringent as other preparations as the tannins have been removed.

WOAD

ISATIS TINCTORIA
Family Brassicaceae, Cabbage

OTHER NAMES: Dyer's woad, garden woad, asp of Jerusalem, pastel (Spanish), wad or waad (Anglo-Saxon), llysiau'r lliw (Welsh for herbs of dye), glaston (this may also be originally a Welsh word, meaning blue tone).

DESCRIPTION: Gerard tells us: '*Glaston or Guadon, Woad is about three feet high, with long, bluish-green leaves growing round and out of the stalk, growing smaller as they reach the top, when they branch out with small yellow flowers, which in turn produce seed like little black tongues.*' It is an attractive back-of-border garden plant.

PROPERTIES AND USES: Gerard again: '*The decoction made of Woad is good for hardness of the spleen, also good for wounds and ulcers to those of strong constitution and those accustomed to much physical labour and coarse fare. It is used as a dye, profitable to some, hurtful to many.*' Culpeper says: '*It is a cold and dry plant of Saturn. Some people affirm the plant to be destructive to bees, and fluxes them, which, if it be, I cannot help it. I should rather think, unless bees be contrary to other creatures, it possesses them with the contrary disease, the herb being exceeding dry and binding. However, if any bees be diseased thereby, the cure is, to set urine by them, but set it in a vessel, that they cannot drown themselves, which may be remedied,*

if you put pieces of cork in it. The herb is so drying and binding, that it is not fit to be given inwardly. An ointment made thereof staunches bleeding. A plaster made thereof, and applied to the region of the spleen which lies on the left side, takes away the hardness and pains thereof. The ointment is excellently good in such ulcers as abound with moisture, and takes away the corroding and fretting humours. It cools inflammations, quenches St. Anthony's Fire [ergot poisoning], *and stays defluxion of the blood to any part of the body. The chief use of this plant is among the dyers, but it is possessed of virtues which claim our regard for their medical effects. The tops of the plant possess those in the greatest perfection, and a strong infusion of them is the best method of giving them. This operates by urine and is excellent against obstruction of the liver and spleen, but its use must be continued a considerable time.*' It is used in Chinese medicine for meningitis, mumps and sore throats, but can be poisonous.

HISTORY: The herb was found to be too astringent to be given internally as a medicine, and has been used medicinally as a plaster, applied to the region of the spleen, and as an ointment for ulcers, inflammation and to staunch bleeding. The dye chemical extracted from woad is indigo, the same dye, but in a far lower concentration as that obtained from the true indigo plant, *Indigofera tinctoria*.

Ancient Dyes

The famous blue dye comes from the leaves of the woad plant, especially those of the first year's growth. It was used for dye as long ago as Neolithic times, and ancient Egyptians used it to dye cloth wrappings for mummies. In Caesar's *Gallic Wars*, he notes that the British stained themselves blue with vitrum, which was translated as woad, but instead seems to have been a copper- or iron-based pigment. The ever unreliable Pliny the Elder wrote that the French called it *Glastum*, and stated that British women and girls coloured themselves with the dye and went naked to some of their sacrifices. It may have been plentiful in Britain, but by the time of the Saxons it was being imported from France to dye home-spun cloth.

Woad was eventually superseded by the arrival of indigo in commercial quantities in the Middle Ages. Laws were passed across Europe to protect the woad industry from the competition of the indigo trade, with woad's supporters claiming that indigo rotted yarns. In Germany, indigo came to be known as the *devil's dye*. However, woad dye 'fixes' and improves the quality and colour of indigo, when mixed in certain proportions. Woad is also used to form a base, or mordant, for a black dye. In the beautifully illuminated *Lindisfarne Gospels*, woad was used for a blue paint throughout the manuscript.

Woad belongs to the same plant family as cabbage, cauliflower and broccoli, and contains very high levels of the organic compound *glucobrassicin*, 20 times more than that found in broccoli. University of Bologna researchers believe that chemicals like these could one day prove to have an important part to play in the prevention and treatment of cancer. They were also able to boost its concentration by damaging the leaves, whereby glucobrassicin is released as a defence mechanism. Studies suggest that glucobrassicin, a type of glucosinolate, flushes out cancer-causing compounds including derivatives of oestrogen, and recent research found that people who ate foods rich in glucosinolates had reduced levels of chemicals linked to smoking-related lung cancer. Researchers have already suggested that eating vegetables rich in chemicals such as glucobrassicin might help protect people against cancer, but it has been difficult for scientists to extract enough glucobrassicin from plants to test its effect. It is thought that its antitumour properties are likely to be particularly effective against breast cancer.

WOOD BETONY

STACHYS OFFICINALIS
Family Lamiaceae/Labiatae, Mint

OTHER NAMES: Common betony, bishop's wort, louse wort, wild hop, purple betony, devil's plaything, *cribau San Ffraid* (St Brigit's combs, Welsh).

DESCRIPTION: This grassland herb grows 2 feet (60 cm) high with a 10-inch (25-cm) spread, and has pointed, toothed leaves and attractive pinkish-purple lipped flowers carried on top of the stem. *Stachys* is the Greek word for 'ear of corn' and refers to the shape of the flower spike.

PROPERTIES AND USES: Antonio Musa, chief physician to Emperor Augustus, wrote a treatise on it listing 47 diseases curable by the use of betony, all of which

Culpeper faithfully relates: '...*it is a very precious herb, that is certain, and most fitting to be kept in a man's house, both in syrup, conserve, oil, ointment and plaister; The flowers are usually conserved...it preserveth the liver and bodies of men from the danger of epidemical diseases, and from witchcraft also; it helpeth those that loath and cannot digest their meat, those that have weak stomachs and sour belchings, or continual rising in their stomach, using it familiarly either green or dry; either the herb, or roots or the flowers, in broth, drink, or meat, or made into conserve, syrup, water, electuary, or powder, as every one may best frame themselves unto, or as the time and*

Serpent Killer, Stag Healer

Maud Grieve tells us that many superstitions grew up around betony. For example, serpents would fight and kill each other if placed within a ring composed of it. Wild beasts recognized its benefits and used it if wounded. Stags, if wounded with an arrow or lance, would search out betony, and, eating it, be cured. Betony was endowed with power against evil spirits, being carefully planted in churchyards and hung about the neck as an amulet or charm. The latter sanctified, according to Erasmus, '...*those that carried it about them,*' and being also '*good against fearful visions*' and an efficacious means of '*driving away devils and despair*'.

season requireth; taken any of the aforesaid ways, it helpeth the jaundice, falling sickness, the palsy, convulsions, or shrinking of the sinews, the gout and those that are inclined to dropsy, those that have continual pains in their heads, although it turn to phrensy. The powder mixed with pure honey, is no less available for all sorts of coughs or colds, wheesing, or shortness of breath, distillations of thin rheum upon the lungs, which causeth consumptions…the decoction thereof made in wine and taken, killeth the worms in the belly, openeth obstructions both of the spleen and liver; cureth stitches, and pains in the back and sides, the torments and griping pains in the bowels, and the wind colic; and mixed with honey, purgeth the belly, helpeth to bring down women's courses, and is of special use to those that are troubled with the falling down of the mother, and pains thereof, and causes an easy and speedy delivery of women in child-birth. It helpeth also to break and expel the stone, either in the bladder or kidneys. The decoction with wine gargled in the mouth, easeth the tooth-ach. It is commended against the stinging and biting of venomous serpents, or mad dogs, being used inwardly and applied outwardly to the place…' Closely related to hedge woundwort *(Stachys sylvatica)* betony was thought to have similar properties when applied to wounds.

HISTORY: From the time of the Ancient Egyptians to the Anglo-Saxons betony was thought to have magical powers, and it was prominent in medieval herb gardens, as it was used almost as a panacea by the herbalists. Wood betony was used to bathe children who were possessed or bewitched, as the bathwater washed away the bad magic. Betony was used to treat chest and lung problems,

Virtues of Betony

The 12th-century Welsh Physicians of Myddfai wrote:

THE FOLLOWING ARE THE VIRTUES OF BETONY
He who will habituate himself to drink the juice, will escape the strangury. If it is boiled in white wine, and drank, it will cure the colic, and swelling of the stomach. Pounding it small, expressing the juice and apply it with a feather to the eye of a man, will clear and strengthen his sight, and remove specks from his eye. The juice is a good thing to drop into the ears of those who are deaf. The powder mixed with honey is useful for those who cough; it will remove the cough and benefit many diseases of the lungs. If boiled with leek seed, it will cure the eye, and brighten as well as strengthen the sight.

worms, fever, gout, uterine bleeding, dizziness and other afflictions, and even as a protection against witchcraft. There was an Italian saying: *'Venda la onica e compra beonica'* (Sell your coat and buy betony). Dried leaves were used in herbal tobaccos and snuffs, for instance Rowley's British Herb Snuff which was used for headaches. In his *Herball*, Richarde Banckes wrote: *'Eat Betony or the powder thereof and you cannot be drunken that day'* whereas Gerard more bluntly states: *'It maketh a man to pisse well'*.

WOOD SORREL

OXALIS ACETOSELLA
Family Oxalidaceae, Wood Sorrel

OTHER NAMES: Wood sour, sour trefoil, stickwort, fairy bells, hallelujah, cuckowes meat, three-leaved grass, surelle, stubwort, shamrock.

DESCRIPTION:
It carpets deciduous woodland with its pale green, heart-shaped leaves, folded through the middle, that occur in groups of three on a slender reddish brown stalk. There are delicate flowers with white papery flowers with pink streaks, and it grows about 6 inches (15 cm) high.

PROPERTIES AND USES: Culpeper: '*Venus owns it. Wood Sorrel serves to all the purposes that the other Sorrels do, and is more effectual in hindering putrefaction of blood, and ulcers in the mouth and body, and to quench thirst, to strengthen a weak stomach, to procure an appetite, to stay vomiting, and very excellent in any contagious sickness or pestilential fevers. The syrup made of the juice, is effectual in all the cases aforesaid, and so is the distilled water of the herb. Sponges or linen cloths wet in the juice and applied outwardly to any hot swelling or inflammations, doth much cool and help them. The same juice taken and gargled in the mouth, and after it is spit forth, taken afresh, doth wonderfully help a foul stinking canker or ulcer therein. It is singularly good to heal wounds, or to stay the bleeding of thrusts or stabs in the body;*

and helps to stay any hot defluxions into the throat and cleanses the viscera.' In Maud Grieve's *Herbal* we read that wood sorrel has '*diuretic, antiscorbutic and refrigerant action, and a decoction made from its pleasant acid leaves is given in high fever, both to quench thirst and to allay the fever.*' Herbalists believe that wood sorrel is more effectual than the true sorrels (*Rumex* species) as a blood cleanser, and will strengthen a weak stomach, produce an appetite, check vomiting and remove obstructions of the

Four-leaf Clovers

In 1620, Sir John Melton wrote, '*If a man walking in the fields find any four-leaved grass, he shall in a small while after find some good thing.*' It is estimated that, on average, there are 10,000 three-leaf clovers for every instance of a true four-leaf clover. Thus, finding a true four-leaf clover needs the proverbial 'luck of the Irish.' Other *Oxalis* species, with four regular leaflets, in particular *Oxalis tetraphylla* (four-leaved pink-sorrel) or *Oxalis deppei* (iron cross) are sometimes misleadingly sold as 'four-leaf clover'.

viscera. The juice of the leaves turns red when clarified and makes a fine, clear syrup, and the juice is gargled as a remedy for ulcers in the mouth, and applied to heal wounds and to stem bleeding. Sponges and linen cloths were saturated with the juice and applied to reduce swellings and inflammation.

HISTORY: Both botanical names *Oxalis* and *acetosella* refer to its acidity, being derived from the Greek *oxys*, meaning sour or acid, and *acetosella*, meaning vinegar salts. It has some folk names as an old herbal outlines: '*The apothecaries and herbalists call it Alleluya and Paniscuculi, or Cuckowes meat, because either the Cuckoo feedeth thereon, or by reason when it springeth forth and flowereth the Cuckoo singeth most, at which time also Alleluya was wont to be sung in Churches.*' In Europe *Conserva Ligulae* used to be made by apothecaries beating the fresh leaves with three times their weight of sugar and orange peel, making a cooling and

acid drink that was a favourite remedy in malignant fevers and scurvy. In Dr James Duke's 1992 *Handbook of Edible Weeds*, he tells us that the Cherokees ate wood sorrel to alleviate mouth sores and sore throats, Kiowas chewed wood sorrel to alleviate thirst on long trips, Potawatomi Indians cooked it with sugar to make a dessert, the Algonquins considered it an aphrodisiac, and the Iroquois ate wood sorrel to help with cramps, fever and nausea. Its leaves have been used in spring salads and for food for centuries. In Henry VIII's time it was held in great repute as a pot-herb, but after the introduction of French sorrel, with its large succulent leaves, wood sorrel gradually lost its position as a salad and pot-herb. Wood sorrel, like spinach, sweet potatoes, rhubarb, beans and broccoli, contains oxalic acid which is considered slightly toxic because it interferes with food digestion and the absorption of some trace minerals. It is known to bind with calcium and inhibit its absorption.

True Shamrock

Traditionally, the wood sorrel was thought to be to be the three-leaved plant by which the missionary Welshman St Patrick demonstrated the Trinity to the Irish pagans. St Patrick filled the Emerald Isle with lush fields of shamrocks, supposedly to keep snakes from ever returning, both the physical reptiles, and metaphorically the heathen beliefs. The symbol was found on early tombs and coins, but the Irish Gaelic word *seamrog*, little clover, the origin of the word shamrock, was not found in writing until the early 1700s. Other candidates for the 'true shamrock' are lesser trefoil (hop clover, *Trifolium dubium*), white clover *(Trifolium repens)*, red clover *(Trifolium pratense)* and black medick *(Medicago lupulina)*.

WOOD AVENS

GEUM URBANUM
Family Rosaceae, Rose

OTHER NAMES: Culpeper names it Colewort, Herb Benet and Avens. Herb bonnet, herb benet, St Benedict's herb, city avens, wild rye, way bennet, goldy star, clove root.

DESCRIPTION: The pretty flowers have five pale yellow petals. The fruits have burrs, which help seed dispersal by getting caught in the fur of rabbits and other passing animals.

PROPERTIES AND USES: Culpeper says: '*It is governed by Jupiter, and that gives hopes of a wholesome healthful herb. It is good for the diseases of the chest or breast, for pains, and stiches in the side, and to expel crude and raw humours from the belly and stomach, by the sweet savour and warming quality. It dissolves the inward congealed blood happening by falls or bruises, and the spitting of blood, if the roots, either green or dry, be boiled in wine and drank; as also all manner of inward wounds or outward, if washed or bathed therewith. The decoction also being drank, comforts the heart, and strengthens the stomach and a cold brain, and therefore is good in the spring-time to open obstructions of the liver, and helps the wind colic; it also helps those that have fluxes, or are bursten, or have a rupture; it takes away spots or marks in the face, being washed therewith. The juice of the fresh root, or powder of the dried root, hath the same effect with the decoction. The root in the spring time steeped in wine, give it delicate savour and taste, and being drank fasting every morning, comforts the heart, and is a good preservative against the plague, or any other poison. It helps digestion, and warms a cold stomach, and opens obstructions of the liver and spleen. It is very safe; you need have no dose prescribed; and is very fit to be kept in every body's house.*' Later herbalists used it to treat diarrhoea, heart disease, halitosis, mouth ulcers and colic.

HISTORY: Paracelsus suggested its use against liver disease, catarrh and stomach upsets. In the 15th century wood avens was credited with the power to drive away evil spirits, and to protect against poison, rabid dogs and venomous snakes. The clove-smelling roots were kept in houses to effect this, and also used as a spice in soups and for flavouring ales.

Blessed Herb

It was associated with Christianity because its leaves grew in threes and its petals in fives (recalling the Holy Trinity and the Five Wounds of Christ). Thus herb benet is a contraction of herba benedicta, blessed herb.

(COMMON) WORMWOOD

ARTEMISIA ABSINTHIUM
Family Asteraceae, Aster

OTHER NAMES: Wormwood, absinthe wormwood, green ginger, crown for a king.

DESCRIPTION: Grows to a height of 3 feet (90 cm) and a spread of 4 feet (1.2 m), with tiny yellow flowers and aromatic grey-green leaves. The leaves and flowers are very bitter, with a musky smell.

PROPERTIES AND USES: Culpeper: *'This is a martial herb, and is governed by Mars. This is the strongest; the Sea Wormwood is the second in bitterness, and the Roman joins a great deal of aromatic flavour, with but a little bitterness: therefore, to acquire and enjoy the full powers they possess, they must be separately known and well distinguished, for each kind has its particularly virtues. The two first grow wild in our country; the third is frequent in the physic garden, and may always be had, but, as not a native, is not particularly considered here. The common Wormwood here described, is very excellent in weakness of the stomach; and, far beyond the common knowledge, is powerful against the gout and gravel. The leaves are commonly used, but the flowery tops are the right part.'* Wormwood became used mainly as a bitter tonic, kept evil spirits at bay. With the exception of rue, wormwood is the bitterest herb in general use, and used to be used by brewers instead of hops. The leaves resist putrefaction, so were used in antiseptics.

HISTORY: Dioscorides and Pliny considered wormwood to be a stomachic tonic, and anthelmintic (to eliminate worms). In Biblical days it was a symbol of calamity and sorrow, and in Proverbs, 5:4 we read: *'her end was as bitter as wormwood'*. *'As bitter as wormwood'* used to be a common saying. Constituents in wormwood are anti-inflammatory and reduce fevers, and small doses of wormwood tea were taken before meals to stimulate digestion and prevent heartburn and flatulence. As its name implies, wormwood is a powerful worming agent that has been used for hundreds of years to expel tapeworms, threadworms, and especially roundworms from dogs, cats, humans and other animals. Bunches of wormwood were hung in chicken coops to deter flies, lice and fleas.

Green Dumplings

Wormwood is the traditional colour agent for green songpyeon (a type of steamed dumpling made from rice flour), eaten during the Korean thanksgiving festival of *Chuseok*. It is picked in the spring when it is still young, and juice extracted from the leaves provides the dye and flavouring required for the dough.

(ROMAN) WORMWOOD

ARTEMISIA PONTICA
Family Asteraceae, Aster

OTHER NAMES: European wormwood, bitter weed.

DESCRIPTION: With blue-green stems it grows to 2 feet (60 cm) tall, and bears tiny yellow flowers.

PROPERTIES AND USES:
Culpeper: '*It is also a martial plant. The fresh tops are used, and the whole plant dried. It is excellent to strengthen the stomach; but that is not all its virtues, the juice of the fresh tops is good against obstructions of the liver and spleen, and has been known singly to cure the jaundice… The flowery tops are the right part. These made into a light infusion, strengthen digestion, correct acidities, and supply the place of gall, where, as in many constitutions, that is deficient. One ounce of the flowers and buds should be put into a vessel, and a pint and a half of boiling water poured on them, and thus to stand all night…This regularly observed for a week, will cure all the complaints arising from indigestion and wind;…An ounce of these flowers put into a pint of brandy, and steeped there for the space of six weeks, will produce a tincture of which a table-spoonful taken in a glass of water twice a day, will, in a great measure, prevent the increase of the gravel, and give great relief in the gout…The Wormwood wine, so famous with the Germans, is made with this Roman Wormwood, put into the juice, and worked with it; it is a strong and an excellent wine,* not unpleasant, yet of such efficacy to give an appetite, that the Germans drink of it so often, that they are capable to eat for hours together, without sickness or indigestion.'

HISTORY: The genus name *Artemisia* comes from Artemis, the Greek name for the goddess Diana. In the Herbarium of Apuleius we read: '*Of these worts that we name Artemisia, it is said that Diana did find them and delivered their powers and leechdom to Chiron the Centaur, who first from these Worts set forth a leechdom, and he named these worts from the name of Diana, Artemis, that is Artemisias.*' Wormwood counteracted the effects of poisoning by hemlock, toadstools and the biting of the 'sea dragon'. Mexicans celebrated their great festival of the goddess of salt with a ceremonial dance by women who wore on their heads garlands of wormwood.

Vermouth

This is the most delicate and the least powerful of the wormwoods, and the aromatic flavour with which its bitterness is mixed has resulted in it being used in making the fortified wine vermouth. The aperitif's name is derived from the German word *Wermut*, wormwood.

(SEA) WORMWOOD

ARTEMISIA MARITIMA
Family Asteraceae, Aster

OTHER NAMES: Old woman (in reference to 'old man' or southernwood, which it resembles).

DESCRIPTION: This plant is common in sea marshes and appears similar to southernwood, but with more delicate grey-green leaves, and yellow flowers. It grows to 18 inches (45 cm) in height.

PROPERTIES AND USES: Culpeper writes: '*It is a very noble bitter, and succeeds in procuring an appetite, better than the common Wormwood which is best to assist digestion...The power and efficacy of Wormwoods in general are scarce to be credited in the vast extent of cases to which they may be applied. Hysteric complaints have been completely cured by the constant use of this tincture. In the scurvy, and in* the hypochondriacal disorders of studious sedentary men, few things have greater effect; for these it is best in strong infusions; and great good has risen from common Wormwood, given in jaundice and dropsies. The whole blood, and all the juices of the body, are affected...Women using it whilst suckling, their milk turns bitter.'

HISTORY: The fragrant branches of the sea wormwood were often put into linen closets and mattresses to drive out fleas. In the Dutch island of Texel its name is actually '*flea herb*'.

From *Five Hundred Points of Good Husbandry*, 1557

*While wormwood have seed, get a
  handful or twain,
To save against March, to make flea
  to refrain:
Where chamber is swept, and
  wormwood is strown,
No flea, for his life, dare abide to be
  known.
What savour is better, if physic be
  true,
For places infected, than wormwood
  and rue?
It is as a comfort, for heart and the
  brain,
And therefore to have it, it is not in
  vain.*

Thomas Tusser

Dreaming of True Love

An old love charm: '*On St. Luke's Day, take marigold flowers, a sprig of marjoram, thyme, and a little Wormwood; dry them before a fire, rub them to powder; then sift it through a fine piece of lawn, and simmer it over a slow fire, adding a small quantity of virgin honey, and vinegar. Anoint yourself with this when you go to bed, saying the following lines three times, and you will dream of your partner that is to be: "St. Luke, St. Luke, be kind to me, / In dreams let me my true-love see."*'

YARROW

ACHILLEA MILLEFOLIUM
Family Asteraceae/Compositae, Aster, Sunflower

OTHER NAMES: Culpeper also calls it: Nose-Bleed, Milfoil, Thousand-Leaf. Woundwort, old man's pepper, old man's mustard, yarroway, seven years' love, arrowroot, bad man's plaything, carpenter's weed, carpenter's plant, death flower, devil's plaything, devil's nettle, evil's nettle, field hops, hundred-leaved gradd, knight's milfoil, knyghten, militaris, military herb, noble yarrow, sanguinary, soldier's woundwort, stanch grass, staunch grass, stanch weed, thousand seal, snake's grass etc.

DESCRIPTION: It grows 12–36 inches (30–90 cm) with a 24-inch (60-cm) spread. Its small flowers vary from greyish-white to pale pink, and are grouped in flat clusters. It has numerous feathery leaves.

PROPERTIES AND USES: Culpeper writes: '*It is under the influence of Venus. As a medicine it is drying and binding. A decoction of it boiled with white wine, is good to stop the running of the reins in men, and whites in women; restrains violent bleedings, and is excellent for the piles. A strong tea in this case should be made of the leaves, and drank plentifully; and equal parts of it, and of toad flax, should be made into a poultice with pomatum, and applied outwardly. This induces sleep, eases the pain, and lessens the bleeding. An ointment of the leaves cures wounds, and is good for inflammations, ulcers, fistulas, and all such runnings as abound with moisture. Some writers of credit take the pains to inform us what plants cattle will not eat; they judge of this by looking at what are left in grounds, where they feed; and all such they direct to be rooted up.*

We have in this an instance, that more care is needful than men commonly take to show what is and what is not valuable. Yarrow is a plant left standing always in fed pasture; for cattle will not eat its dry stalk, nor have the leaves any great virtue after this rises; but Yarrow still is useful. It should be sown on barren grass ground, and while the leaves are tender, the cows and horses will eat it heartily. Nothing is more welcome for them, and it doubles the

---

Plant Doctor

Yarrow is known as a '*plant doctor*'. Planted near unhealthy plants, its root secretions help the ailing plant by triggering disease resistance. Its leaves are one of the best compost accelerators, and they can be infused to make a fertilizer and fungicide that cures downy mildew and preventing fungal disease.

natural produce. *On cutting down the stalks as they rise, it keeps the leaf fresh and they will eat it as it grows.*' If you cut yourself on a walk, chew or crush yarrow leaves or flowers and press them on the wound – the bleeding will stop. It has been used for regulating the menstrual cycle, and helping with poor circulation and high blood pressure. A hot cup of yarrow tea induces a therapeutic sweat which cools fevers and helps the body expels toxins. The dried flowers are long-lasting, and the leaves are good in salads. The chemical make-up of yarrow is complex, and it contains many active medicinal compounds in addition to the tannins and volatile oil azulene.

HISTORY: The Greeks used it to stop haemorrhaging and the Roman armies used it to stop blood pouring from wounds inflicted during battle. The Druids made amulets from yarrow to protect the home from evil. The English name, yarrow, comes from the Saxon word '*gearwe*'. It has been used as a cold cure since before the early medieval period. In the Middle Ages, yarrow was one of the ingredients in *gruit*, a selection of herbs that were used to make beer, before the widespread use of hops. Folk tales tell how yarrow can prevent, but not cure, baldness, and it was recommended for nervous headaches. Leaves held over the eyes gave the gift of second sight. Albertus Magnus (*c.*1206–80) wrote in his *Book of Secrets* that if one's hands are smeared with yarrow juice and then plunged into a river they will act as magnets to fish. Put into sachets, yarrow is said to attract friends and distant relations to you and to ensure that love will last for at least seven years. Yarrow

Achilles's Healer

Chiron, the centaur in Greek mythology, taught its virtues to Achilles so he might make an ointment to heal his warrior Myrmidons who were wounded in the siege of Troy. Chiron then named the plant for this favourite pupil, giving his own name to the blue cornflower *(Centaurea cyanus)*. Alternatively, Achilles scraped the rust from his spear, which grew into yarrow which helped him to cure the wounded, hence the species name *achillea*.

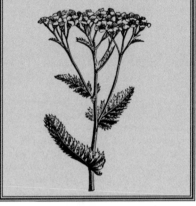

could also help you to find your true love, either by sleeping with yarrow under your pillow to bring dreams of your true love or by cutting the stems across the middle, which would supposedly reveal the initials of your future spouse. Yarrow was tied to an infant's cradle to stop its soul being stolen. Originally the Chinese system of divination described in the *I-Ching* was practised by throwing dried yarrow stalks to divine the future, before coins were invented.

References

The following of Nicholas Culpeper's copious works were consulted:

A Physical Directory, or a Translation of the London Directory, 1649 (A translation of the *Pharmacopoeia Londonesis* of the Royal College of Physicians)

Directory for Midwives, 1651

Semeiotica Uranica, or An Astrological Judgement of Diseases, 1651

Introduction to the Reader, Galen's Art of Physick, 1652

Catastrophe Magnatum or The Fall of Monarchy, 1652

The English Physitian, 1652

The Compleat Herball, 1653

Astrological Judgement of Diseases from the Decumbiture of the Sick, 1655

BHMA (British Herbal Medicine Association), *British Herbal Pharmacopoeia*, BHMA 1983, Bournemouth

Blunt, Wilfrid, and Raphael, Sandra, *The Illustrated Herbal*, Frances Lincoln 1979, London

Boehme, Jacob, *De Signatura Rerum: The Signature of All Things*, 1621, reprinted James Clarke & Co. Ltd. 1969, Cambridge

Clarkson, Rosetta, *Green Enchantment: The Golden Age of Herbs and Herbalists*, Macmillan 1940, New York

Clarkson, Rosetta, *Magic Gardens: A modern chronicle of herbs, and savory seeds*, Macmillan 1939, New York

Dioscorides, Pedanius, *De Materia Medica: Being an Herbal with many other medicinal materials*, 65 CE, translated by Tess Anne Osbaldeston, Ibidis Press 2000, Johannesburg

Gerard, John, *The Great Herball or Generall Historie of Plants*, 1621 reprinted Dover Publications Inc. 1975, New York

Grieve, M., *A Modern Herbal* (ed. Hilda Leyel), 1931, London, Penguin reprint 1982

Hensel, Wolfgang, *Medicinal Plants of Britain and Europe*, Black's Nature Guides, A&C Black 2008, London

Hoffmann D., *The New Holistic Herbal*, second edition, Element 1990, Shaftesbury

Junius, Manfred M., *Practical Handbook of Plant Alchemy*, Inner Traditions International Ltd. 1985, New York

Lust, J., *The Herb Book*, Bantam 1990, London

Mabey, R. (ed.), *The Complete New Herbal*, Penguin 1991, London

Mabey, Richard and McIntyre, Michael, *The New Age Herbalist: How to Use Herbs for Healing, Nutrition, Body Care, and Relaxation*, Prentice Hall 1988, London

Mills, S.Y., *The A-Z of Modern Herbalism*, Diamond Books 1993, London

Ody, P., *The Herb Society's Complete Medicinal Herbal*, Dorling Kindersley 1993, London

Parkinson, John, *A Garden of Pleasant Flowers: Paradisi in Sole*, 1629, reprinted Dover Publications Inc. 1991, New York

Pliny the Elder, *Naturalis Historia* (The Natural History), 77–79 CE, translated John Bostock, Taylor and Francis 1855, London, available on the Tufts University website www.perseus.tufts.edu

W. Ryves, *The Life of the admired physician and astrologer of our times, Mr Nicholas Culpeper. In Culpeper's School of Physic*, London 1659

Thulesius, O., *Nicholas Culpeper, English Physician and Astrologer*, Macmillan Press 1992, London

Tusser, Thomas, *His Good Points of Husbandry*, 1557, reprinted Country Life Limited, 1931 London

Weiss, R.F., *Herbal Medicine*, Beaconsfield Arcanum 1991, Beaconsfield

Wren, R.C., *Potter's New Cyclopaedia of Botanical Drugs and Preparations*, C.W. Daniel 1988, Saffron Walden

Index

Index

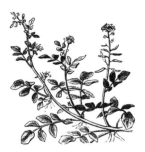

Copyright © 2011 by Quercus Publishing Plc 2011

First Lyons Press edition, 2011

Lyons Press is an imprint of Globe Pequot Press

Text by Terry Breverton
Edited by Philip de Ste. Croix
Designed by Paul Turner and Sue Pressley, Stonecastle Graphics Ltd
Index by Philip de Ste. Croix

All pictures © Dover Publications Inc., with the exception of those on the following pages,
which are in the Public Domain: 8, 9, 12, 14, 15, 16, 17, 26, 27, 30, 31, 41, 53 (below), 59,
60, 63, 69, 75, 76, 77, 80, 84, 89, 91, 92 (below), 101, 106, 110, 112, 122, 129 (above), 145,
147, 157, 161, 165, 169, 173, 179, 182, 183 (right), 191, 197, 207, 208, 209, 210, 215, 217
(above left), 229, 233, 240, 254, 263, 265, 266, 267 (above), 271, 273, 279, 281, 287, 289,
290, 291, 301, 305, 307, 309 (below left), 312, 315, 317 (above), 320, 324, 325, 327, 328,
331, 333, 334, 342, 346 (below right), 349, 351, 364, 365, 368, 372, 374.
Page 49 Extract © Dr Arthur Hollman and The Worshipful Company of Barbers.

Library of Congress Cataloging-in-Publication Data is available on file.

ISBN 978-0-7627-7022-9

Printed and bound in China

10 9 8 7 6 5 4 3 2 1

This book is intended for entertainment and reference purposes, and is in no way to be
considered as a substitute for consultation with a recognized health-care professional. As such
the author and others associated with this book accept no responsibility for any claims arising
from the use of any treatment mentioned here.